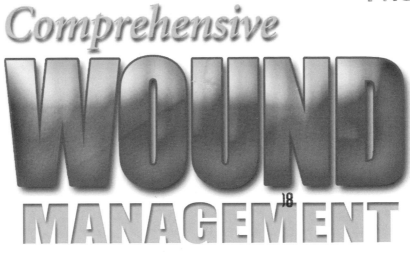

Comprehensive WOUND MANAGEMENT

Comprehensive WOUND MANAGEMENT

Glenn L. Irion, PhD, PT, CWS

University of South Alabama
Mobile, Alabama

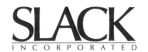

SLACK
INCORPORATED

An innovative information, education and management company
6900 Grove Road • Thorofare, NJ 08086

The procedures and practices described in this book should be implemented in a manner consistent with the professional standards set for the circumstances that apply in each specific situation. Every effort has been made to confirm the accuracy of the information presented and to correctly relate generally accepted practices. The author, editor, and publisher cannot accept responsibility for errors or exclusions or for the outcome of the application of the material presented herein. There is no expressed or implied warranty of this book or information imparted by it.

The work SLACK publishes is peer reviewed. Prior to publication, recognized leaders in the field, educators, and clinicians provide important feedback on the concepts and content that we publish. We welcome feedback on this work.

Printed in the United States of America.

Library of Congress Cataloging-in-Publication Data
Irion, Glenn
    Comprehensive wound management / Glenn L. Irion,
        p, ; cm.
    Includes bibliographical references and index.
    ISBN 1-55642-477-9 (alk. paper)
      1. Wounds and injuries--Treatment. 2. Wound healing. I. Title.
    [DNLM: 1. Wounds and Injuries--diagnosis. 2. Wounds and Injuries--therapy.
    3. Physical Therapy Techniques--methods. 4. Wound Healing--physiology. WO 700 I68c 2002]
    RD93 .I75 2002
    617.1--dc21

                                                                    2002017651

Published by: SLACK Incorporated
               6900 Grove Road
               Thorofare, NJ 08086 USA
               Telephone: 856-848-1000
               Fax: 856-853-5991
               www.slackbooks.com

Contact SLACK Incorporated for more information about other books in this field or about the availability of our books from distributors outside the United States.

For permission to reprint material in another publication, contact SLACK Incorporated. Authorization to photocopy items for internal, personal, or academic use is granted by SLACK Incorporated provided that the appropriate fee is paid directly to Copyright Clearance Center. Prior to photocopying items, please contact the Copyright Clearance Center at 222 Rosewood Drive, Danvers, MA 01923 USA; phone: 978-750-8400; website: www.copyright.com; email: info@copyright.com.

For further information on CCC, check CCC Online at the following address: http://www.copyright.com.

Last digit is print number: 10 9 8 7 6 5 4 3 2 1

DEDICATION

This textbook is dedicated to my children, Lindsay, Kyle, Christina, Phillip, and Connor and my wife, Jean, who managed to deal with "Daddy" on the computer all night.

CONTENTS

Instructors: *Comprehensive Wound Management Instructor's Manual* is also available from SLACK Incorporated. Don't miss this important companion to *Comprehensive Wound Management* available at *http://www.efacultylounge.com*.

ACKNOWLEDGMENTS

The author wishes to acknowledge the assistance of several individuals and organizations in the preparation of this text. Laura Gibbs assisted by proof-reading. Kyle Irion, Laura Gibbs, Amanda Whitehead, and Cory Van Meter contributed in the production of photographs of techniques. Chad Lairamore photographed the original pictures of patient wounds. Kim Taylor, Jennie Gregory, Dana Beggs, and Angie Young assisted by providing many of the patients who were photographed at Saint Vincent's Infirmary Medical Center in Little Rock, Baptist Medical Center in Little Rock, and Baptist Memorial Medical Center in North Little Rock. Both the Little Rock Medical Center and the Burn Unit of Arkansas Children's Hospital graciously provided photographs of wounds. I am also grateful to the patients who were willing to allow their health problems to be a source of help to others with wounds. Finally, the author gratefully acknowledges the assistance of those at SLACK Incorporated, including Olivia Lenahan, Carrie Kotlar, and John Bond.

ABOUT THE AUTHOR

Dr. Irion is certified as a Wound Specialist through the American Academy of Wound Management and is Associate Professor at the University of South Alabama where he teaches wound management, neuroscience, pathology, and cardiopulmonary physical therapy. He is actively engaged in wound healing research and clinical practice. The author received a PhD in Physiology at Temple University School of Medicine and further developed his research skills during postdoctoral fellowships at the Medical College of Virginia and the University of Cincinnati. The author of more than 30 research articles, Dr. Irion is also author of the textbook *Physiology: The Basis of Clinical Practice*, published by SLACK Incorporated.

PREFACE

This text is divided into four units in an effort to develop a systematic understanding of normal and abnormal integumentary physiology, factors involving the patient, causes of wounds, and to develop a rational plan of care based on this understanding. For the most part, this process is that described in the *Guide to Physical Therapist Practice*. Emphasis is placed on a systematic approach in taking a history, performing a physical examination, and performing special tests based on data collected from the history and physical examination. An assessment of the patient's condition and a diagnosis are developed based on the results, along with a prognosis. A plan of care is developed based on a subjective report, objective findings, and the patient's unique set of circumstances, including occupation, social support, dwelling, and level of understanding of the condition and its care.

Based on this organization, the first unit consists of a description of the anatomy and physiology of the skin, normal wound healing, and abnormal wound healing. The second unit addresses characteristics of the patient. Chapters in this unit cover history taking and tests & measures, physical examination, and nutrition. The third unit is focused on the wound and consists of chapters on acute wounds, neuropathic ulcers, pressure ulcers, vascular insufficiency, and assessment of wounds. When these concepts are understood, a plan of care can be developed. For this reason, the fourth unit addresses the interventions carried out in the plan of care. These include debridement, sharp debridement, physical agents, dressings, topical agents, pain management, infection control, burn management, documentation, and administrative concerns. The Appendix lists and discusses Agency for Health Care Policy and Research (AHCPR) Guidelines.

It is my hope that the readers of this text will learn to develop a systematic approach based on history, physical examination, special tests, and assessment of individual patients, rather than relying on referral/diagnosis-driven protocols, and that the reader will learn to adjust the plan of care as the patient and the wound change.

- Glenn L. Irion, PhD, PT, CWS

Normal and Abnormal Skin and Wound Physiology

The purpose of this unit is to provide background information that will guide history taking and physical examination to develop an assessment, diagnosis, prognosis, and plan of care. Analogous to chess, we wish to understand the layout of the board, the pieces, and the moves that are allowed. To continue with this analogy, in chess we are allowed many possible moves, but based upon the opposition, certain moves will be more fruitful than others. Understanding normal anatomy and physiology of skin, how unimpeded wound healing occurs, and understanding common problems with healing will help us make the right moves for our patients.

Anatomy and Physiology of Skin

OBJECTIVES

- Identify the layers of the skin and subcutaneous tissues and their roles in health.
- Identify the components of the epidermis, including cells, accessory structures, and layers.
- Identify the components of the dermis, including cells, fibers, ground substance, and other structures.
- Describe changes in the skin of the elderly.

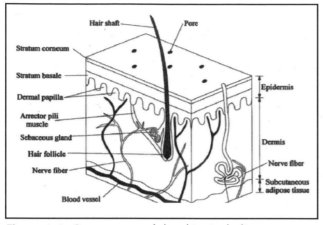

Figure 1-1. Components of the skin, including accessory structures of the epidermis. Note how deeply the hair follicles and sweat glands are surrounded by dermis.

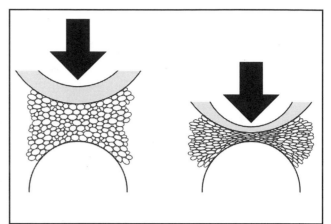

Figure 1-2. The cushioning effect of subcutaneous fat. Pressure between the skin and bony prominences is dissipated by the deformation of subcutaneous fat, rather than damage to the skin and other subcutaneous tissues.

SKIN STRUCTURE

The average person is enclosed in approximately 2 m^2 of skin, which on average is 2 mm thick. This makes the skin the largest organ of the body. The skin also carries out several important functions beyond the obvious function of physically separating the internal environment within the body from the harsh external environment. The skin acts as a physical barrier against microorganisms, trauma, ultraviolet light, and many (but not all) parasites. In addition, the skin has a major role in thermoregulation and vitamin D metabolism. The skin also has cellular and humoral components of the immune system and a variety of molecular defense systems against microorganisms. Unfortunately, the immune system on occasion is a source of injury to the skin and may cause devastating loss of skin integrity in diseases such as Stevens-Johnson syndrome and pemphigus.

The skin consists of two primary layers, the epidermis and dermis (Figure 1-1). A subcutaneous fat layer is also critical to skin function. Subcutaneous fat increases the thermal insulation of the skin and protects it from injury by pressure or shearing forces between bony prominences below the skin and the surface on which a person rests, as depicted in Figure 1-2. Below subcutaneous fat, other structures including muscle, tendon, ligaments, and bone may be found. The epidermis consists of organized layers of stratified epithelium with a well-defined transition of cell shape and structure as cells proceed from deeper layers to more superficial layers. The epidermis is generally 75 to 150 microns (μm) thick, but becomes 400 to 600 μm thick in palms and soles, which have an epidermal layer not found in other parts of the body. The dermis is much thicker than the epidermis but is not as regularly organized. Within the dermis is dense fibroelastic connective tissue that encloses accessory structures of the epidermis, fibrous bands that connect to fascia and bone, and below it a subcutaneous loose areolar or fatty connective tissue.

COMPONENTS OF EPIDERMIS

Keratinocytes are the major cells in terms of number and function in the epidermis (Figure 1-3). They are considered by researchers to be the native cells of the epidermis to distinguish them from cells believed to migrate into the outer layer of skin during development. The cells are termed *keratinocytes* due to their production of filaments made of keratins (in addition to other proteins). The keratinocytes provide the physical, including waterproof, barrier of the skin.

Immigrant cells include melanocytes (neural crest cells), Langerhans cells (immune cells), and Merkel cells (sensory receptors). Melanocytes have physical features common to neural cells, including dendrites. Approximately 3% of epidermal cells are melanocytes. These cells produce and distribute melanin, the brown pigment of skin and other tissues that provides protection against ultraviolet radiation. On average, each melanocyte distributes melanin to 30 keratinocytes via dendrites. Exposure to ultraviolet radiation stimulates melanin production and leads to the phenomenon known as tanning.

Langerhans cells are resident macrophages of the skin and provide the functions generally attributed to macrophages, including presentation of antigen to T cells. Different individuals become sensitized to a variety of foreign antigens, some of which are presented by Langerhans cells and manifest themselves as type IV immune reactions (delayed hypersensitivity). These include reactions to poison ivy and latex. Latex, in particular, is a major concern in wound management and will be addressed extensively in Chapter 18 on infection control. Merkel cells are interest-

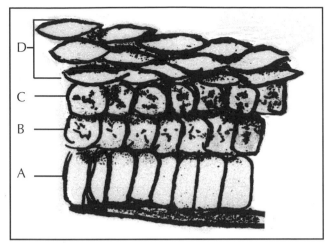

Figure 1-3. Cells and layers of the epidermis. The epidermis consists of four layers: (A) stratum basale, (B) stratum spinosum, (C) stratum granulosum, (D) stratum corneum.

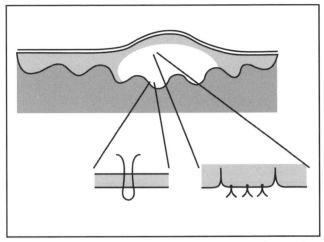

Figure 1-4. Formation of blisters. Fluid accumulation due to inflammation causes rupture of desmosomes and separation of the epidermis from the dermis.

ing sensory receptors in the sense that they consist of a separate receptive element at the junction of the epidermis and dermis, and a sensory neuron, whereas other mechanoreceptors consist of a specialized ending of the neuron and other sensory neurons carrying pain and temperature have nonspecific endings.

Accessory structures of the epidermis dwell in invaginations of epidermis into the dermis (see Figure 1-1). These structures may carry epidermal cells deeply into the dermis. The significance of the invagination of these structures is evident in partial-thickness burns. Although thermal injury may destroy the epidermis and some dermal depth, epidermal cells lining the accessory structures may provide cells to resurface the injured skin. These structures, which include pilosebaceous and sweat glands, are discussed more fully near the end of this chapter.

Layers of the Epidermis

Upon inspection of the epidermis by microscopy, distinct layering can be observed. From deep to superficial, the layers are termed the *stratum basale* (basal layer), *stratum spinosum* (spiny layer), *stratum granulosum* (granular layer), and *stratum corneum* (the hornlike layer). In addition, a layer termed the *stratum lucidum* (clear layer) is observed in the palms and soles, creating a much thicker epidermal layer. These layers are depicted in Figure 1-3.

The stratum basale consists of cuboidal/low columnar epithelium and is considered the germinative layer of the epidermis. It creates an undulating layer that rides along the surface of the dermis. This undulation increases the surface of contact between the dermis and epidermis, and provides greater resistance to shear stress. The height of these undulations on palms and soles produces the unique patterns of fingerprints and footprints. Excessive shearing

forces between the dermis and epidermis damage this area, creating blisters (Figure 1-4). As the germinative layer of the epidermis, markers of cell replication are abundant as well as organelles of very active cells, including mitochondria, Golgi apparatus, endoplasmic reticulum, and ribosomes. As the cells mature, they migrate superficially. The stratum spinosum consists of several layers of cells with keratin aggregation observed in bundles. As the cells migrate through the stratum spinosum, they become progressively flatter and begin to produce intracellular granules. The next layer, the stratum granulosum, exhibits continued flattening with extrusion of granules into the intercellular space. The granules consist of different lipid molecules. The lipid components of the extruded granules act as a permeability barrier between cells that act in a fashion similar to caulk or grout. As the cells continue to mature and migrate through the stratum granulosum, one can observe an accumulation of keratohyaline on filament meshwork within the cells, which is most developed in the superficial layer, the stratum corneum. This accumulation of a filamentous network gives rise to the name of this layer. As cells mature within this layer, degradation of mitochondria, the nucleus, and other organelles as well as gradual flattening of cells occur. On microscopy one can observe 15 to 20 layers of flattened cells filled with keratohyaline. The lower layers of cells demonstrate lipid layering and desmosomes, which provide physical linkage of adjacent cells. Upper cells of this layer, in contrast, demonstrate a loss of desmosomes and lipid layering. On average, approximately 14 days are required for a cell to migrate from the stratum basale to the stratum corneum, and each cell lasts about 14 days within the stratum corneum.

Cell Envelope

The cell envelope is a structure unique to keratinocytes. It develops beneath the cell membrane as cells mature and migrate superficially through the epidermis. It is constructed of several cross-linked proteins. These proteins are first detectible in the stratum spinosum. The envelope forms in the stratum granulosum and is complete in the stratum corneum. The enzymes required to synthesize the cell envelope develop as the cell matures.

Lipids

Lipids within the epidermis form the permeability barrier between adjacent keratinocytes. A distinct layering of lipid is observable in the stratum corneum. Sources of lipid within the stratum corneum include sebaceous glands, cell membranes, and lamellar granules. Lamellar granules develop in the stratum spinosum and are extruded in the stratum granulosum. The lack of essential fatty acids results in dry, scaly skin and increased skin permeability.

Growth Factors

A number of growth factors affect skin, including epidermal growth factor (EGF), acidic and basic fibroblast growth factor (aFGF and bFGF), insulin, insulin-like growth factor I and II (ILGF I and ILGF II), interleukin 2 (IL-2), colony-stimulating factors, nerve growth factor, platelet-derived growth factor (PDGF), and transforming growth factor α and β and (TGFα and TGFβ). These growth factors have multiple sites of action. Receptors for EGF and TGFα are found on basal keratinocytes, sweat duct cells, hair follicles, sheath cells, basal sebocytes, vascular smooth muscle cells, and arrector pilorum muscle cells. Growth factors EGF and FGF increase fibroblast number, TGFα has been linked to angiogenesis and fibroplasia, and PDGF has been linked to chemotaxis, DNA synthesis, collagen deposition, and wound contraction. Experimentally, PDGF normalizes wound repair in diabetic animals but is also suspected to be involved in atherosclerosis and neoplasia. Signals for release of growth factors have been studied. These include phospholipase C/protein kinase C, which is activated by bradykinin, histamine, thrombin, EGF, and PDGF. Phospholipase C/protein kinase C is implicated in both proliferation and differentiation of skin cells, the release of prostaglandins, and increased gene expression. Another signaling mechanism, tyrosine kinase, has been associated with TGFα, insulin, and bFGF to promote proliferation of skin cells. Prostaglandins and leukotrienes are associated with inflammation, which, as discussed later, is an important component of normal healing, but if prolonged impedes healing.

Accessory Structures

Hair follicles, sebaceous glands, sweat glands including eccrine and apocrine, and sensory receptors are described below and depicted in Figure 1-1.

Hair Follicles

Hairs are constructed of intermediate filaments, primarily keratins. This is basically the same material that makes up nails, horns, and claws. Each hair consists of microfibrils embedded in a matrix. In turn, each filament consists of coils of polymerized α-helices of protein molecules. Hairs grow cyclically with random cycles, so within a population of hairs, various hairs are at different phases at any given time. Hair follicles are dynamic tubular invaginations of epidermis lined with epithelial cells. Two major types of hairs are found on the human body. Vellus hairs are soft, unpigmented hairs that cover nearly the entire body and are often termed "under hairs." The other type are terminal hairs, which are firm, long, coarse, pigmented, and easily observable with the unaided eye. These are found on the scalp of both sexes, and beginning at puberty with tremendous variability on the trunk and extremities, more so on men than women.

During the growth cycle, hair follicles extend more deeply into the dermis, then gradually shorten as growth stops. The typical terminal hair grows about 0.5 mm/day on the head and about 0.4 mm/day on the body.

Nails

A nail plate sits on a rectangular epidermal bed with ridged surfaces that interdigitate and provide adherence of the nail to the nail bed. In contrast to keratinocytes, no keratohyaline granules develop in nail cells. The cuticle is continuous with digit epidermis and grows along with the nail. The nail itself, defined as devitalized cells, begins 7 to 8 mm proximal to the cuticle and the nail thickens as its plate migrates distally. The living cells develop in the matrix of the nail bed and cells move from the matrix into the nail plate, losing their organelles and becoming hard and waterproof.

Sebaceous Glands

These glands are found everywhere on the body surface except on the palm, sole, and dorsum of the foot, producing the substance known as sebum. The glands are the most dense and largest on scalp and face. These glands are not isolated but appear with and share a common opening onto the skin surface with hair follicles. Sebum flows through a short canal into the follicular canal, then onto skin. On mucous membranes, the sebaceous glands open directly onto skin. These glands remain small until puberty. Within sebaceous glands, cells replicate at the base of

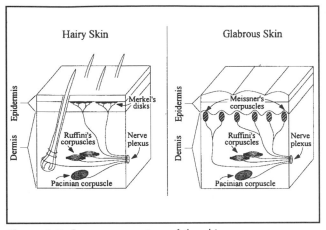

Figure 1-5. Sensory receptors of the skin.

the gland and migrate as lipid accumulation occurs within the duct. The cells themselves eventually become the excretory product (holocrine gland). Cells lose their nuclei and degrade, resulting in oil deposition onto the skin. The cells within the gland have a turnover time of 14 days. Although no short-term regulatory mechanisms are known (several old-wives' tales exist, however), androgens increase sebum production and estrogens decrease production. The rapid increase in androgen production with puberty predisposes these glands to occlusion and infection, resulting in acne.

Sweat Glands

Two types of sweat glands have been described. Eccrine glands have a thermoregulatory function, whereas apocrine glands have a "social" or emotional component. Both exist as coiled epithelial tubes. Apocrine glands are associated with hair follicles, whereas eccrine glands are distributed throughout the body surface. A tremendous variation in gland size and secretory rate exists from person-to-person. Centrally, sweating is stimulated at a threshold central temperature and increases with body temperature. Sweat glands also respond to local skin temperature. Central temperature is nine times more effective in stimulating sweat production than local skin temperature. Eccrine glands are innervated by cholinergic sympathetic nerves. These glands secrete plasma-like fluid, but reabsorb ions including Na, Cl, and HCO_3 along their length in response to aldosterone. Thus sweat is hypotonic at a low secretion rate, but increases in tonicity as sweat rate increases. Apocrine glands, in contrast, have adrenergic innervation and are stimulated by events that produce nonspecific activation of the sympathetic nervous system, including anxiety. These glands are found primarily in the axillary and perineal areas. The secretion of apocrine glands in certain animals is believed to be a chemoattractant. Whether this occurs in humans is still debated.

Sensory Receptors

Receptors present in the skin include mechanoreceptors that are sensitive to touch, particularly to vibration, thermoreceptors that are sensitive to warmth and cold, and nociceptors that are sensitive to painful stimuli and particular types of chemicals. Four major receptors are involved in producing the simple sensation of touch and are depicted in Figure 1-5. These include Pacinian corpuscles, Meissner's corpuscles, Ruffini endings, and Merkel disks. Pacinian corpuscles and Meissner corpuscles are rapidly adapting receptors with specialized endings. Pacinian receptors are found deep in the skin and respond to high-frequency vibration within a range of 60 to 500 Hz and to deep pressure. Pacinian corpuscles are particularly important in the evaluation of thermal injuries. The ability to detect deep pressure following deep burns indicates the survival of the deepest region of the dermis, whereas anesthesia to pinprick indicates a full-thickness injury. Meissner corpuscles respond to lower-frequency vibration up to 80 Hz and may be used to detect movement of the skin. Meissner corpuscles are located in nonhairy (glabrous) skin. In hairy skin, the Meissner corpuscle is replaced by hair receptors with similar properties. Ruffini endings and Merkel disks are slowly adapting receptors. Merkel disks have small receptive fields, are superficial, and are useful for localizing continuous pressure. Ruffini receptors are found deep in the skin and respond to deep pressure and stretch. These receptors are also directionally sensitive and are useful in proprioception and kinesthesia.

Thermoreceptors are found both peripherally in the skin and within deep structures. Skin thermoreceptors provide information used to sense environmental temperature, to determine the level of thermal comfort, and to regulate body temperature. Cutaneous receptors serve as warnings to avoid damaging the skin and feed information forward concerning the environmental temperature so that the thermoregulatory system can prevent a fall in internal temperature. Both cold and warm sensations are derived from neurons without specialized end-organs. Temperature information is transmitted by slowly conducting C and $A\delta$ neurons. Warmth and cold receptors are slowly adapting so they can convey both changes in temperature and develop a steady action potential frequency when temperature is held constant. Cold receptors respond within a range of approximately 5° to 45°C with a peak action potential frequency of about 25°C. Warm fibers respond within a range of about 30° to 45°C with a peak response at about 42°C. A combination of information from both types of receptors is necessary to detect temperature over a range of 5° to 45°C. Very high or low temperatures stimulate pain receptors and, therefore, give the same sensation.

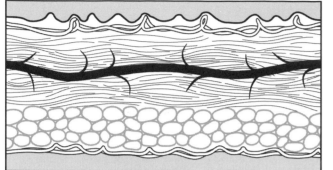

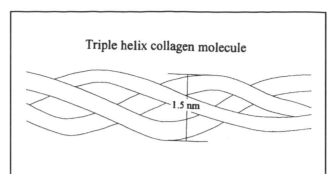

Figure 1-6. Structure of the dermis.

Figure 1-7. Structure of collagen fibers.

Nociceptors are receptors for "noxious" stimuli. They have no specialized endings and are distributed throughout the skin, muscle, bones, joints, dura, and capsules of organs. Two different types of neurons transmit different types of information. Neurons of the Aδ class transmit pain information that is localized, graded to intensity, and lasts as long as the stimulus is applied. The older type of neuron, the C fiber, transmits a more diffuse, poorly localized, and persistent pain associated with tissue damage or inflammation. These receptors respond to a number of chemical messengers including capsaicin, substance P, potassium, serotonin, bradykinin, histamine, and prostaglandins. Nociceptors also convey a discomfort in response to ischemia that motivates individuals to unconsciously shift weight. The lack of nociception places individuals at risk for pressure ulcers on skin beneath weight-bearing bony prominences.

Basal Lamina

The basal lamina is the junction of the dermis and epidermis. It consists of the clear, 20-nm-thick lamina lucida and the lamina densa. The two layers of the basal lamina are named based on their microscopic appearance. Within the lamina lucida, anchoring filaments pass from the basal layer. In the lamina densa, filamentous glycoproteins and type IV collagen are found. To increase the adherence of the epidermis to the dermis, collagen fibers pass through loops of anchoring filaments within the lamina densa. In certain diseases, the filamentous attachments of the epidermis to the dermis are selectively destroyed, resulting in a loss of large sheets of epidermis.

Dermis

The dermis consists of two major layers with important functional differences and three basic components, which are depicted in Figure 1-6. Fibroblasts are the principal cells of the dermis. Although they are not tremendously numerous or active in stable skin, fibroblasts are capable of secreting important macromolecules during the healing process. Fibers, especially collagen and elastic fibers, are

common in the dermis and are described further below. The third component is the ground substance, a gel of glycosaminoglycans and water.

Papillary Layer

The papillary dermis (pars papillaris) is thin and molded against the epidermal ridges/grooves. It consists of smaller, more loosely distributed collagen fibers than the deeper reticular dermis. In contrast to the reticular dermis, its fibers consist mainly of type III and IV collagen. The major feature of this layer is the network of blood and lymphatic vessels organized into plexuses. This layer is important in regulation of heat loss. Increased blood flow through the papillary dermis results in greater loss of heat to the environment.

Reticular Dermis

This layer of dermis has a much greater thickness than the papillary layer and is relatively acellular and avascular compared to other tissues. It is characterized by denser fibers and less gel than the papillary layer and type I collagen with a mesh-like organization with preferential direction. This organization of the reticular fibers gives rise to the structures known as Langer's lines, forming a grain-like nature to the skin. Langer's lines are important in performing body composition analysis with skin-fold calipers. A proper skin fold results only when the skin is pinched such that Langer's lines run perpendicular to the calipers. They are also important in understanding preferential direction of skin contraction following injury.

Fibers of the Dermis

Collagen fibers (Figure 1-7) are the principal fibers of the dermis, representing 77% of fat-free, dry weight. Collagen provides tensile strength in many tissues, including the skin. Different types of collagen, based on subtle variations in the molecular structure of the individual collagen molecules, are found in the body. Type I is predominant in reticular dermis, providing high tensile strength (ability to withstand traction). Other types of collagen are

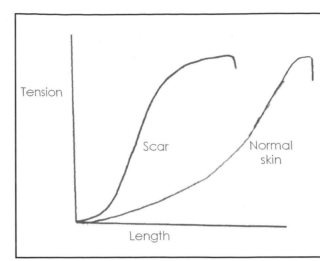

Figure 1-8. Stress-strain relationship of tendon and skin. Note four regions: In the first region, lengthening occurs with little stress. In the second region, a linear relationship between lengthening and stress can be observed. With further stress, fibers are damaged and elasticity is lost. Also note the greater extensibility of skin for a given stress. Scar tissue extensibility is similar to tendon.

characterized by their ability to withstand compression or are more elastic.

Elastic fibers consist of a fibrillar component termed *fibrillin* and an amorphous component named *elastin*. Elastic fibers are characterized by their wavy nature and springlike quality, thereby providing elasticity to skin. In Marfan's syndrome, fibrillin is defective, resulting in the physical characteristics of the disease as well as aortic insufficiency and risk of aortic aneurysm.

Ground Substance

Ground substance refers to the viscoelastic sol-gel of hydrophilic polymers found between cells and fibers of the dermis. The multiple branches of proteins with their charges are able to hold tremendous quantities of interstitial water in place. Overwhelming of the ground substance due to fluid balance derangement (ie, increased capillary pressure due to tissue injury or heart failure) produces free water movement in the interstitial space, manifested as pitting edema. Ground substance both lubricates and separates the fibers of the dermis, allowing them to move freely across each other. The binding of these molecules to collagen fibers also increases the tensile strength of collagen fibers.

Glycosaminoglycans are the primary type of molecule in ground substance. These molecules consist of chains of polysaccharides linked to protein that are metabolized and degraded by fibroblasts. Different proportions of glycosaminoglycans are present in different tissues and contribute to the biomechanical properties of these tissues. The more common glycosaminoglycans are hyaluronic

acid, chondroitin-4 sulfate, dermatan sulfate, and sulfate. Different connective tissues of the body different proportions of these specific molecules. mal skin, hyaluronic acid, chondroitin sulfate, a matan sulfate represent about 42%, 5%, and 54% glycosaminoglycans. In scar tissue, hyaluron decreases dramatically, and chondroitin sulfate in to proportions similar to those of tendon and bone

Biomechanics of Skin

Skin is much more elastic than the dense connect sue of bone, ligament, and tendon. Some of the diffe are due to the components, and some are due arrangements of these components. Tendons are ve and elongate very little with applied force. This stiff primarily due to the parallel arrangement of very bundles of collagen but, as discussed above, tendo different proportions of glycosaminoglycans than cartilage or skin. In addition to its elastic nature, n skin has tensile and viscous properties. Much of the ticity comes from viscous elements; therefore, sk described as having a viscoelastic property. In a si model, collagen fibers may be ascribed the role of pr ing tensile strength (ie, the ability to resist lengthen However, collagen fibers are both coiled and undula As stretch is applied to collagen fibers, they bec straightened, and at several points along each bundl collagen fibers, a number of elastic fibers attach to other and other collagen bundles. Further stretch strai ens the alignment of collagen and elastic fibers. The th dimensional interaction of collagen fibers and the atta ment of elastic fibers made of elastin provide the ability the skin to recoil when a stretch is applied to it. Grou substance, made of glycosaminoglycans and water, a provides some elasticity to the skin. Dehydration of t skin, as occurs with aging, diminishes skin turgor a allows the fibers of the skin to become lax. This is ma fested as tenting, in which a pinch of skin does not rec when released.

The response of material to an applied force is graph cally represented as a stress-strain curve (Figure 1-8). Th force applied to the tissue represents the stress (dependen variable on the y axis), and the length of the tissue repre sents the strain as the independent variable plotted on th x axis. Therefore, these measurements represent a meas urement of force across the tissue as its length is changed. Five areas subdivided within two major regions are characteristic of connective tissue. In the elastic region, no permanent change in tissue length occurs with stretch. If force is plotted with both increase and release of the stretch, a somewhat different path is followed. This phenomenon is termed *hysteresis* and is due chiefly to the viscoelastic nature of connective tissue.

the structure of the fibers within the dermis and their arrangement provide tensile strength and elasticity of the dermis. Excessive stretch applied to the skin results in tearing. Tearing occurs much more readily in the skin of the elderly. Subcutaneous fat provides thermal insulation and cushions bony prominences. Emaciated individuals are at much higher risk of pressure ulcers because of the lack of soft tissue between the bony prominences and skin.

STUDY QUESTIONS

1. List the functions performed by the skin.
2. Contrast the complexity and thickness of the dermis and epidermis.
3. Contrast the functions of the papillary and reticular dermis.
4. How does knowledge of the layers of the skin assist in determining the depth of skin injury?
5. In terms of healing, what is the benefit of the depth of the appendages of the skin?

BIBLIOGRAPHY

Irion G. *Physiology: The Basis of Clinical Practice*. Thorofare, NJ: SLACK Incorporated; 2000:181-188.

Normal Wound Healing

2

- List the phases of normal wound healing and their time frames.
- List the six processes that occur in a healing wound.
- Describe events of the inflammatory (lag) phase, including hemostasis and roles of immune cells.
- Describe the events of granulation tissue formation.
- Describe the need for coordination of granulation tissue formation and re-epithelialization.
- Describe the events of the remodeling phases and factors determining wound strength.
- Contrast the injury and healing of superficial, partial-thickness, and full-thickness wounds with subcutaneous tissue involvement.
- Describe features distinguishing fetal wound healing from adult wound healing.

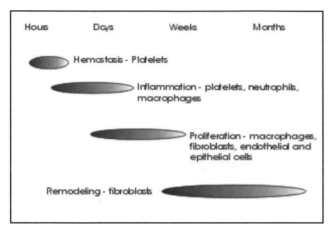

Figure 2-1. Time frames of the phases of wound healing by secondary intention. The relative length of each phase is depicted as the length of each ellipse. Note the time scale, the overlapping of phases, and the cells responsible for each phase.

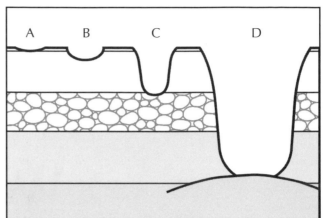

Figure 2-2. Skin structures involved in different depths of wounds.

Upon injury, a stereotypical sequence of events occurs, leading to the bridging of the defect and resurfacing. The depth of injury to the skin determines the sequence of events. Wounds may injure only in the epidermis (superficial), only some of the depth of dermis (partial-thickness), or the wound may damage the complete thickness of the dermis (full-thickness) and even extend into subcutaneous tissue. Most, but not all, of the wounds referred to individuals reading this text will involve full-thickness with subcutaneous involvement and healing by the secondary intent. The bulk of this chapter is a discussion of secondary intent.

Following a full-thickness injury, a programmed sequence of events unfolds, which the clinician may either facilitate or disturb with interventions. In this chapter, a description of these events is given. In subsequent chapters the ways we can facilitate and avoid interfering with the processes will be described. In sequence, these phases of normal wound healing by secondary intent are hemostasis, inflammation, proliferation, and remodeling (Figure 2-1). During these phases an overlapping, orderly sequence of six processes occurs: activation of hemostasis, activation of inflammation, re-epithelialization, granulation tissue formation, contraction, and remodeling.

TYPES OF WOUND HEALING

Superficial-thickness wounds are caused by shearing, friction, and mild burn (first degree). Healing occurs by regeneration of epithelial cells on the wound surface due to loss of contact inhibition, and migration of epidermal cells across the surface. Because no defect in skin continuity occurs, this type of healing does not cause scars, and accessory structures remain intact (Figure 2-2A). However,

this type of injury can mask a serious deeper injury. In many cases of pressure and shear injury, necrotic tissue may be hidden below an intact epidermis. Erosion of the epidermis (iceberg/volcano analogy) may lead to expulsion of necrotic tissue, creating a large void.

Partial-thickness wounds (Figure 2-2B) heal in a similar fashion as superficial thickness wounds. Damage to the dermis occurs, but accessory structures are spared. Eschar may form on the wound (desiccated necrotic tissue, similar to a scab). Partial-thickness wounds have similar causes to superficial wounds but generally with greater intensity of insult and may be caused by pressure.

Full-thickness wounds (Figure 2-2C) and wounds with subcutaneous involvement (Figure 2-2D) may be closed by primary intent, delayed primary intent (also known as tertiary intent), or by secondary intent. Primary -closure (Figure 2-3A) is used for surgical wounds or other incisions or lacerations that have clean, smooth edges and minimal subcutaneous tissue loss. Delayed primary closure uses sutures or staples later, often after irrigation and drainage of an abscess or osteomyelitis (Figure 2-3C). This type of closure is chosen when contamination, tissue loss, or risk of infection is present. Secondary intent (Figure 2-3B) is used for wounds with tissue loss, irregular edges, tissue necrosis, high microbial count, or presence of other debris. The phases of healing by secondary intent are described later.

Hemostasis and Inflammation

The first phase, hemostasis and inflammation, is initiated with blood vessel disruption and the extravasation of blood constituents. Injury to blood vessels is followed rapidly by activation of platelet aggregation and the coagulation cascade, resulting in the formation of the insoluble fibrin molecule and hemostasis. During this process, activation of complement occurs, leading to the sequence of

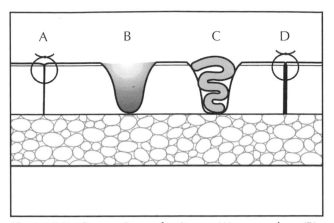

Figure 2-3. Comparison of primary (A), secondary (B), and delayed primary (C and D) (tertiary) healing. C depicts packing of wound to be closed later. D depicts wound in C closed with sutures. Note the clean edges and minimal granulation tissue of primary healing. Secondary healing is characterized by the production of granulation tissue and wound contraction. Delayed primary healing may be associated with some amount of granulation tissue and contraction depending on the amount of tissue lost to necrosis.

events of inflammation, including the recruitment of macrophages and neutrophils.

Platelets

With tissue injury, platelets are activated by collagen and thrombin. A positive feedback of secretion and aggregation ensues, amplifying the platelet response to injury. With platelet activation, platelet-derived growth factor (PDGF) release occurs. As discussed in Chapter 1, PDGF plays a major role in healing and is frequently defective in poorly controlled diabetes mellitus.

Coagulation Cascade

The series of chemical reactions leading to the production of fibrin is stimulated by the Hageman factor, which is activated either by exposure to collagen or by the release of tissue factor by injured cells. In addition, complement and other proteins activated by Hageman factor intensify the inflammatory response to injury.

Neutrophils

An influx of white cells begins with neutrophils early and macrophages later. Neutrophils increase the permeability of undamaged vessels, causing the leakage of plasma and proteins and the swelling associated with inflammation. The basic sequence used by neutrophils to clear bacterial contamination consists of opsonization of bacteria by complement, generation of chemotactic factors, adhesion of white blood cells to endothelium, emigration of white blood cells through vessels, attachment of opsonized bacteria to white blood cells, phagocytosis, and killing and digestion of bacteria.

Due to the nonspecific nature of neutrophil action, neutrophil recruitment also leads to tissue damage caused by release of enzymes and free radicals. Neutrophils are recruited by numerous factors related to the injury and, under normal circumstances, largely leave the area of injury when bacteria and dead cells are removed. The activation of neutrophils causes release of elastase and collagenase, which degrade the connective tissue surrounding the injury. Their primary function in an injury site is the destruction of bacteria via phagocytosis, and enzyme and free radical release. Neutrophil infiltration ceases in a few days if a wound becomes clean. At this time, programmed death of the neutrophils (apoptosis) occurs, which limits the destruction of cells in the area of injury. The appearance of spent neutrophils phagocytized by macrophages marks the end of early inflammation. However, contamination of wounds causes persistence of neutrophil immigration. Foreign surfaces initiate complement activity; therefore, repeated trauma by harsh treatment of wounds may also cause persistence of neutrophils.

Macrophages

Macrophages have the dual roles of destruction of nonviable material and the stimulation of growth of new tissue. The macrophage is both the garbage collector and the architect. The accumulation of macrophages continues regardless of neutrophil activity due to the presence of selective chemoattractants for macrophages. Initially, macrophages are responsible for phagocytosis of bacteria, spent neutrophils, and cell debris. In addition, they release numerous substances, including prostaglandins and leukotrienes, a variety of chemoattractants for cells to repair the defect, and the release of the growth factors PDGF, basic fibroblast growth factor (bFGF), and transforming growth factor β and α (TGFβ and TGFα). Macrophages, like neutrophils, also release proteases to aid in the degradation of devitalized tissue. The presence of macrophages is necessary for both the initiation and propagation of granulation tissue.

Mast Cells

Recently, mast cell-nerve interaction has drawn attention in wound healing and various other signaling mechanisms. During trauma, mast cells are degranulated, causing the release of a large number of chemical signals. Degranulation appears to be mediated by both an immediate sensory nerve-mediated response to injury and direct trauma. Although the chemical messengers are released in the immediate area of injury, the importance of mast cell degranulation with release of substances including histamine, heparin, bFGF, interleukin 4, tumor necrosis factor α (TNFα), and TGFβ is believed to be more immediately important in the tissue surrounding the wound.[1, 2]

In the immediate area of the wound, hemostasis prevents the loss of fluid, cells, and proteins; however, thrombosis of vessels may interfere with supply of nutrients to surrounding areas and increase the necrosis of tissue beyond the area of injury. Histamine produces vasodilation and increased permeability, thereby maintaining blood flow to adjacent tissue, as well as allowing cells responsible for immunity and repair into the area of injury. Heparin controls hemostasis, preventing excessive coagulation and damage to surrounding tissue. Basic FGF stimulates attraction and reproduction of epidermal cells, interleukin 4 increases synthesis of types I and III of collagen, laminin, and fibronectin. Mast cell release of TNFα and TGFβ provides a strong stimulus for the production of collagen. Capsaicin, the active ingredient in chili peppers, has been studied as a means of decreasing pain through the release of substance P and the downregulation of capsaicin receptors. Release of substance P and related compounds causes degranulation of mast cells, the release of endothelial adhesion molecules, and other cytokines that promote healing.

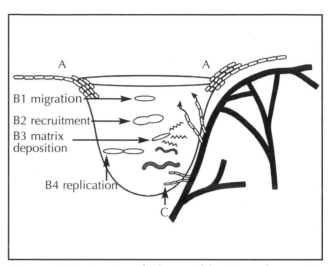

Figure 2-4. Events of the proliferative phase. (A) Proliferation and migration of epithelial cells from wound margins. (B) Proliferation of fibroblasts and production of collagen fibers. (C) Proliferation of angioblasts and angiogenesis.

Proliferative Phase

During the proliferative phase (Figure 2-4), both re-epithelialization and granulation tissue formation occur. In some types of wounds, wound contraction also occurs. Re-epithelialization begins within 24 hours, although it may not be observable for the first 3 days. This perceived delay at the macroscopic level is the basis for the term *lag phase*, which is sometimes used in the place of the term *inflammatory phase*. Granulation tissue formation begins in 3 to 5 days. During this time, re-epithelialization and granulation occur concurrently. Re-epithelialization provides protection, whereas granulation and contraction fill defects in tissue.

A variety of signals for initiation of new tissue growth are responsible for the proliferative phase, including chemotactic factors and growth factors released by the accumulation of macrophages and degranulation of mast cells in the injured tissue. In addition, the loss of neighboring cells (loss of cell restraint or contact inhibition) stimulates the replication of epidermal cells.

Granulation Tissue Formation

The production of granulation tissue is dependent on macrophage accumulation. Macrophages stimulate fibroblast ingrowth, deposition of loose connective tissue, and angiogenesis (formation of new capillaries in the wound). These processes, termed *fibroplasia* and *angiogenesis*, are also stimulated by chemotactic factors released by platelets in addition to those of the macrophages. Stimulation of fibroblasts by growth factors results in proliferation of fibroblasts, migration of fibroblasts to the area of injury, connective tissue matrix deposition, and wound contraction. Granulation tissue formation is stimulated by

low levels of bacteria in the wound but inhibited by high levels of bacteria.

Connective Tissue Matrix

The connective tissue matrix deposited by macrophages provides substrate for migration into the wound by other macrophages, angioblasts (immature cells of capillary walls), and fibroblasts. Angiogenesis is the process of forming new blood vessels, in this case in the area of a wound. During angiogenesis, endothelial cells respond to chemotactic and growth factors, and enzymes are released to degrade the basement membrane of existing blood vessels. As angioblasts are attracted to the distal end of blood vessels, they are stimulated to extend pseudopods through existing vessels, leading to the migration of angioblasts. The proliferation of angioblasts to form tube-like extensions from existing capillaries creates new capillaries. These new vessels allow healing to continue by supplying the cells with nutrients to support an increased metabolic rate and the materials to construct granulation tissue. The loops of vessels and matrix produce a shiny, reddish-pink tissue into pebbly mounds, which leads to the term *granulation tissue*.

Re-epithelialization

Resurfacing of the injured tissue is accomplished by the movement of keratinocytes from free edges, including those surrounding hair follicles and sweat glands, into the wound. As new cells are formed at the wound's edge, they adhere to the granulation tissue beneath, and replicated cells migrate by a means called *epiboly*, which has been described as a "leap frog" or "pouring over" of cells to reach the advancing wound edge (see Figure 2-4). With the loss of contact inhibition and the presence of growth factors, an alteration of the phenotype of cells occurs. A retraction of internal keratin filaments occurs along with dissolution of desmosomes to allow mobility of keratinocytes toward the wound edge. The newly unrestrained keratinocytes develop actin filaments and mobility, they lose apical/basal polarity, and extend pseudopods toward the wound. These cells will produce a provisional matrix consisting of fibrin, fibronectin, and type V collagen if the basement membrane is damaged. Cells also change the composition of undamaged basement membrane by incorporating more fibronectin as it is stimulated by the release of TGFβ. Cells are transformed to a normal phenotype when the wound is covered, and the keratinocytes are again constrained. Normal composition of the basement membrane is restored and desmosomes are re-established to secure keratinocytes through the basement membrane to the dermis.

Fibroplasia and Contraction

Fibroblasts undergo a phenotypic change following injury. Migration into the wound is aided by fibronectin. The fibroblasts retract their endoplasmic reticulum and Golgi bodies and begin to synthesize large quantities of collagen. In addition, they form actin filaments, transforming into myofibroblasts. The molecules deposited by fibroblasts, in particular fibronectin, result in the production of a loose extracellular matrix. An amplification of granulation tissue growth results as fibronectin and allows fibroblast movement across it, fibronectin links multiple fibroblasts into network, and greater quantities of matrix molecules are released into the wound site. The process of contraction produces radial movement of intact skin around the wound toward the center of the wound. Contraction of full-thickness wounds reduces the quantity of new tissue required to fill the wound.

Remodeling

The process of remodeling is typically thought of as a long-term response to wounding. However, extracellular matrix changes continually. Extracellular matrix and fibroblasts control each other until a stable matrix is formed in months to years. As a result, the extracellular matrix is different in the periphery and center of a wound. Although wound strength increases with deposition of collagen, strength increases by a greater magnitude than what can be attributed to the accumulation of collagen. The reasons suggested for this phenomenon include selective degradation of unstressed collagen fibers, reinforcement of stressed fibers, and reinforcement of collagen fibers by glycosaminoglycans.

Effects of Oxygen

Oxygen is believed to be important to several aspects of wound healing, including the competence of the immune cells, development of new blood vessels, and the production of collagen.[3] Tissue partial pressure of oxygen (PO_2) has been shown to vary with distance from a wound from a value close to 0 mmHg at the wound site and areas of vessel injury and to a value near arterial PO_2 near uninjured vessels. Hypoxia along with hypercapnia (excessive carbon dioxide) and acidosis may impair both immunity and collagen synthesis.[4] However, hypoxia is a strong stimulus for the angiogenesis. Lactate produced by either aerobic or anaerobic metabolism stimulates angiogenesis. Because macrophages produce lactate even under aerobic conditions, the stimulation of angiogenesis occurs even in a normoxic condition.

Much of the antimicrobial effect of immune cells is mediated by oxidative killing by neutrophils. The rate of oxidative killing by neutrophils is directly dependent on the production of superoxide radicals from molecular oxygen, which in turn is dependent on the PO_2 of tissue surrounding the neutrophil.[5]

Fetal Wound Healing

Differences in fetal incisional wound healing have been described for several years. Incisional wounds heal rapidly, with normal skin morphology and without scarring. Other features of scarless fetal repair include a lack of neutrophils and acute inflammation, rapid epithelialization, low vascularity, highly organized collagen, and a hyaluronan-rich matrix.[6,7] Discovery of the exact mechanism allowing scarless healing is hoped to lead to application to abnormal wound healing in the adult. One factor that is clearly delineated is the rich hyaluronic acid environment of the fetal wound. Hyaluronidase introduced into a fetal wound results in fibrosis and angiogenesis characteristic of adult wound healing.[8] Thus, a high level of hyaluronic acid and low hyaluronidase detected experimentally may be necessary for scarless healing.

Adult skin transplanted to a fetus and then wounded heals with scarring.[9] Fetal tissue transplanted to a subcutaneous location on an adult and wounded heals without scarring, but when transplanted to a cutaneous location does scar. When transplanted to a subcutaneous location, the graft heals with collagen generated by the fetal fibroblasts, whereas the cutaneous transplants heal with collagen from the host, leading to scarring. Moreover, adult skin transplanted to fetuses heals with scar formation, indicative that fetal cells, not the environment of the wounded tissue, determines whether scarring occurs. As the fetus approaches full-term, wounds heal with inflammation, granulation tissue formation, wound contraction, and scarring. Excisional wounds differ from incisional wounds in that tissue must be generated to fill a gap between edges of the wound. With this type of wound, both the size and gestational age increase the likelihood of adult-like scar formation.[10,11] The most promising strategy to mimic fetal healing at this time is manipulation of TGFβ. This cytokine has several roles in wound healing, particularly as a chemoattractant for cells involved in inflammation. TGFβ does not increase with fetal wounding as it does in adults. Moreover, the addition of antibodies to TGFβ significantly reduces scarring in adult skin, whereas application of TGFβ increases scarring.[12]

SUMMARY

Normal wound healing differs with the depth of injury. Simple partial-thickness wounds heal by re-epithelization, whereas full-thickness wounds may heal by either primary intention or secondary intention. Primary intention refers to surgical closure of clean, narrow wounds. Delayed primary or healing by third intent is used after a wound is sufficiently clean and narrow, to be closed later. Healing by secondary intent requires a coordination of hemostasis, inflammation, re-epithelialization, production of granulation tissue, wound contraction, and remodeling of the scar tissue. Fetal incisional wounds heal without scarring, although the risk of scarring increases with both the size of the wound and age. The greater proportion of hyaluronic acid and lower TGFβ activity appears to be important in scarless fetal wound healing. Transplant studies indicate that cells that are active in healing, rather than the wound environment, determines whether scarless healing occurs.

STUDY QUESTIONS

1. Contrast healing of superficial and partial-thickness wounds to full-thickness wounds.

2. Why does inflammation only occur in vascularized tissues?

3. Why might harsh treatment of wounds resulting in bleeding slow wound healing?

4. What benefit does exercise provide in preventing loss of range of motion following large, full-thickness skin injuries?

REFERENCES

1. Bauer O, Razin E. Mast cell-nerve interactions. *News in Physiological Sciences.* 2000;15:213-218.
2. Gottwald T, Coerper S, Schaffer M, Koveker G, Stead RH. The mast cell-nerve axis in wound healing: a hypothesis. *Wound Repair and Regeneration.* 1998;6:8-20.
3. Byl NN, Hopf H. The use of oxygen in wound healing. In: McCulloch JM, Kloth LC, Feedar JA, ed. *Wound Healing: Alternatives in Management,* 2nd ed., Philadelphia, Pa: F.A. Davis; 1995.
4. Allen DB, Maguire JJ, Mahdavian M, et al. Wound hypoxia and acidosis limit neutrophil bacterial killing mechanisms. *Arch Surg.* 1997;132:991-996.
5. Greif R, Akca O, Horn E-P, Kurz A, Sessler DI. Supplemental perioperative oxygen to reduce the incidence of surgical-wound infection. *N Engl J Med.* 2000;342:161-167.
6. Lorenz HP, Lin RY, Longaker MT, Whitby DJ, Adzick NS. The fetal fibroblast: the effector cell of scarless fetal skin repair. *Plast Reconstr Surg.* 1995;96:1251-1259.
7. Estes JM, Adzick NS, Harrison MR, Longaker MT, Stern R. Hyaluronate metabolism undergoes an ontogenic transition during fetal development: implications for scar-free wound healing. *J Pediatr Surg.* 1993;28:1227-1231.
8. West DC, Shaw DM, Lorenz P, Adzick NS, Longaker MT. Fibrotic healing of adult and late gestation fetal wound correlates with increased hyaluronidasae activity and removal of hyaluron. *International Journal of Biochemistry and Cell Biology.* 1997;29:201-210.
9. Longaker MG, Whitby DJ, Ferguson MWJ, Lorenz HP, Harrison MR, Adzick NS. Adult skin wounds in the fetal environment heal with scar formation. *Ann Surg.* 1994;219:65-72.
10. Cass DL, et al. Wound size and gestational age modulate scar formation in fetal wound repair. *J Pediatr Surg.* 1997;32:411-415.
11. Cass DL, Meuli M, Adzick NS. Scar wars: implications of fetal wound healing for the pediatric burn patient. *Pediatric Surgery International.* 1997;12:484-489.
12. Shah M, Foreman DM, Ferguson MWJ. Neutralisation of TGF-β1 and TGF-β2 or exogenous addition of TGF-β3 to cutaneous rat wounds reduces scarring. *J Cell Sci.* 1995;108:985-1002.

Abnormal Wound Healing

3

OBJECTIVES

- Define abnormal wound healing. List common causes.
- List signs of infection.
- Describe the appearance of necrotic tissue and its influence on wound healing.
- Describe the appearance of epiboly, the problems it causes with healing, and means of correcting it.
- Define maceration; describe its appearance, and list its cause and means of correcting it.
- Define desiccation; discuss its impact on healing, and list means of correcting it.
- Describe the appearance of wounds with chronic inflammation and chronic proliferation.

Abnormal wound healing refers to the failure of a wound to progress through the phases of wound healing described in the previous chapter, including the potential failure of inflammation, re-epithelialization, granulation tissue formation, and remodeling. Abnormal healing may manifest itself as chronicity of the phases of either inflammation or proliferation. Other manifestations may include abnormal granulation, re-epithelialization, or remodeling.

CHRONIC INFLAMMATION

Typical problems in wound healing include chronic inflammation, infection, hypergranulation, slow granulation, epiboly, maceration, desiccation, and chronic proliferation. Chronic inflammation generally results from the failure to optimize the wound and surrounding skin environment and protection of the wound from forces that initially produced the wound. Inability to remove necrotic tissue from a wound, clear infection, prevent repeated trauma to a wound, optimize wound and skin moisture[1], or addition of foreign surfaces are likely culprits.[2] These problems arise because of insufficient debridement, occlusion, or protection of the wound. Other problems include failure to correct the underlying causes of the wound such as arterial insufficiency, venous hypertension, pressure, shear, and inappropriate temperature and moisture.

Debridement refers to the removal of devitalized (dead) tissue by one of several mechanisms described in Chapters 12 and 13. Chronic inflammation may also be caused by repeated trauma due to inadequate occlusion or protection. Occlusion of a wound refers to the process of creating a separate environment around the wound (a microenvironment) by using special dressings that retain a combination of fluid, macromolecules, and heat within the wound. Protection may be achieved by simple dressings, bulky bandages, or splints, depending on the location and extent of the wound.

Chronic inflammation is characterized by discoloration of the surrounding skin with evidence of microvascular bleeding such as hemosiderin staining, ecchymosis, and induration, with possible undermining or tunneling. The wound itself will consist of necrotic tissue, fibrinous eschar, and produce moderate to maximum drainage (Figure 3-1). Because the initial phase of wound healing is dependent on inflammation to prepare the wound site, anti-inflammatory and other drugs that decrease the effectiveness of the immune system, such as anticancer drugs, chelating drugs (drugs that bind metal ions), and immunosuppressive drugs used for either preventing transplant rejection or treating autoimmune diseases, delay wound healing. Individuals with compromised immunity due to either a primary immunodeficiency (one of several genetic diseases) or secondary immune deficiency (eg, poorly controlled diabetes mellitus, alcoholism, or acquired

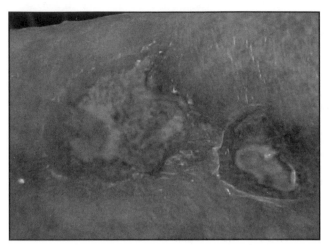

Figure 3-1. Appearance of chronic inflammation. Note the cardinal signs of inflammation in the surrounding skin: redness, swelling, and edema. Also note the presence of necrotic tissue within the wound bed. (Also shown in Color Atlas following page 274.)

immune deficiency syndrome) may experience a lack of inflammation to start the healing process. These wounds may also have damage to the surrounding skin with hemosiderin staining and ecchymosis. Because the lack of inflammation is often associated with arterial insufficiency, the surrounding skin may be an ashen gray or even a purple color. A wound lacking inflammation will be dry and cool, covered in eschar, usually hard and black, with little or no drainage (Figure 3-2).

INFECTION

In the case of the acute wound, the presence of bacteria is believed to cause chronicity. Persistence of bacteria in an acute wound is believed to increase the production of inflammatory cytokines such as interleukin-1 and TNFα.[3] Treatment of wound infection is directed at restoring the balance of bacteria in the wound through debridement, drainage, and appropriately timed wound closure. Closure of a wound with greater than 100,000 bacteria per gram is nearly certain to result in infection in adults in most areas of the body, although well-vascularized tissues, such as the face, are able to tolerate a greater bacterial burden.[4] Necrotic tissue, hematoma, and foreign bodies, including sutures, may need to be removed to restore a proper balance of bacteria in an infected wound.

Certainly in the acute wound, infection is the major concern in terms of delayed wound healing. Unfortunately, many topical (locally applied) treatments to control wound infection are cytotoxic (poisonous to cells) and by themselves delay wound healing. Povidone-iodine and Dakin's solution, in particular, have been recommended against use in pressure ulcers because of their cytotoxicity.

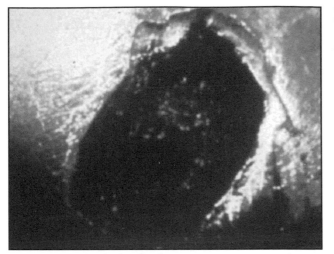

Figure 3-2. The lack of inflammation in a wound covered with black eschar. Also note the desiccation of the surrounding skin. Lack of inflammation prevents the proliferation of epidermal cells and fibroblasts necessary to close this wound. Courtesy of Little Rock Veteran's Administration Hospital. (Also shown in Color Atlas following page 274.)

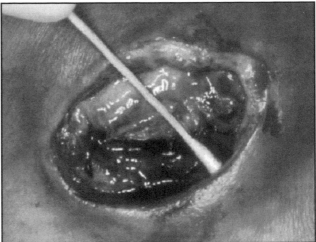

Figure 3-3a. Subcutaneous tissue defects. Undermining is an area of subcutaneous tissue loss beneath the wound edge, as demonstrated by the cotton-tipped applicator, usually in the form of an arc. Also note the presence of rolled edges, known as epiboly. The rolling under the edge prevents closure of the wound. Courtesy of Little Rock Veteran's Administration Hospital. (Also shown in Color Atlas following page 274.)

Although infection (see Chapter 18) delays wound healing, treating a wound that is not infected as if it were is not harmless but significantly delays what would be otherwise normal healing. Infection refers to the unchecked replication of bacteria. Normally, small quantities of a number of bacteria and fungi may be present on the surface of a wound. However, in analogy to a community aquarium, the proper mix, amounts, and different bacteria and fungi are usually benign. With introduction of a new species or even strains of bacteria or fungus, or a change in the microenvironment of a wound, a particular type of microorganism may grow out of control. Generally, clinical infection capable of slowing wound healing has been defined by the presence of greater than 100,000 organisms per gram. Infection is also characterized by invasion of tissue below wound surfaces. Degrading the tissue beneath the skin surface produces the phenomena of undermining, tunnels, and sinus tracts, which are depicted in Figures 3-3a and 3-3b.

Undermining is the development of a wound configuration of a "cliff," in which the size of the wound beneath the skin exceeds the opening of the visible wound. This is determined by probing the wound during the physical examination. A *sinus tract* is caused by the degradation of subcutaneous tissue in a linear manner with another wound opening at the other end of the tunnel. *Tunneling* usually implies a blind linear area of subcutaneous necrosis without a wound opening at the other end of the tunnel.

Signs of Infection

One of the major problems in diagnosing wound infection is that the same characteristics are present in both infection and inflammation. Both infection and inflammation are characterized by heat, tenderness, erythema, and swelling. Part of the problem is that release of cytokines occurs in response to the presence of both necrotic tissue and bacteria. Several descriptions of wound infections exist in the literature. In surgical wounds, a definitive diagnosis of infection requires the presence of purulent drainage or a spreading inflammation beyond what is expected of normal healing. Additionally, a quantitative culture obtained by tissue biopsy demonstrating greater than 100,000 organisms per gram or the presence of beta-hemolytic streptococci may be necessary to diagnose a wound infection. For surgical wounds, the prevailing belief is that a wound that heals primarily without discharge is uninfected and is infected if purulent discharge occurs.[3] The problem with culturing the purulent discharge is that bacteria may not be detected because the purulent drainage consists of dead bacteria, neutrophils, and tissue debris. Biopsy cultures of the wound, as opposed to swab cultures, are more likely to contain the bacteria causing the infection. In chronic wounds, infection may sometimes be detected visually as a dark discoloration (often brown) surrounded by normal reddish tissue, indicating an invasion

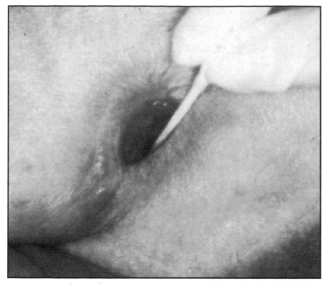

Figure 3-3b. Subcutaneous tissue defects. Tunneling is demonstrated with a cotton-tipped applicator as a linear subcutaneous defect. Courtesy of Little Rock Veteran's Administration Hospital. (Also shown in Color Atlas following page 274.)

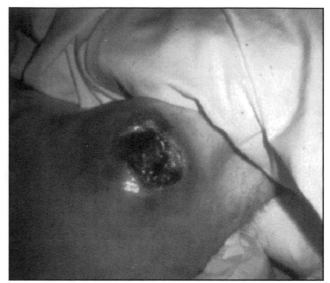

Figure 3-4. Infected trochanteric wound. As compared to the wound in Figure 3-1, inflammation greatly exceeds the edges of the wound and profound edema is present. Also note the presence of necrotic tissue and the emaciated condition of the patient. Courtesy of Little Rock Veteran's Administration Hospital. (Also shown in Color Atlas following page 274.)

of bacteria into healthy surrounding tissue (Figure 3-4). Infection can cause necrosis of what had been healthy tissue, degrading it and expanding the size of the wound. This is particularly apparent in the cases of what has been termed "flesh-eating bacteria" that invade along fascial planes, continuing to expand into and destroy healthy tissue.

Recommendations for treatment of infected pressure ulcers include the use of systemic antibiotics and a trial of topical antibiotics, which must be prescribed by a physician. The persistence of inflammation occurs in the presence of either necrotic tissue or bacteria. Cytokines such as interleukin-1 and TNF increase in response to bacteria in a wound, increase matrix metalloproteinases, and inhibit growth factors. Another risk factor for wound infection is the innervation of the tissue. Experimentally, the loss of innervation increases the bacterial growth in a wound 100-fold.[5] Subsequent research indicates that denervation decreases leukocyte function and increases the number of septic areas within the wound. Therefore, wounds accompanied by nerve injuries can be expected to have a higher risk of infection.[6]

A critical cause of delayed wound healing that can be addressed by the therapist or nurse is the presence of necrotic tissue. Necrotic tissue causes the mutual problems of increased risk of infection and slow wound healing. By their natures, infection increases the risk of delayed healing, and delayed healing increases the risk of infection. Removal of necrotic tissue through the process of debridement removes much of the risk of infection. In the case of

infected wounds, nonocclusive wound dressings are recommended. Microenvironmental dressings are conducive to cell growth and replication. Unfortunately, this may include bacteria; therefore, nonocclusive dressings and frequent cleansing are recommended for infected wounds.

SUBOPTIMAL WOUND ENVIRONMENT

Slow granulation describes the situation in which re-epithelialization exceeds granulation, forming a crater in a skin surface. There are two basic options to correct this problem. One is to slow the progression of re-epithelialization by burning the epithelial edge with silver nitrate. Silver nitrate sticks are available for this purpose (Figure 3-5). These sticks need to be moistened with normal saline before application, and the wound needs to be flushed with normal saline to prevent burning other areas of the wound. Another possibility is to investigate the cause of delayed granulation. One may wish to optimize the environment for granulation by using an occlusive dressing to retain moisture content, temperature, and growth factors within the wound microenvironment.

Epiboly is a condition in which the epithelial edge of a wound rolls under itself (see Figures 3-3a and 3-3b). When the margin of a wound rolls under itself, epithelial cells contact each other, causing contact inhibition, and re-epithelialization ceases. Epiboly is corrected by burning

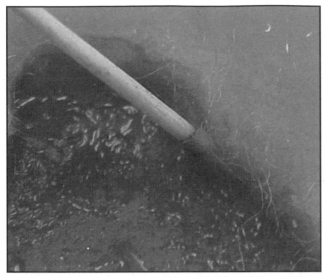

Figure 3-5. Silver nitrate stick, which may be used to burn rolled-over edges to aid epithelialization in a wound slowed by epiboly.

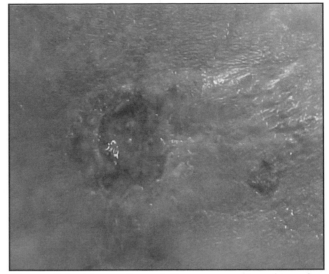

Figure 3-6. Maceration of the surrounding skin of a wound. Note the swollen, bleached out, and very wet appearance of the wound. (Also shown in Color Atlas following page 274.)

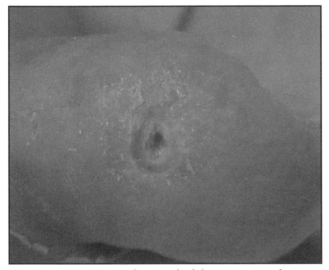

Figure 3-7. Desiccated wound of the great toe of a neuropathic foot. Also note the dryness of the surrounding skin and large margin of callus surrounding the wound, which is characteristic of neuropathic ulcers. (Also shown in Color Atlas following page 274.)

with silver nitrate or cutting the rolled edges from the wound to reestablish a free edge, and optimizing the wound environment.

Maceration (Figure 3-6) is the result of excessive moisture on epithelial surfaces, giving the appearance of a tissue that is swollen and "bleached out." Normal skin may become macerated even under seemingly trivial circumstances such as swimming or staying in a bath tub too long. During maceration, swelling of epithelial cells with disruption of desmosomes and death or loss of attachment of epithelial edges occurs. Application of a protective sub-

stance such as barrier cream or skin sealant on the surface of the wound can often protect the surrounding skin from maceration (see Chapter 16). Using a dressing with increased absorbency to keep moisture off the surrounding skin or more frequent dressing changes may also reduce maceration. Decreasing the handling of a wound to minimize trauma and inflammation may reduce the amount of fluid released from the wound, thereby decreasing the risk of maceration.

Desiccation is the drying out of a wound (Figure 3-7). It is caused by one or more of the following in combination: nonocclusive dressing that allows fluid to evaporate uncontrollably from a wound, excessive dressing changes with loss of fluid from the wound, or fluid disorders. Desiccation can be prevented by using an occlusive dressing to retain moisture in the wound bed, decreasing the frequency of dressing changes, or the use of a hydrogel filler or sheet (a gel substance) that can release moisture into a wound. When treating desiccation, however, one must be alert to the possibility of causing maceration of surrounding skin!

Hypergranulation refers to growth of granulation tissue in excess of the surface of the wound (Figure 3-8). Hypergranulation is usually caused by interference with re-epithelialization of wounds because of epiboly, maceration, or unrelieved pressure on the surrounding skin. Hypergranulation allows the wound to develop a "mound" exceeding the height of the surrounding skin and producing a cosmetically unacceptable scar. Steps may be taken to correct slow epithelialization by protecting the wound margin from maceration, removing any rolled-over edges (epiboly) by burning the affected wound margin with a sil-

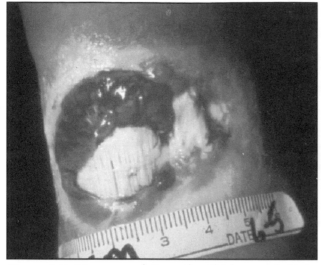

Figure 3-8. Hypergranulation of a tibial wound. Note the maceration of the surrounding skin, the height of the granulation tissue above the surrounding skin, bleeding of the granulation tissue, and the appearance of the tendon in the wound. Courtesy of Little Rock Veteran's Administration Hospital. (Also shown in Color Atlas following page 274.)

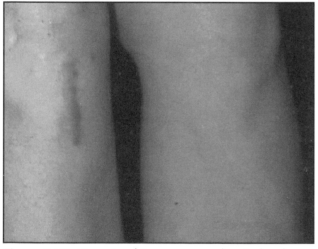

Figure 3-10. Hypertrophic scars secondary to hardware removal several months after arthroscopic surgery for anterior cruciate ligament repair. Note the presence of faint white resolved hypertrophic scars. (Also shown in Color Atlas following page 274.)

ver nitrate stick, or surgically cutting the epiboly. This condition of chronic proliferation occurs frequently with venous insufficiency. Damage to periwound skin with hemosiderin staining or ecchymosis and contraction of the skin is frequently observed. In venous insufficiency, the granulation tissue is a bright, healthy red color. Treatment includes reducing edema (swelling), if present, by techniques described in Chapter 10, including massage, compression pumping, and compression bandaging. Chronic

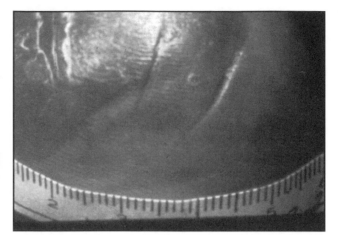

Figure 3-9. Subcutaneous hematoma of the heel. The clinician cannot determine the extent of subcutaneous necrosis in this case. Several authorities have suggested protecting this type of wound as long as it is stable. Courtesy of Little Rock Veteran's Administration Hospital. (Also shown in Color Atlas following page 274.)

proliferation may also be attributable to arterial insufficiency, which is obvious from the pink color of the granulation tissue. However, arterial insufficiency can be concurrent with venous insufficiency. Generally, little is available other than medicine, which must be prescribed by a physician to either dilate arterial vessels or improve the flow of blood through narrowed vessels, or surgery to repair or bypass narrowed arterial vessels. Arterial insufficiency frequently fails to produce inflammation or proliferation in addition to a failure of re-epithelialization.

Another complication of wound healing is subcutaneous hematoma due to chronic insult to underlying tissue (Figure 3-9). With this condition, the extent of necrosis cannot be determined easily.

OVER-REPAIR

Classically, two types of over-repair have been described: hypertrophic scars (Figure 3-10) and keloids. These phenomena result in susceptible individuals following wounding and are often discussed as part of the remodeling process of normal wound healing. Rather, these responses to wounding represent a failure to terminate the remodeling of a wound. Both types of wounds have the characteristic gross appearance of "three R's": red, raised, and rigid. In addition, keloids are more persistent, tend to regrow if excised, and extend beyond the area of injury. Hypertrophic scars may rise above the level of the surrounding skin, but generally do not extend beyond the area of injury. With time, these scars decrease in size, height, and vascularity. In many cases, the hypertrophic scars become white, flat, and avascular after several weeks to months. Keloid scars have been associated with diminished levels of interferon alpha and gamma and increased levels of interleukin-6 and TNFα, which is consistent with loss of inhibition on fibroblast metabolism and runaway collagen accumulation.[7]

Recently, a differentiation has been made between hypertrophic scars caused by surgical wounds and proliferative scars associated with burn injuries. Proliferative scarring associated with burn injuries does not appear until the patient is healthy and has reached a normal immunocompetence. Individuals susceptible to proliferative scarring following burn injury demonstrate increased interleukin-1, interleukin-6, TNFα, and TGFβ2 activity in blood cells. In particular, TGFβ stimulates a number of processes related to excessive repair and inappropriate scarring in many conditions, in addition to proliferative scarring. Treatment of proliferative scarring is described in Chapter 19.[8]

SUMMARY

Wound healing can be delayed by a number of factors either due to the patient's condition or due to inappropriate care of the wound. The wound fails to progress through the normal stages described in the previous chapter, either due to chronicity of a phase or failure of a phase to begin. Conditions that either prevent or sustain inflammation are common culprits. These include the presence of necrotic tissue, infection, placing gauze or cytotoxic agents in the wound, rough handling, and compromised immunity. Undermining, tunneling, and sinus tracts may occur as a result of compromised healing. Optimal care is provided by maintaining a moist wound bed and keeping the surrounding skin moist. Failure to do these also slows wound healing, causing desiccation, hypergranulation, or maceration. Excessive moisture caused by venous insufficiency needs to be addressed by appropriate compression therapy. Lack of inflammation due to arterial insufficiency needs to be addressed by a vascular surgeon.

STUDY QUESTIONS

1. If infection is a cause of slow wound healing, why are we so concerned about the effects of topically applied antimicrobial agents to wounds?

2. Why do wounds with epiboly fail to re-epithelialize and often have hypergranulation?

3. Why must the excessive moisture of venous insufficiency be treated to optimize wound healing?

4. Why does inflammation often fail in the presence of arterial insufficiency?

5. What products are available to keep surrounding skin dry in the presence of high levels of drainage?

REFERENCES

1. Winter GD, Scales JT. Effect of air drying and dressings on the surface of a wound. *Nature.* 1963;197:91-92.

2. Himel HN. Wound healing: focus on the chronic wound. *Wounds.* 1995;7 Suppl A (5):70A-77A.

3. Robson MC, Mannari RJ, Smith PD, Payne WG. Maintenance of wound bacterial balance. *Am J Surg.* 1999;178:399-402.

4. Robson MC. Wound infection. A failure of wound healing caused by an imbalance of bacteria. *Surg Clin North Am.* 1997; 77:637-650.

5. Alison WE, Phillips LG, Linares HA, et al. The effect of denervation on soft tissue infection pathophysiology. *Plastic and Reconstructive Surgery.* 1992;90:1031-1035.

6. Hui P-S, Pu LL, Kucukceleki A, et al. The effect of denervation on leukocyte function in soft tissue infection. *Surgery.* 1999;126:933-938.

7. McCauley RL, Chopra V, Li YY, Herndon DN, Robson MC. Altered cytokine production in black patients with keloids. *J Clin Immunol.* 1992;12:300-308.

8. Polo M, Ko F, Busillo F, et al. Cytokine production in patients with hypertrophic burn scars. *J Burn Care Rehabil.* 1997;18:477-482.

The Patient

A patient is wheeled up to the whirlpool. The dressing is removed and the wound is measured. A few observations are made and a few questions are asked about how the wound came about. The wound is put in the whirlpool every day for 2 months and never gets better. What went wrong?

A wound represents an impairment in the integumentary system. What occurs within the patient happens to the wound. A host of problems, some of which might seem remote to the cause of the wound, led to the wound or its slow healing. If the unique characteristics of the patient and lifestyle are not understood, optimizing wound healing cannot be understood. This unit is focused on discovering characteristics of the patient that either contribute to the etiology of the wound or impair wound healing. This unit includes three chapters that describe the vital information to prevent wounds from occurring and optimizing healing.

History Taking & Tests and Measures

4

OBJECTIVES

- Describe the six integumentary patterns described in the *Guide to Physical Therapist Practice*.[1]
- List critical elements in taking a history to aid in diagnosis and prognosis.
- List risk factors for developing wounds and slow healing of wounds that may be elicited by a history.
- Describe lab studies that may aid in the development of a diagnosis and prognosis.
- Describe the impact of social and work history on wound management.
- Describe how mobility impacts wound management.
- Describe how various types of equipment may affect wound management.

THE *GUIDE TO PHYSICAL THERAPIST PRACTICE*

The guide was published in its original form in the November 1997 issue of *Physical Therapy*[1] as a means of improving the uniformity of physical therapist practice. The guide consisted, at that time, of two parts: a description of the practice of physical therapy and a series of preferred practice patterns. The guide was revised in 2001, with little change to the integumentary practice patterns. The preferred practice patterns are grouped by body systems into musculoskeletal, neuromuscular, cardiopulmonary, and integumentary. Within each body system, a different number of patterns are described. Musculoskeletal refers mainly to the areas typically described previously as orthopedic, including disease or injury to the muscles and their structural supports such as bone, ligament, and tendon. Neuromuscular includes a number of injuries or diseases of the nervous system, ranging from the input to the nervous system, processing of sensory input, and output to the effectors. Cardiopulmonary patterns, especially in the first revision of the guide, represent disease or injury affecting the heart, blood vessels, and lungs. The integumentary patterns include:

- Pattern A: Primary Prevention/Risk Factor Reduction for Integumentary Disorders.
- Pattern B: Impaired Integumentary Integrity Secondary to Superficial Skin Involvement.
- Pattern C: Impaired Integumentary Integrity Secondary to Partial-Thickness Skin Involvement and Scar Formation.
- Pattern D: Impaired Integumentary Integrity Secondary to Full-Thickness Skin Involvement and Scar Formation.
- Pattern E: Impaired Integumentary Integrity Secondary to Skin Involvement Extending into Fascia, Muscle, or Bone.
- Pattern F of the original version, dealing with lymphedema, was moved to the cardiopulmonary section in the second edition and is not covered specifically in this text. A number of other sources, including several continuing education programs, are available to learn more about management of lymphedema.

The guide makes explicit use of terminology not previously used uniformly by physical therapists. In particular, the terms *examination*, *evaluation*, *diagnosis*, *prognosis*, *plan of care*, *intervention*, and *outcomes* are defined in the guide as used in physical therapy. Examination includes taking a history from the patient verbally or on a history form, or a combination of the two. Taking a history is the major emphasis of this chapter. A physical examination guided by the history of the patient is then performed.

The physical examination consists of a pertinent systems review examining components of the cardiopulmonary, neuromuscular, musculoskeletal, and integumentary systems; determining ability to communicate; and performing specific tests and measures as the history, systems review, and other tests and measures dictate.

In the past, the terms *evaluation* and *assessment* have been used interchangeably. To some, the terms convey different meanings. According to the guide, evaluation is the mental process by which the clinician makes judgments regarding diagnosis and prognosis. Diagnosis is "a label encompassing a cluster of signs and symptoms, syndromes, or categories" resulting from evaluating the data collected from the examination. Typically, the diagnosis encompasses one of the preferred practice patterns. Rather than reiterating the referring diagnosis, which is pathology-driven, the process is meant to establish which preferred practice pattern best fits the individual patient to produce an impairment-driven diagnosis. In many cases, two or more patterns may seem to fit a given individual. However, we are usually able to select one pattern that includes the most appropriate outcomes for that individual. In certain cases, especially involving multiple trauma or multisystem involvement, two or more patterns may be necessary.

Prognosis refers to the clinician's estimate of optimal level of function that could be attained given the unique combination of diagnosis and characteristics of the individual patient. A prognosis also includes a time frame quantified either as a number of visits or number of weeks/months. A combination of time and visits may also be used. For example, one may have a prognosis that a wound will be clean and stable in 2 weeks, requiring 20 visits.

The plan of care lists specifically the goals, expected outcomes, interventions to be used, duration (a time frame) and frequency of visits needed, and criteria for discharge. Interventions are divided among three categories:

1. Communication, coordination, and documentation
2. Patient education
3. Procedural interventions such as debridement and dressing changes

Outcomes are the measurable or observable products of intervention and are generally related to goals and discharge criteria.

Each pattern includes a uniform set of headings. The first heading is Patient Diagnostic Group. Under this heading, a number of medical diagnostic categories are listed, followed by a listing of possible diagnoses included in and excluded from the specific pattern. Also given is a listing of possible ICD9 (International Classification of Disease, Version 9) codes that might apply to patients/clients described by the pattern. Examination is defined as the collection of information including taking a history, performing a systems review, and performing tests and measures. Under the examination heading, an exhaustive list of possible items to be discovered by the history is listed. Systems review includes determination of the physiological and anatomical status of the cardiopulmonary, integumentary, musculoskeletal, and neuromuscular systems, as well as communication, affect, cognition, language, and learning style. An alphabetical listing of pertinent tests and measures for the practice pattern follows. Typical for the integumentary patterns are assessments of integumentary integrity; analysis and assessment of orthotic, protective, and supportive devices; analysis and assessment of pain; and tests and measures of ventilation, respiration, and circulation.

The next major heading is Evaluation, Diagnosis, and Prognosis. Each of these terms is defined, followed by a prognosis for the pattern based on an 80% confidence limit (ie, 80% of patients/clients described by a pattern will achieve the stated outcomes within the time limits listed). Also listed under this heading is a list of factors that either may require a new episode of care or may modify the time limits stated in the prognosis. The next major heading is Intervention. Interventions are discussed throughout Unit 4 of this text.

Pattern A is the primary prevention and risk factor reduction pattern. The primary health problems that fit this pattern include those with a low or moderate risk assessment score (Braden or Norton scale, discussed in Chapter 9), amputations, diabetes mellitus, and spinal cord injury.

Pattern B refers primarily to superficial wounds, including first-degree (superficial) burns, grade 0 neuropathic ulcers (ulcers due to decreased sensation, motor, or autonomic nerve function), and stage I pressure ulcers. As a progression, pattern C deals with partial-thickness wounds and scar formation. This pattern is used mainly for patients with second-degree (superficial partial-thickness) burns, certain blistering dermatological disorders, grade 1 neuropathic ulcers, and stage II pressure ulcers. Pattern D progresses to full-thickness wounds and includes full-thickness burns, necrotizing fasciitis, grade 2 neuropathic ulcers, stage III pressure ulcers, venous insufficiency, abscess, and frostbite. Pattern E includes wounds with subcutaneous tissue involvement. These may include abscess; necrotizing fasciitis; grade 3, 4, or 5 neuropathic ulcers; stage IV pressure ulcers; surgical wounds; arterial insufficiency; acute amputation; chronic surgical wounds; electrical burns; and frostbite.

ELEMENTS OF A HISTORY

History must be complete enough to guide the clinician to the proper tests and measures to determine the cause of the wound and to identify any characteristics of the wound, patient, family, caregivers, living arrangements, work/school, and resources that would affect the outcomes of different intervention strategies so that an optimal plan of care can be devised.

Demographic data include age, sex, race/ethnicity, and primary language. The age of the patient has an impact on the rate of healing, the typical daily activities of the patient, and the probability of certain etiologies of the wound. Hand and foot dominance are often overlooked unless the wound is located on a hand. With wounds on a hand or foot, the patient needs to be questioned about activities involving those extremities and a discussion concerning alternatives for accomplishing tasks with any limitations placed on the extremities. It may also be important in terms of any home program to ensure that the patient has sufficient dexterity to perform self-care.

Developmental history includes any disorders that may aggravate the wound, create difficulty in carrying out a home program, or impede the patient's ability to protect the wound.

A history of present condition should include the date of onset (if known), course of events, and pattern of symptoms of what the patient thinks caused the wound. In the case of an acute wound, the cause is usually obvious, such as a burn or laceration. In the case of a chronic wound, it is imperative to ascertain how the wound was managed. For example, was the underlying venous insufficiency treated? What preventive measures have been undertaken to alleviate pressure? Is the present treatment causing chronic inflammation? The specific concerns that led the patient to seek services and concerns or needs of the patient need to be explored. The plan of care may need to be modified to match the priorities of the patient, rather than forcing the clinician's priorities on the patient. Many times, optimal treatment for the wound is not the optimal treatment for the individual patient because of work, home, or other concerns. The plan of care will also need to accommodate the patient's, family's, and caregiver's emotional response to the current clinical situation and possible treatments. The functional status and activity level prior to the problem and expectation of return to this function and activity are critical areas for an interview to ascertain. Functional status and activity level may be a cause or complicating factor for a wound. For example, the person with a neuropathic ulcer on the plantar surface whose work requires walking or the person with venous insufficiency who is on his or her feet all day can both cause and slow healing of ulcerations. The clinician must determine the current and prior functional status in self-care and home management activities, including activities of daily living (ADLs) and instrumental activities of daily living (IADLs), and who is available to assist with activities if the patient is not able or needs to desist from the activities to allow wound healing. Moreover, recreational or leisure activities and degree of physical fitness need to be considered in both developing a diagnosis and tailoring a plan of care that matches the patient's needs.

A list of medications being taken for the current condition, as well as other conditions, is critical information. Unfortunately, for many individuals the list is long and can be forgotten in the outpatient situation. A strategy of asking the patient to bring all prescriptions can aid in an accurate list. Inpatient or home therapy can be easier, but patients may take nonprescription drugs, including over-the-counter, street drugs, herbs, or other substances that can also affect wound healing. The past history of the current condition needs to include prior therapeutic interventions and careful questioning to determine why previous therapy was ineffective. Was the underlying problem addressed? Was the intervention not carried through? Was the intervention performed incorrectly? These can be delicate questions, especially when the clinician thinks the cause of the wound is obvious. The clinician needs to be prudent in implying incompetence of other health care providers, especially before a clear diagnosis can be made.

RISK FACTORS FOR DEVELOPING WOUNDS AND SLOWING THE HEALING OF WOUNDS

The risk factors listed below should always be explored. A simple means is to have the patient fill out a health history form. A thorough history should be available on the chart of an inpatient; moreover, often the medications taken by the patient alert the clinician to a possible disease. Given the prevalence of diabetes mellitus and its impact on wounding and healing, every patient should be asked about diabetes and family history for diabetes. Other risk factors include gastrointestinal disorders as well as cardiopulmonary and vascular disorders that may impede the flow of nutrients to tissue, resulting in ulceration. Incontinence, impaired mobility, and immune system status can both allow wounds to develop and impede wound healing.

LAB STUDIES

Results from basic lab studies can be found on the charts of inpatients. It is unlikely that an outpatient will be able to provide much assistance to the clinician in providing results of lab studies. Results that are useful to the clinician include blood counts to determine if anemia, thrombocytopenia (lack of platelets), or leukopenia (lack of white blood cells) is present. Blood chemistry including electrolytes (potassium, sodium, chloride, and bicarbonate), blood urea nitrogen (BUN) and creatinine for renal function, and blood glucose should be present on the chart

of an inpatient and may be available from the referring physicians.

Blood Counts

Both total white blood cell (WBC) count and differential white cell counts may be important in certain cases. In terms of risk for infection or diagnosis of infection, neutrophil counts are also critical. Normal WBCs range from 4500 to 11,000/mm^3 in both men and women.[2] Leukocytosis is commonly defined as a count exceeding this range. Of particular importance in the context of wound management is the diagnosis of infection. Other causes of leukocytosis that should be considered include leukemia or another form of cancer, tissue injury, and some other source of inflammation. Leukocytosis is frequently accompanied by fever, somnolence, and anorexia produced by elevated cytokines released in these conditions. As discussed in subsequent chapters, wound infection has a profound effect on decision making. Leukopenia, defined as a count less than the range listed above, can be produced by a number of causes, including bone marrow disease (aplastic anemia), viral infection, and cancer chemotherapy. As the white cell count falls, the clinician must become more careful with technique. A WBC below 1000 or neutrophil count below 500 usually requires reverse isolation with gloving, gowning, donning a mask, and sterile technique even for routine wound care.[3]

Neutrophils observed in a differential count may be termed either segmented (mature) or banded (immature). Neutrophil counts are generally elevated in the presence of bacterial infection. A large number of bands is particularly diagnostic of bacterial infection. Lymphocytes are divided into B cells and T cells, and further divided into categories. B cells are responsible for antibody-mediated immunity, whereas T cells are involved in specific cell-mediated immunity against specific antigens. T cell immunity is associated particularly with neoplasms and viral infection but is involved in delayed hypersensitivity reactions, including skin reactions (eg, poison ivy). Monocytes are blood cells equivalent to the tissue macrophage. These cells are responsible for later destruction of marked cells and destruction of debris following neutrophil infiltration. Eosinophils are involved in defenses against worms and are implicated in allergic responses, including asthma. Basophils are the blood equivalent of mast cells, which release mediators of inflammation, particularly histamine. Normal differential counts are 50% to 60% neutrophils, 30% to 40% lymphocytes, 1% to 9% monocytes, 0% to 3% eosinophils, and 0% to 1% basophils. In addition, bands (immature neutrophils) range from 0% to 7%. Elevations in neutrophils, termed *neutrophilia*, and especially bands are usually indicative of infection by pyogenic organisms such as Staph or Strep species. Lymphocytosis (excessive B or T lymphocytes) is indicative of viral infection. Monocytosis (elevated monocyte count) may occur in severe infections. Excessive numbers of eosinophils (eosinophilia) are indicative of severe allergic reactions or worm infestation, and basophilia indicates parasitic infection or hypersensitivity reactions. *Neutropenia*, defined as a neutrophil count of less than 500, along with leukopenia requires reverse isolation.[3]

The normal red cell count is greater in men than women. For men, the normal ranges are 4.7 to 6.1 million per μL, a hematocrit of 42% to 52%, and a hemoglobin concentration of 14 to 18 g/dL. These ranges for women are 4.2 to 5.4 million per μL, 37% to 47%, and 12 to 16 g/dL, respectively.[2] During pregnancy, these numbers decrease. The importance of red cells, regardless of which parameters are used, is their ability to transport oxygen to aid in wound healing. Elevations in red cell parameters (polycythemia) are rare but clinically significant. Much more common are conditions that lower these numbers, producing anemia. Causes of anemia include bleeding, diseases of red cell production (aplastic anemia, pernicious anemia, iron and vitamin deficiencies), diseases characterized by excessive destruction of red cells (hemolytic anemias, including several autoimmune diseases, and sickle cell anemia), and genetic diseases of hemoglobin synthesis (thalassemias). Several lab tests are available for determining the cause of anemia. Another major cause is cancer chemotherapy. Regardless of the cause of anemia, decreased oxygen transport capacity of blood has a deleterious effect on wound healing. Improving red cell and elevating red cell parameters by correcting the cause, by transfusion, or by administration of endogenous erythropoietin is important to assist wound healing.

Platelets are fragments of cells called *megakaryocytes*. Platelets have a major role in hemostasis, which is usually the first step in acute wound healing. The normal range for platelets is 150,000 to 400,000 per μL. *Thrombocytosis* is the term for an elevated count, whereas a deficiency is termed *thrombocytopenia*. In terms of wound healing, the normal concern is thrombocytopenia rather than thrombocytosis. Thrombocytopenia, like anemia and leukopenia, occurs with aplastic anemia and cancer chemotherapy. Platelets can be diminished by a number of autoimmune diseases or consumed in disseminated vascular coagulation. Thrombocytopenia reduces the initial reaction to wounding and proliferation by decreasing the availability of platelet-derived growth factor (PDGF). The effectiveness of platelets is also reduced in von Willebrand's disease, a genetic disorder that prevents the platelet from adhering at the site of injury.

Tests related to hemostasis are the International Normalized Ratio (INR), prothrombin time (PT), and partial thromboplastin time (PTT). Inadequate hemostasis is a concern for several aspects of wound management, and these values and their interpretation should be understood.

Thrombin is produced in the coagulation cascade as the final enzyme of the processes, converting fibrinogen to fibrin, augmenting the strength of the platelet aggregate, and trapping red cells in the thrombus. PTT is an index of the effectiveness of the coagulation cascade only, whereas PT is affected by clotting factors, prothrombin, and fibrinogen. PT is prolonged with anticoagulation therapy, vitamin K deficiency, and genetic defects in the coagulation cascade, such as hemophilia and von Willebrand's disease. PT is tested both to screen for coagulation disorders and to determine the effectiveness of anticoagulation therapy. Because of variation in PT in different labs, the INR was developed. This index corrects for variations in testing materials and compares results of PT to reference values; therefore, INR should be identical in different labs for the same person. Normal values for PT range from 12 to 15 seconds, PTT ranges from 25 to 40 seconds, and INR should be between 0.9 and 1.1. Note INR does not have units; it is a ratio of PT to PT reference values. Values of PT 1.5 to 2.5 times normal are desirable for patients with hypercoagulability concerns such as history of deep venous thrombosis, coronary artery disease, or cerebrovascular disease. A PT greater than 2.5 times normal presents a risk of spontaneous bleeding, but particular care must be taken even with a therapeutic PT. Using INR numbers, concern for bleeding occurs at a value greater than 2.0. A value of 3.0 places the patient at risk of spontaneous bleeding.[3]

Electrolytes

The electrolytes routinely analyzed are serum sodium, potassium, chloride, bicarbonate, and sometimes calcium and magnesium. Because these are electrolytes, alterations from normal ranges can have profound effects on excitable tissues—muscle, nerve, and myocardial cells. Normal serum sodium has a range of 135 to 145 mEq/L, potassium is 3.5 to 5.0, chloride is 98 to 109, bicarbonate is 20 to 30, calcium is 9.0 to 10.5, and magnesium is 1.2 to 2.0 mEq/L.[2,3] The amount of sodium in the body determines fluid volumes, and alterations can cause swelling or shrinkage of cells. Potassium is the primary determinant of membrane potentials. Excessive potassium in the extracellular fluid depolarizes cells, whereas depleted extracellular potassium hyperpolarizes cells. Potentially life-threatening arrhythmias can develop with either hyper- or hypokalemia. Hypokalemia can produce muscle tetany due to depolarization of muscle and nerve cells, whereas hyperkalemia leads to hyperpolarization and muscle weakness. Alterations of chloride are diagnostic for fluid balance disorders, and bicarbonate changes are diagnostic of acid-base disorders. Both calcium and magnesium are intimately involved with neuromuscular function. Ionized calcium decreases the probability of neuromuscular excitation and, as such, both hypocalcemia and hypomagnesemia cause tetany and arrhythmias. Hypercalcemia and hypermagnesemia cause muscle weakness and arrhythmias.

Renal Function

The two lab values of BUN and creatinine are routinely measured. Normal kidney function eliminates these substances within a given range of these values. Failure of the kidneys allows nitrogen and creatinine to accumulate in the blood. Normal values of BUN range from 10 to 20 mg/dL in adults. Because BUN represents a balance between production of urea from breakdown of proteins and excretion by the kidney, a sharp increase in protein intake may increase BUN. Increased BUN may also result from gastrointestinal bleeding and dehydration. Decreases in BUN may be seen with liver disease because of a diminished ability of the liver to produce urea, and with overhydration. Creatinine is a product of muscle tissue. The normal range for creatinine is 0.5 to 1.2 mg/dL. Creatinine excretion decreases with renal disease, causing plasma creatinine to increase above this concentration. Plasma concentration may decline with decreasing muscle mass or increase with muscle injury. Of concern with renal disease are the accompanying cardiovascular problems, including hypertension and anemia. Because erythropoietin is synthesized by renal cells, administration of exogenous erythropoietin may be used to treat the anemia of end-stage renal failure.

Blood Glucose

Normal fasting blood glucose is considered to be less than 110 mg/dL. Blood glucose rises with eating and decreases with insulin and exercise. A person with normal glucose metabolism will return blood glucose to the normal range within 2 hours of consumption of 75 g of glucose. A person with diabetes mellitus (DM) will have a blood glucose in excess of 200 mg/dL at the end of the test, and a person with impaired glucose tolerance will have a blood glucose between 140 and 200 mg/dL. Either an oral glucose tolerance test or an elevated fasting blood sugar is indicative of DM. By the older definition, hyperglycemia is present with a blood glucose in excess of 150 mg/dL. Newer definitions have lowered the threshold. In 1998, a new category called impaired fasting glucose was defined by the American Diabetes Association. Impaired fasting glucose is considered to exist at a value of 110 to 125 mg/dL. This state has been referred to as a prediabetic state. Some experts suggest that interventions at this point might be able to prevent the development of type 2 DM. A blood glucose in excess of 126 mg/dL on at least two measurements is diagnostic of DM.

Impaired glucose metabolism is considered a risk factor for future DM and macrovascular disease. A person with a fasting blood glucose between 120 and 150 mg/dL is con-

sidered to have impaired glucose tolerance. As such, clinicians should be concerned about wound management for an individual with any impairment in glucose uptake. Another test commonly performed is the 2-hour postprandial blood sugar. In this test, blood glucose is measured 2 hours after eating. A normal value should be obtained within this time frame. Short-term, elevated blood glucose values up to 250 mg/dL are not considered to be dangerous. When blood glucose concentration exceeds this level, the ability of the renal tubules to reabsorb glucose is saturated and glucose appears in the urine. Over the long-term, elevations of blood glucose above 120 mg/dL are considered a health risk. A means of monitoring long-term glucose control is to measure glycated hemoglobin. The percentage of glycated hemoglobin is an index of how glucose has been controlled over the 120-day life span of the average red blood cell. Poor glucose control causes glycated hemoglobin (HbA1c) to exceed 9%. This corresponds to an average blood glucose of greater than 210 mg/dL. Optimal control produces HbA1c values of less than 6.1%, which represents an average blood glucose of less than 120 mg/dL.

An additional concern and potential medical emergency is hypoglycemia. Hypoglycemia results from an imbalance of eating, insulin, and exercise, and is not uncommon in ill individuals. Symptoms of hypoglycemia may manifest at a wide range of blood glucose values. At a value of 70 or less, corrective action should be taken, usually by providing oral carbohydrates in various forms such as sugar tablets, carbohydrate snacks, or concentrated sugar drinks such as orange juice—but not diet drinks! Symptoms of hypoglycemia are basically those of generalized sympathetic nervous system activation. This includes tachycardia, shaking, and excessive sweating. The patient may also complain of a headache or be apathetic and uncoordinated. Maintaining a balance of eating, insulin, and activity needs to be stressed with a patient with diabetes, especially an individual who is sick or has wounds. Illness or surgery can lead to wild fluctuations in blood glucose. Frequently, stress elevates corticosteroids, which in turn elevate blood glucose. Insulin doses are increased, but often patients fail to eat regularly and blood glucose can plummet. Clinicians must be constantly aware of this possibility and should be able to test for blood glucose and take corrective action themselves in addition to reporting the episode to the physician responsible for managing the patient's diabetes.

SOCIAL AND WORK HISTORY

Cultural beliefs and behaviors may profoundly affect the patient's ability to heal from a wound and may also directly or indirectly be the cause of a wound. Some religious beliefs will limit the range of interventions available for a plan of care. Moreover, the use of home remedies that are a part of a person's heritage but are unknown to the clinician may affect wound healing.

A frank discussion of family and caregiver resources, including time—not just financial resources—is important in determining what interventions are likely to be successful. Social interactions, social activities, and support systems may affect the patient's willingness to adhere to a treatment plan. Current and prior community and work (job/school) activities need to be analyzed in terms of possible causes of wounds and whether these activities are likely to help or hinder wound healing.

Living environment, community characteristics, and projected discharge destination must be discussed. Frequently, the living environment and discharge destination must be considered together. A patient with little support and living in an environment that is physically challenging may need to be admitted to a facility that provides the support necessary, whereas a person under identical clinical conditions living in a one-floor efficiency apartment on the ground floor may be discharged to home.

Social habits can be difficult to ascertain. Unfortunately, many of these social habits profoundly slow wound healing. Habits such as smoking, excessive alcohol consumption, and drug abuse are important pieces of information to allow the clinician to make an appropriate plan of care.

MOBILITY

The patient needs to be asked about mobility and to demonstrate mobility to the clinician. How mobile is the person in a bed or in a chair? Can the patient shift weight or get into and out of a bed or a chair independently, or is assistance needed? Is a referral to physical therapy or occupational therapy needed to aid in the prevention of more wounds or to promote healing of existing ulcers?

EQUIPMENT

What equipment does the patient have? Does he or she know how to use it? Does the equipment suit the impairment or disability of the patient? For example, does a person with weightbearing restrictions use a rolling walker? Does a person with diminished vision or poor balance use a rolling walker or standard walker? Why was the patient given the equipment? In many cases the patient may have borrowed a cane, walker, or crutches from a friend or family member without being instructed in its use and is simply using the wrong type of equipment. Patients may have a piece of equipment but not use it for cosmetic reasons or forget to use it. Asking a patient why he or she was given a walker may elicit a response that the patient was supposed to have weightbearing restrictions but those were not communicated to you.

SUMMARY

A number of factors related to the patient's health status and history can either cause a wound or impair the healing of a wound. The *Guide to Physical Therapist Practice* is used to structure the history and physical examination of the patient. The terms *history*, *physical examination*, *review of systems*, *diagnosis*, *prognosis*, *plan of care*, and *outcomes* are defined. Deviations from normal lab values need to be interpreted for a potential influence on wound healing, especially blood cells and glucose. The clinician must also understand the social/work/play history of the patient and any medications, either prescribed by a physician or self-prescribed.

STUDY QUESTIONS

1. Why are we concerned about the use of anti-inflammatory drugs in wound management?

2. What is the importance of an elevated white cell count?

3. Contrast the pathology-driven medical diagnosis with the impairment-driven diagnosis described in the *Guide to Physical Therapist Practice*.

4. Why is it important to have a patient show you all of the medications being taken?

5. Why should you observe a patient using any assistive or adaptive devices?

REFERENCES

1. American Physical Therapy Association. Guide to Physical Therapist Practice. *Physical Therapy*. 1997;77:1177-1619.

2. Garritan S, Jones P, Kornberg T, Parkin C. Laboratory values in the intensive care unit. *Acute Care Perspectives*. 1995;3(4):7-11.

3. Goodman CC, Boissonnault WG, Fuller KS. Laboratory tests and values. In: Goodman CC, Boissonnault WG, eds. *Pathology: Implications for the Physical Therapist*. WB Saunders; Philadelphia, Pa: 1998.

Physical Examination

5

The history helps direct the physical examination. Obviously, a thorough physical examination may take several hours to complete. The history and careful observation, however, narrow the focus of the physical examination. For most patients, all aspects of the physical exam can be addressed within a few minutes if the history is done well. For other patients, a very thorough examination will be required even if the cause of the wound is very clear. An example is the patient with a history of diabetes mellitus. A very thorough examination of the strength and sensation of the lower extremities is in order, regardless of the physical appearance of the wound. On the other hand, a person with a partial-thickness burn on the forearm may be examined in 10 to 15 minutes.

GROSS APPEARANCE

Along with the risk factors and history, the gross appearance of a wound may offer several important clues concerning the cause of the wound and the prognosis for healing. Details of wound examination are explored in greater detail in Chapter 11. In particular, one should examine the wound for color, odor, drainage, and shape. Wound color is a strong indication of the vascular supply of the tissue within the wound. A bright, beefy red color indicates good circulation. A pink color is a sign of diminished arterial blood flow. Worse yet is a dusky, dark color indicative of tissue at high risk of necrosis or severe infection.

An infected wound generally has a detectible odor; however, a wound with large amounts of solubilized necrotic tissue will have an odor even in the absence of infection. This situation arises with appropriate use of occlusive dressings. When an occlusive dressing is used to promote autolytic debridement (allowing natural enzymes to degrade necrotic tissue) and is left in place the proper length of time, a brownish, soupy drainage with an odor may be observed within the wound bed. However, the odor will not persist beyond wound cleansing, whereas an odor persists with the cleansing of an infected wound. The appearance of the drainage will be addressed in more detail in Chapter 11. A thin, clear fluid is considered normal. A thick, creamy drainage with an odor is indicative of localized wound infection. Moreover, certain organisms produce distinctive odors. *Pseudomonas* species produce an unforgettable fruity odor, frequently accompanied by a greenish coloration of the wound bed and pus. *Proteus* produces a urea-like smell, and other infections usually produce a foul odor that causes a withdrawal reflex.

The shape of a wound may indicate the cause of a wound. A highly regularly shaped round/oval wound is typically associated with pressure (Figure 5-1a). Wounds caused by vascular insufficiency will have irregular shapes due to the variation in anatomical supply of the tissue

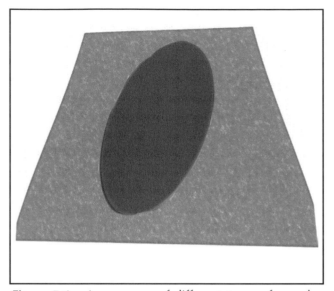

Figure 5-1a. Appearance of different types of vascular ulcers. Mechanical forces tend to produce round or elliptical ulcers, as in neuropathic or pressure ulcers.

involved (Figure 5-1b). In particular, venous insufficiency ulcers tend to be extremely irregular and may have a shape resembling a coast line, with numerous peninsulas or bays of healthier tissue surrounded by necrosis.

Skin Color

Melanin and hemoglobin are the two primary determinants of skin color. Melanin is the brown pigment produced by melanocytes. In individuals of sub-Saharan African descent, melanin pigmentation may be so great that variation in hemoglobin content of the skin becomes obscured. Saturated hemoglobin with good arterial supply produces the pinkish hue typical of Caucasian skin. Differences in blood flow can vary skin color from a ghostly pallor to a bright red.

Pallor suggests arterial insufficiency. Worse yet is a purplish hue produced by the presence of desaturated hemoglobin circulating through an extremity. This indicates severe arterial insufficiency, severe congestive heart failure, or severe pulmonary disease. A bright red color is produced by hyperemia (excessive blood flow). Reddish color (erythema) is an indication of inflammation and perhaps infection. Because blood flow also brings warm blood from the body's core to the surface, erythema is usually accompanied by skin warmth, also an indication of inflammation or infection. The two possibilities of inflammation and infection are discussed in greater detail in Chapter 11. In heavily melanin-pigmented skin, hyperemia produces a violet or eggplant color that may be missed by the inexperienced clinician.

The loss of brown pigmentation may be manifested in two important ways. In vitiligo, patches of hypopigment-

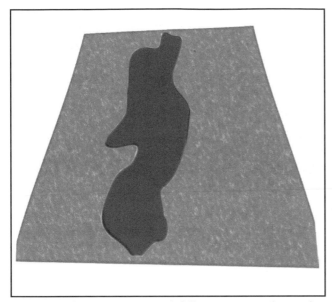

Figure 5-1b. Appearance of different types of vascular ulcers. Vascular insufficiency produces ulcers with irregular borders corresponding to tissue deprived of nutrition.

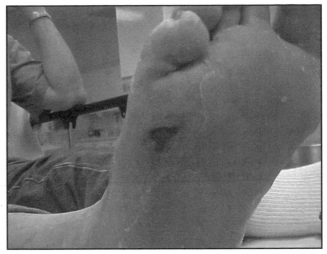

Figure 5-2. Appearance of a diabetic foot. Note the dryness of the skin and thickened nails. (Also shown in Color Atlas following page 274.)

ed skin, usually a few centimeters across with somewhat irregular borders, are observed. Albinism produces a uniform hypopigmentation with accompanying hypopigmentation of the hair and irises of the eyes. Increased brown pigmentation occurs with stimulation of melanocytes with adrenocorticotrophic hormone (ACTH). The structure of ACTH closely resembles the hormone melanocyte-stimulating hormone. High concentrations of ACTH occur with Addison's disease and pregnancy. In pregnancy, increased brown pigmentation occurs in characteristic locations such as the face, nipples, and the linea nigra along the vertical centerline of the abdomen and extending to the umbilicus.

Hair and Nails

Loss of hair and thickening of nails are characteristic of arterial insufficiency but also occur with aging. A change in hair and nail appearance can be established by asking the patient or comparing left and right sides. In the case of bilateral changes, the clinician may need to rely on patient recollection and personal judgment of normal hair and nail appearance. Thick, multilayered, yellowed nails are common with poorly controlled diabetes, along with thick, rough skin on the soles (Figure 5-2).

Temperature

As discussed, skin temperature is altered by the magnitude of blood flow to the skin. Decreased skin temperature and pallor accompany lack of blood flow to the skin. The clinician must determine whether the diminished temperature is localized to an area of an extremity or perhaps to the entirety of the extremity by comparing two extremities. In addition, one must account for the ambient temperature, amount of clothing, and physical activity of the limb prior to examination. A single foot that feels cool compared with the other foot and the rest of the body is a clear sign of arterial insufficiency. At the other extreme, an area of skin that is warmer than expected based on a bilateral comparison or, in the judgment of the clinician, warmer than it should be based on ambient temperature, clothing, and physical activity is a sign of inflammation or infection and is usually accompanied by hyperemia.

In many cases, temperature can be assessed easily by the clinician's touch. Very poor arterial circulation and fever are readily detected by most clinicians. Quantification of local temperature is often desirable, however. Tools available to perform this quantification include thermistors and radiometers. A *thermistor* is a temperature-sensitive probe that alters its resistance with changes in temperature. Typically, a thermistor is plugged into a display unit with either an analog needle or digital display to allow temperature to be read in both Celsius and Fahrenheit scales (Figure 5-3). The probe is put in contact with the skin for a minimum of a few seconds (depending on the particular unit used, read instructions) to determine temperature. Thermistors are generally very accurate and reliable but require direct contact with the tissue of interest. *Radiometers* are based on detection of infrared radiation emitted by the object of interest. Heat is exchanged from an object to surrounding objects not in direct contact by infrared radiation. The amount of infrared radiation is directly proportional to the temperature of the object.

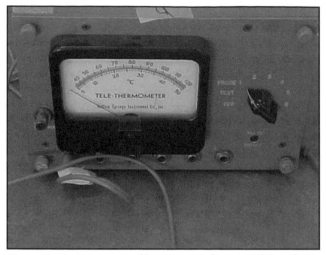

Figure 5-3. One type of instrument for use with a thermistor to detect skin temperature.

Therefore, a radiometer is capable of determining skin temperature without direct contact with a wound. However, these devices are used infrequently because of their price.

In addition, the patient's body temperature should be measured using a device approved by the facility. Increased temperature is indicative of systemic infection. However, the clinician should be aware of factors that may affect temperature, including the temperature of the room, previous activity, excessive clothing, and recent exposure to a hot environment.

ACCUMULATIONS

Various materials may accumulate in the skin as a result of disease processes. When these disease processes are also the causes of wounds, identification of the accumulation in the skin is useful in determining the etiology of a wound. Hemosiderin is a particularly important accumulation. *Hemosiderin* (literally "blood-iron") is an accumulation of iron that results from the degradation of red blood cells. Hemosiderin is a storage form of iron in the tissue. Macrophages eventually pick up hemosiderin from the tissues and recycle the iron to the bone marrow. Hemosiderin produces a brownish-yellow discoloration, usually referred to as *hemosiderin staining*. Hemosiderin staining, particularly just superior to the medial malleolus, is very predictive of venous hypertension. Many chronic wounds will have hemosiderin accumulating in the skin immediately adjacent to the wound due to repetitive trauma.

Bilirubin and its precursor biliverdin are also the result of the breakdown of hemoglobin. Bilirubin and biliverdin are seen in bruises. Shortly after the loss of blood directly beneath the skin (eg, a contusion) the purplish hue is due

to biliverdin. As biliverdin is broken down into bilirubin, the skin takes on a yellowish tint (jaundice). Later, as bilirubin is removed by the circulation from the site of injury, the brownish-yellow hemosiderin remaining at the site of injury becomes obvious. Generalized jaundice indicates systemic overload of bilirubin. Jaundice occurs frequently in newborns due to the destruction of red cells carrying fetal hemoglobin. In adults, jaundice represents the imbalance of hemoglobin breakdown and bilirubin excretion. Jaundice may result from either hemolytic anemia (excessive breakdown of hemoglobin) or the inability to excrete bilirubin due to hepatic disease (hepatitis) or biliary obstruction.

Lipodermatosclerosis and Lymphatic Disease

Lymphatic disease results in rough, tough skin with increased pigmentation. To some, the appearance resembles that of the skin of an orange, thus the term *peau d'orange*. The fluid and protein accumulating in the interstitial space causes fibrosis and puckering. In contrast to the mobilizable accumulation of fluid in venous insufficiency, lymphatic edema is difficult to mobilize. Lipodermatosclerosis may also occur in severe venous insufficiency.

HYDRATION, TURGOR, AND ELASTICITY

These three are grouped together due to their association with the aging process. In senescent skin, a loss of all three occurs. With normal hydration, a firm gel is evident in the dermal portion of the skin. Hydration, turgor, and elasticity can be tested by pinching the skin. With a pinch, a firm, rounded skin fold can be gently lifted from the surface. This skin fold immediately retracts to its former position when released. In senescent skin, a dry, triangular skin fold can be observed, which does not immediately retract to its position upon release but remains elevated in the shape of a tent, thus the term *tenting*. Tenting can be seen at certain locations, especially the neck, without pinching the skin. Turgor refers specifically to the firmness of skin as it is pinched. This firmness is caused by the gel-like property of a normally hydrated dermis, in which water molecules are trapped by the glycosaminoglycans of the ground substance of the dermis. With insufficient hydration, turgor is lost, as is the firm feel to the skin fold. Elasticity refers to the snapping back of healthy skin as the skin fold is released. It is partially due to skin turgor but, as the name implies, is also due to the presence of elastic fibers constructed of the protein elastin in the skin. The number and thickness of elastic fibers decrease with age. However, the skin of otherwise younger healthy skin can lose hydration, turgor, and elasticity in environments with low humidity, especially in the winter. Skin can rapidly lose moisture to dry, cold air and even crack in winter, requiring the use of moisturizing lotions to maintain hydration, turgor, and elasticity.

Overhydrated skin occurs with derangements of fluid balance, resulting in edema. Edema can result from many causes but basically results from excessive hydrostatic pressure in capillaries or the imbalance of osmotic pressure across the capillary walls. Edema results from congestive heart failure, venous insufficiency, and hyperemia producing excessive capillary hydrostatic pressure from too great a fluid volume, failure to pump blood from veins back to the heart, or excessive dilation of arterial vessels such that pressure does not fall as much as normal as blood moves through dilated vessels into the capillaries. Lack of plasma proteins because of lack of production in liver disease or malnutrition and loss of plasma proteins by kidney disease allows excessive movement of water out of capillaries. Finally, excessive quantities of proteins in the interstitial space due to injury, especially burns, or due to very high capillary pressure, encourages the movement of water out of capillaries into the interstitial space, a phenomenon known as *third spacing*.

VASCULAR TESTING

Because of the potentially serious nature of arterial insufficiency and the treatments used for venous and lymphatic diseases, the importance of arterial testing cannot be overemphasized. Compression and elevation used to treat venous and lymphatic disease are likely to exacerbate the already compromised circulation. Several tests for arterial sufficiency are available and range from highly sophisticated and expensive testing to cheap and easy, but questionably valid, tests. The most cost-effective test in most facilities is measurement of the *ankle brachial index* (ABI), also called *ankle pressure index* (API) in some geographical regions. This test is based on the idea that obstruction of peripheral arteries diminishes the pressure of arterial blood as it passes distally into an extremity. Normal, healthy arteries produce little drop in arterial pressure; therefore, arterial pressure measured in the brachial artery is very close to aortic pressure. Even in the arteries of the legs, very little pressure is lost. This discussion assumes that pressure is measured at the same height. For example, when blood pressure is measured with a sphygmomanometer, the cuff is placed at the same level as the heart. By the same token, blood pressure measured in the leg needs to be done with the leg slightly elevated to raise it to the same level as the heart when the patient is lying in supine.

Unlike the brachial artery, which is sufficiently superficial to allow one to hear changes in flow pattern with a stethoscope as vessels become occluded and free to flow, the vessels of the lower extremity are generally not amenable to this technique. In the arm, we can closely approximate true systolic pressure as the pressure in the cuff at the point that blood can be heard spurting under the cuff only at the peak systolic pressure. The lack of noise heard through the stethoscope then approximates diastolic pressure when blood is free to flow continually under the cuff through the cardiac cycle. For the lower extremities, an instrument called a *Doppler stethoscope* is used, typically over either the dorsalis pedis or posterior tibial arteries. The *Doppler effect* is typically described as the change in pitch made as a train approaches and then moves away. As the train approaches, sound waves are compressed, increasing frequency, and as the train moves away, the sound waves are rarefied, decreasing frequency. A Doppler stethoscope emits ultrasound at 5 to 8 megaHertz (MHz). When the ultrasound strikes a moving medium, such as flowing blood, the shift in frequency is converted to a sound transmitted either to a speaker or ear pieces. Older models used ear pieces. Most modern devices have built-in speakers to allow the Doppler shift to be heard.

The technique involves finding either the dorsalis pedis (Figure 5-4) or posterior tibial artery by palpation, then holding the probe at a 45-degree angle along the length of the artery, as confirmed by a swishing sound. A blood pressure cuff is placed on the calf and inflated until the swishing sound is lost. The lack of sound indicates that arterial flow is occluded. The cuff is slowly deflated, as is done in sphygmomanometry. Resumption of the swishing sound indicates that pressure in the artery is just greater than pressure in the cuff. Note the lack of a unique sound to indicate diastolic pressure. The Doppler stethoscope does not work on the principle of Korotkoff sounds. It indicates either the presence or absence of blood flow; therefore, only systolic pressure can be determined. The same technique with the Doppler device is done on the brachial artery. If done at the same height relative to the heart, the values should be very close. Generally, the value in the leg is 5% to 10% greater due to the reflection of pressure waves along the longer vessels of the leg. Therefore, we expect the ABI to be 1.05 to 1.10 in a healthy person. When ABI falls below 0.8 (ankle systolic pressure is 80% of brachial systolic pressure) some experts recommend that compression therapy not be used. Other individuals are more liberal, using a limit of 0.7. A value of 0.75 to 0.9 is indicative of moderate arterial disease. A patient with an ABI of 0.5 to 0.75 is considered to have severe arterial disease, and a value 0.5 or lower is considered dangerous for the health of the limb[1,2] and requires referral to a vascular surgeon. The performance of ABI testing is shown in Figures 5-5a and 5-5b. A value of greater than 1.1 may indicate calcification of arterial ves-

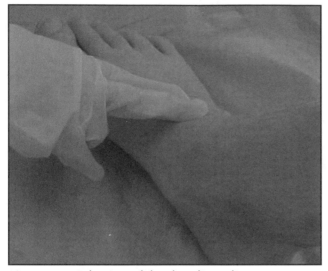

Figure 5-4. Palpation of the dorsalis pedis.

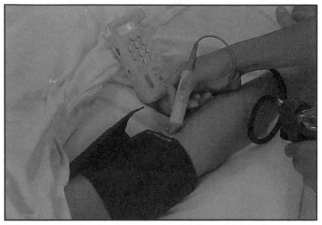

Figure 5-5a. Performance of ankle brachial index measurement. Doppler probe is held at a 45-degree angle over the brachial artery to determine systolic pressure in the arm.

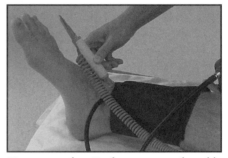

Figure 5-5b. Performance of ankle brachial index measurement. Same technique is used over the dorsalis pedis artery with elevation of the leg to the same height as the brachial artery and the heart.

sels. Calcification prevents the collapse of arterial vessels when cuff pressure exceeds arterial pressure. Therefore, a value greater than 1.1 must be viewed with suspicion, and other forms of arterial testing will be needed to conclusively diagnose arterial disease.

Pneumoplethysmography is a more sophisticated means of determining the same phenomenon. The principle underlying this technique is that diastolic pressure becomes insufficient to drive flow through diseased arteries. The technique measures relative blood flow during systole and diastole. As the ratio of systolic blood flow to diastolic blood flow increases, the risk to the limb increases. In severe disease, the ratio may become infinite as blood flow ceases during diastole with severe occlusion. The device consists of an air chamber surrounding the lower extremity and a device to measure changes in volume through the cardiac cycle. The device must be put through a calibration sequence and is expensive to obtain.

Simple tests include the palpation of dorsalis pedis and posterior tibial pulses (see Figure 5-4) correlated with signs of arterial insufficiency already discussed, such as temperature, color of the limb, and the appearance of hair and nails on the extremity. This examination lacks both sensitivity and specificity. Moderate arterial disease can be easily overlooked (lack of sensitivity) and many individuals with perfectly fine lower extremity blood flow may have pulses that are difficult to palpate (low specificity). An old standby is the rubor of dependency test (Figure 5-6). It is based on gravitational challenge to the arterial circulation and observation. With the patient placed in supine (on the back), the lower extremity is raised 60 degrees for 1 minute. Signs of arterial insufficiency may be present in this first phase as complaints of pain with elevation and an ashen appearance to the extremity. In a healthy person, a decrease in the pinkness occurs and returns as the leg is

lowered to the table. In a person with arterial disease, the color of the leg goes beyond the normal pink and becomes quite red due to the phenomenon termed *reactive hyperemia*. Reactive hyperemia refers to the dilation of vessels in response to occlusion of vessels. When the occlusion is released, blood flow is increased markedly above normal, producing the rubor of dependency.[3]

Several tests for venous insufficiency are also available. Often venous disease is grossly obvious by the presence of dilated superficial veins, especially if the dilated vessels are tortuous (following a twisting path, rather than a relatively straight line). Dilation of venous vessels occurs in response to increased pressure in them. Pressure within venous vessels is normally only a few mmHg of pressure. Pressure is kept low even in the lower extremities by the presence of a venous pump. A pump in general consists of an energy source, valves to ensure one-way flow, and clear conduits to carry the flow to and from the pump. With this in mind, the causes of venous insufficiency become clear: occlusion of the vessels, failure of the valves, or loss of the source of energy for the pumping mechanism. Occlusion of venous vessels may occur from within, usually a blood clot or thrombus, or from outside the vessels by obesity, pregnancy, neoplasms, or improperly applied compression devices. Failure of venous valves is very common. The venous valves act to break the column of fluid into small columns. When one valve fails, the valve below is subjected to greater pressure than normal and is at risk for failure, thereby putting each valve below at great risk to fail. Neuromuscular diseases or injuries such as spinal cord injury, peripheral nerve injury, immobilization of an extremity, or following a fracture, decreases the ability of the calf muscle to exert pressure on the outside of leg veins to assist pumping of blood from the leg veins to maintain a low venous pressure. Leg vein pressure increases significantly as one changes from a sitting to standing posture but decreases during walking to a pressure actually less than that measured in sitting.

Available tests include the percussion test, venous filling time test, and venous plethysmography. The percussion test examines the patency of valves. A normal valve does not allow backflow from above the knee to below the knee. During this test, the examiner palpates a superficial vein below the knee and strikes the same vein above the knee. With normal valves, the pressure wave generated is baffled at the valve below. With insufficient valves, the pressure wave is transmitted distally and can be palpated below the knee.

The venous filling time test superficially resembles the rubor of dependency test. The patient is placed in supine and the lower extremity is elevated to 60 degrees for 1 minute. The leg is massaged to reduce leg volume as much as possible. The patient is then asked to stand and the volume of the leg is observed. With normal circulation, the leg volume increases gradually through arterial inflow. Lack of filling within 10 to 15 seconds indicates arterial insufficiency. With venous insufficiency, leg volume increases rapidly through both arterial inflow and venous backflow. In addition, peripheral veins should become obvious. The Trendelenberg test is performed in a similar manner except a tourniquet is placed around the thigh, occluding venous but not arterial flow. The patient stands, and the examiner observes for filling of superficial veins. Immediate filling indicates incompetent valves of communicating veins. The tourniquet is then removed. Rapid filling of superficial veins demonstrates incompetence of the saphenous vein.

Venous plethysmography is a technological improvement of the venous filling time test. Similar to the arterial test, a plastic air chamber is placed over the lower extremity. A simpler pressure-detecting device is attached to the chamber. The patient is asked to stand with the lower

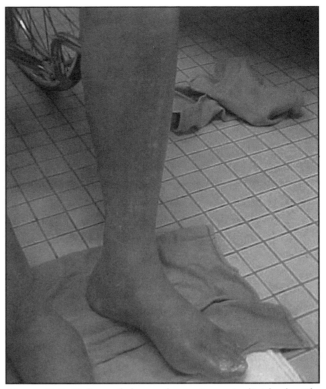

Figure 5-6. Rubor of dependency in an individual with arterial insufficiency. Note the ruddy color of the lower half of both legs; shiny, hairless skin; and the thickened, yellow toenails. (Also shown in Color Atlas following page 274.)

extremity in the chamber to provide a baseline volume. The decrease in volume that occurs in the supine position with the leg elevated is recorded. When a new baseline is reached, the patient is asked to stand rapidly. A progressive increase in lower extremity volume is considered normal. A rapid increase beyond the original standing baseline indicates venous insufficiency.

Transcutaneous oxygen (tcPO$_2$) measurements can be made in specialized vascular labs. The device, as the name implies, measures tissue oxygen through the skin. This measurement is performed with a special airtight sensor that heats the skin to 41°C to allow equilibration between capillary PO$_2$ and the sensor, taking approximately 20 minutes to perform. In particular, the device is used to determine appropriate amputation level but can also be used to predict the likelihood of wound healing. A value of less than 20 mmHg carries a poor prognosis for healing, whereas a value greater than 30 mmHg predicts proper healing. This information can also aid the decision to debride wounds. Using the same criteria, one may decide to debride a wound with a tcPO$_2$ reading of greater than 30 mmHg, but not if the surrounding skin produces a value of 20 mmHg. In any case, when in doubt, a vascular surgeon should be consulted.

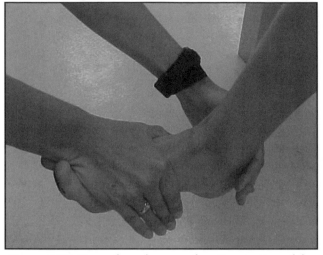

Figure 5-7a. Strength and range of motion testing of the foot and ankle. Long muscles innervated in the leg are tested.

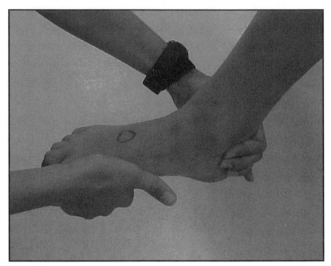

Figure 5-7b. Strength and range of motion testing of the foot and ankle. Intrinsic muscles of the foot are tested.

STRENGTH AND RANGE OF MOTION

These tests are frequently ignored when focus is totally on the wound, rather than on the patient. We need to remember that we are working with a person who needs to function in a particular environment. For most patients, a rudimentary test can be conducted in less than 1 minute. Specific muscle tests can be performed as the examination or history dictate. A brief sequence can consist simply of squeezing the examiner's hand, asking the patient to raise the arms over the head then back to shoulder level. The examiner then asks the patient to resist movement as the examiner attempts to move the shoulders, elbows, and wrists through the different possible planes of movement. The examiner then asks the patient to move the lower extremities through the normal range of motion and then to attempt to resist the examiner's attempts to move the hips, knees, and ankles through their available planes of movement (Figures 5-7a and 5-7b). Those with suspected neuropathy should be more carefully examined for strength, range of motion, and for deformities of the feet. This examination is described more thoroughly in Chapter 8. Individuals with spinal cord injuries and other neuromuscular diseases or injuries should have a more thorough examination for range of motion and strength. Several textbooks are available for guiding a full strength and range of motion examination.

SENSORY TESTING

Rudimentary sensory testing should also be done routinely with every patient. Again, more detailed testing of the distal extremities is required for anyone with suspected peripheral neuropathy or other neuromuscular diseases or injuries. Several textbooks are also available to provide a detailed approach. Often, a simple test of light touch with a cotton-tipped applicator or pinprick (Figures 5-8a and 5-8b) and the patient's eyes closed is sufficient to rule out sensory deficits. A detailed description of the use of monofilaments of different thickness for evaluation of diabetic feet is described in Chapter 8.

REFLEX TESTING

Reflex testing includes the deep tendon reflexes of the biceps, triceps, brachioradialis for the upper extremities, and quadriceps (knee jerk) and gastrocnemius/soleus (ankle jerk) with a reflex hammer (Figures 5-9a and 5-9b). The Babinski hammer is recommended for this procedure for ease of use. The long handle and weighted head allow the hammer's head to be simply dropped onto the tendon of interest as opposed to the Buck or Taylor (tomahawk) hammers, which require more skill in striking the tendon. In addition, testing the Babinski or related reflex on the sole may be necessary given a history of upper motor neuron lesion. Testing for resistance to quick movement and the presence of clonus with quick movement of the wrists and ankles should also be done for individuals with upper motor neuron lesions. Increased tone manifested as either spasticity or rigidity predisposes this individual to pressure ulcers.

MOBILITY, COORDINATION, AND BALANCE

A brief assessment of the patient's bed mobility, transfers, and gait correlated with history including home and work environment is also commonly overlooked. Examine

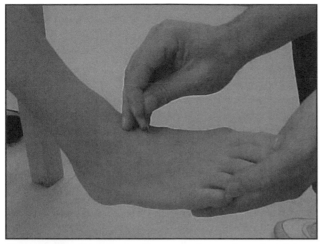

Figure 5-8a. Sensory testing on a foot using pinprick.

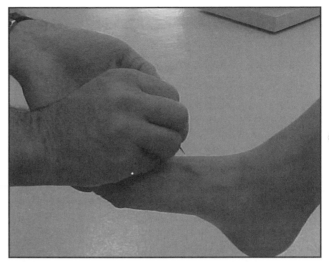

Figure 5-8b. Sensory testing on a foot using pinprick.

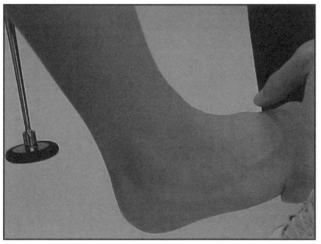

Figure 5-9a. Reflex testing using the ankle jerk: Babinski hammer.

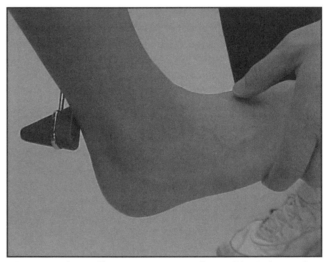

Figure 5-9b. Reflex testing using the ankle jerk: Taylor hammer.

how the individual bears weight on different bony prominences when resting in bed, sitting, moving in bed, coming to sit, coming to stand, and when ambulating. Ask about the use of assistive devices and assess the patient's ability to use the assistive device. Inquire about weight-bearing restrictions, especially those involving the wounded body part. Discussion of footwear is also covered in Chapter 8. Poor balance or coordination may require compensations that have either created or exacerbated the wound. In some cases, simply providing a walker may alleviate the problem. Other cases may require more involved interventions, such as the use of total contact casts (also discussed in Chapter 8). A patient with deficits in mobility should be referred to physical therapy to improve mobility to the level consistent with the patient's desired lifestyle.

AEROBIC/CARDIOPULMONARY

Every patient should be evaluated at least in terms of vital signs: heart rate, blood pressure, respiratory rate, and ideally oxyhemoglobin saturation using a pulse oximeter. Although expensive (~$1000), when used on every patient entering the clinical facility, this measurement adds negligibly to the cost. Simple tests of aerobic function such as upper extremity ergometry or the Balke test may be used. The Balke test consists of setting a treadmill at 3.3 mph and increasing the grade of the treadmill 1% every minute. A treadmill test, whether the Balke, Bruce, or other protocol, is particularly useful for the patient with suspected arterial insufficiency. Intermittent claudication manifested as calf pain at a given intensity of exercise can be monitored through the course of treatment.

Summary

Basic tests performed during the physical examination are described in this chapter. The selection of tests is driven by the history and review of systems described in the previous chapter. A general inspection of the skin is followed by more specific tests of the vascular system, sensation, strength, reflexes, and cardiovascular system. Tests are used to develop a diagnosis; and using the information from the history, a meaningful prognosis is developed.

Study Questions

1. Contrast the appearance of wounds caused by vascular disease and those caused by unrelieved mechanical forces. What creates the different shapes?

2. Define skin turgor; what happens to skin turgor with age? Why does this happen?

3. What are the benefits of measuring skin temperature?

4. What does an elevated or depressed skin temperature indicate?

5. What other tests would confirm suspicions raised by a decreased skin temperature?

6. Name several tests available to evaluate the neuromuscular aspects of the lower extremity.

References

1. Carpenter JP. Noninvasive assessment of peripheral vascular disease. *Advances in Skin and Wound Care.* 2000;13:84-85.

2. Sloan H, Wills EM. Ankle-brachial index: calculating your patient's vascular risk. *Nursing99.* 1999;29(10):58-59.

3. Sieggreen MY, Maklebust J. Managing leg ulcers. *Nursing96.* 1996;26(12):41-46.

Nutrition 6

- Describe the essential nutrients to prevent wounds and promote healing.
- Describe the need for caloric intake to prevent wounds and how the need increases with integumentary injury.
- Describe the normal protein requirement and how it needs to change to promote healing.
- Describe the roles of fatty acids, trace elements, and vitamins in wound prevention and healing.
- Discuss the relationships among obesity, wound healing, and weight loss.
- Discuss means of supplementing nutrition to promote wound healing.

IMPORTANCE OF NUTRITION

Nutrition may break down at many levels, putting a person at increased risk of developing wounds or slow healing of existing wounds. In the healthy individual, many of these potential pitfalls are taken for granted. An individual needs the cognitive abilities to choose appropriate foods, the cognitive and physical abilities to prepare it, and the desire to consume it. Once consumed, proper functioning of the digestive system is needed. The person must be able to mechanically reduce the food to digestible forms, secrete enzymes into the gastrointestinal tract, and absorb the reduced forms. After absorption, the simple nutrients require processing, metabolic control, and delivery to cells. With delivery to cells, the nutrients derived from food need other nutrients to provide energy and structures for the cell. Disease or aging of the gastrointestinal tract, liver, heart, blood vessels, and respiratory system, and diabetes mellitus can undermine optimal diet. Elderly individuals living alone with poor mobility and diminished cognition are at tremendous risk of malnourishment and development of wounds.

Dietary needs may be divided into three basic categories:

1. Energy quantified by the number of calories consumed
2. Protein to regenerate necessary enzymes and other structures
3. Cofactors necessary for metabolism, notably vitamins and trace minerals.

Nutrition of the skin requires a healthy vascular supply through the dermis, which provides a rich supply to the papillary dermis. Blood flow through the papillary dermis provides nourishment to the metabolically active stratum basale where new cells of the epidermis are generated. Diffusion of nutrients occurs from the papillary dermis to the stratum basale to support its metabolic needs. In addition, these plexuses are involved in thermoregulation. However, the blood supply to the relatively acellular reticular dermis is rather low due to its low metabolic rate.

Nutrition is frequently poor in ill or injured individuals, with an estimated 30% to 55% rate of malnutrition in the hospital patient population. Impaired nutritional intake, lower dietary protein intake, impaired ability to feed oneself, and recent weight loss have been shown to be independent predictors of pressure ulcer development. Moreover, these factors are likely to occur in combination in many individuals. A key question is how common malnutrition may be for others with some of the risk factors listed above related to obtaining, preparing, digesting, and delivering nutrients to cells. It is clear that malnutrition is a major risk factor for pressure ulcers and delayed wound healing. Two basic types of malnutrition described in the literature are *marasmius* (total calorie malnutrition) and *hypoalbuminemia* (protein malnutrition), although many individuals may have a combination. Marasmius presents as long-term inadequate intake with chronic weight loss and wasted adipose and muscle tissue but intact visceral protein stores. Hypoalbuminemia is generally a result of an acute insult such as surgery or illness. Protein malnutrition may have a rapid onset and may be difficult to detect without appropriate lab tests. Hypoalbuminemia is characterized by a preservation of fat and somatic protein. Combination malnutrition generally results from an underlying chronic malnourishment with a superimposed acute insult, resulting in loss of fat, muscle, and visceral protein. Nutritional status may be assessed by a combination of anthropometric and biochemical data (Table 6-1).

ANTHROPOMETRIC ASSESSMENT OF NUTRITION

Ideal body weight (IBW) may be computed in a number of ways. A commonly used set of equations is as follows. For men, the equation is 106 pounds for the first 5 feet plus 6 pounds for each additional inch above 5 feet of height (106 pounds for 5' + 6 pounds per inch). For women, the equation is 100 pounds for the first 5 feet and 5 pounds for each additional inch (100 pounds for 5' + 5 pounds per inch). Adjustments are made for body types by subtracting 10% for a small frame and adding 10% for a large frame. For example, a 6 foot 1 inch man has an ideal body weight of 106 + 6 x 13 = 184 pounds, and a 5 foot 3 inch woman has an ideal body weight of 100 + 5 x 3 = 115 pounds. Computing percent of IBW provides an index of risk of either malnutrition or overnutrition. Overnutrition is also an important risk factor due to the relationships among obesity, type 2 diabetes mellitus, and atherosclerosis. Percent IBW is computed by dividing current body weight (CBW) by IBW as: percent IBW = CBW/IBW x 100. Normal is considered to be between 90% to 110% IBW. A value of 80% to 90% is considered to be underweight and a value of 79% or less defines marasmius.[1]

BIOCHEMICAL ASSESSMENT OF NUTRITION

Albumin is considered the gold standard for assessing protein malnutrition. A normal value of albumin is considered to be 3.5 to 5.0 g/dL. Moderate depletion is considered to be a value between 3.2 and 3.5 g/dL, and severe hypoalbuminemia is defined as a value less than 2.8 g/dL. Evaluation of albumin is particularly important for the person with a chronic wound due to the potential for albumin and other plasma proteins to be lost in wound exudate. The problem with low albumin is compounded by its effect on fluid distribution. Albumin loss leads to edema,

---

Table 6-1

RISK FACTORS FOR MALNUTRITION

Self-report of poor intake

Weight less than 80% of ideal body weight

Loss of greater than 10% of usual body weight within last 6 months

Alcoholism

Elderly

Impaired cognitive status

Malabsorption syndromes

Hemodialysis

Multiple trauma

Burns

Heavily draining wounds

Edema unrelated to cardiac or venous disease

Low serum albumin

---

which in turn causes decreased diffusion of nutrients through the interstitial space. In acute protein malnutrition, however, albumin may not be indicative of an inadequate intake early on. Instead, pre-albumin should be analyzed as an indicator of short-term protein intake. Mild, moderate, and severe depletion are defined as less than 17 g/dL, less than 12 g/dL, and less than 7 g/dL of pre-albumin, respectively.[1]

COMPUTING NUTRITIONAL REQUIREMENTS

Both total calories and protein intake need to be computed to meet an individual's nutritional needs. If at all possible, a thorough assessment by a licensed clinical dietician should be done. A simple guideline is to provide 30 to 35 calories per kilogram to maintain current body weight and 40 to 45 calories per kilogram to promote anabolism. For a more precise determination of the nutritional requirements, the Harris-Benedict equation is frequently used.

The equation for basal energy expenditure (BEE) for men is as follows:

BEE (kcal) = 66 + (13.7 x mass in kg) + (5 x height in cm) – (6.8 x age in years)

For women the equation is:

BEE (kcal) = 665 + (9.6 x mass in kg) + (1.8 x height in cm) – (4.7 x age in years)

To calculate total daily expenditure (TDE), one must take account for the patient's activity (activity factor [AF]) and severity of injury (injury factory [IF]). The basal energy expenditure is adjusted to derive total daily expenditure as: TDE = BEE x AF x IF, where AF ranges from 1.2 for bed rest to 2.0 for an extremely active person, and IF ranges from 1.2 for minor surgery to 2.5 for extreme thermal injury. Using the conversions of 2.54 cm per inch and 2.2 lbs per kg, the following examples are given:

Example 1: 160 lb male, 73 inches tall, 40 years old, low activity

30-35 kcal/kg x 160 lbs/2.2 kg/lb = 2182 – 2545 kcal/day

Or using the Harris-Benedict formula:

TDE = (66 + 996.4 + 927.1 – 272) x 1.5 (AF) = 2576 kcal/day

Example 2: 120 lb female, 63 inches tall, 38 years old, extremely active

30-35 kcal/kg x 120lbs/2.2 kg/lb = 1636 – 1909 kcal/day

Or using the Harris-Benedict formula:

TDE = (665 + 523.6 + 288.0 – 178.6) x 2 (AF) = 2596 kcal/day[1]

Required protein intake is computed as 0.8 to 2.0 g of protein per kg. The effectiveness of this intake can be monitored by calculating nitrogen balance. This is done by estimating the number of protein calories ingested in a 24-hour calorie count and the protein used for metabolism by calculating urine urea output. The appearance of urea in the urine indicates the use of protein for purposes other than replacing protein stores of the body, such as supplying energy after the protein is deaminated and urea is produced. Urea indicates a positive protein balance, indicating a sufficient protein intake.

Although weight reduction is an important long-term goal to maintain overall health, the person with a wound should not be placed on a weight reduction diet until the person is no longer at risk for developing a wound or having slow wound healing. Therefore, adjusting the diet to promote weight loss should not be a goal during wound healing. Even the obese individual needs a positive nitrogen balance, sufficient calories, and trace elements to promote wound healing.[2]

DIETARY SUPPLEMENTATION

Depending on several factors, notably the ability to ingest adequate calories and protein, the diet may need to be manipulated by the clinician. The least invasive dietary intervention sufficient for some patients is to increase food intake by increasing intake of nutrient-dense foods such as cheese, nuts, peanut butter, eggs, ice cream, and milkshakes. A further step is the use of commercial supplements such as Sustacal and Ensure. More extreme and invasive interventions include enteral and parenteral feeding. Enteral feeding refers to the delivery of nutrients artificially to the gastrointestinal tract, usually utilizing a pump and a line placed into the gastrointestinal tract. For short-term feeding, a tube may be placed through the nose into the stomach (nasogastric tube). Long-term feeding requires a surgically placed tube either through the skin into the stomach or into the jejunum. A line placed into the stomach is called a PEG (percutaneous endoscopic gastrostomy) tube. A J-tube is surgically placed into the jejunum to provide nutrients for the individual who cannot ingest a sufficient diet.

Vitamins

Vitamins, as originally described, were the presumed fat-soluble factor (vitamin A) and water-soluble factor (vitamin B) necessary for energy metabolism. Vitamin A (retinol) is stored in the liver and obtained in the diet as β–carotene from plants and retinyl esters from animals. Retinoic acid binds to receptors to affect gene expression. Vitamin A acts as a morphogen to regulate epidermal development and is teratogenic. Pregnant women must avoid exposure to high doses of vitamin A and its analogs (eg, retin-A used for treating skin diseases such as acne). Retinol suppresses the maturation of keratinocytes. An excess of retinol causes thinning and drying of the skin. Deficiency of vitamin A causes hyperkeratosis and metaplasia of glands of the epidermis. Retinol and chemicals of similar structure are used therapeutically for acne to suppress oil production of sebaceous glands. Deficiency of vitamin A has been shown to delay wound healing as well as increasing susceptibility to infection, presumably because of a requirement of vitamin A by the immune system.

Deficiency of niacin or tryptophan produces pellagra, a condition characterized by hyperkeratotic eruptions of sun-exposed skin and damage to other organs. Deficiency of vitamin B6 (pyroxidine) or essential fatty acid deficiency causes scaling. Both riboflavin and thiamine are required for collagen synthesis, but no link can be made directly to impairment of wound healing.

Vitamin C is essential for collagen development. Vitamin C deficiency (scurvy) causes diminished tensile strength and slows wound healing but does not prevent wound healing. Vitamin C deficiency in Western civilization is rare, and supertherapeutic doses of vitamin C have not been demonstrated to enhance healing of either acute or chronic wounds.

Vitamin E has been attributed to antioxidant properties and is thought to have a protective effect on the skin by reducing sun and other types of damage. It is frequently used as an additive to over-the-counter skin products with a suggestion of improved skin integrity. However, vitamin E has also been shown to decrease wound healing, possibly by interference with collagen synthesis, and vitamin E has not been demonstrated to be important to wound repair.[2]

Minerals and Trace Elements

Several minerals are required in low concentrations for healthy skin. Copper, manganese, and iron, although appearing to be necessary for tissue regeneration, have not been directly related to impaired wound healing. Selenium is part of an enzyme system (glutathione) that reduces oxidative damage by free radicals. Zinc is a part of many metalloenzyme systems, notably DNA and RNA polymerase. Zinc deficiency leads to dermatitis and slow healing. Supplemental zinc, however, has not been shown to aid wound healing, and excessive zinc may slow healing as well as have deleterious effects on immune function and copper metabolism. Unna's boots applied directly over venous insufficiency ulcers have been demonstrated to slow healing, which may be attributable to the zinc oxide in the material. Copper is also essential to the production of collagen, as well as elastin and melanin. It is present in the enzymes that produce cross-linking of collagen, elastin, and keratin.

SUMMARY

Adequate nutrition depends on a chain of factors, including financial and other resources for obtaining food, cognition, taste, choice of appropriate food, ability to prepare meals, gastrointestinal function, and diseases that alter appetite and cardiovascular function. Both caloric and protein consumption need to be assessed. Equations are available for determining appropriate intake of protein and calories. Assessment of nutritional status can be determined many ways, including simple anthropometric calculations and biochemical tests. The function of key vitamins and minerals for wound healing are discussed.

STUDY QUESTIONS

1. Why must both caloric and protein intake be considered in the assessment of nutrition?

2. Why do diseases such as cancer and infectious disease retard wound healing?

3. How does arterial insufficiency produce malnutrition at the cellular level?

4. How does cognitive status affect nutrition?

5. Describe how a patient may enter a vicious cycle of poor nutrition and immobility.

REFERENCES

1. Shils ME, James A, Olson JA, Shike M. *Modern Nutrition in Health and Disease*. 9th ed. Baltimore, Md: Williams & Wilkens; 1999.

2. Thomas DR. Specific nutritional factors in wound healing. *Advances in Wound Care*. 1997;10:40-43.

Characteristics of Wounds

Once an appropriate history and physical examination have been performed, the clinician next focuses on the wound itself. The cause of an acute wound is often easy to identify. Chapter 7 addresses acute wounds to give perspective on how these tend to be managed and understand how problems may develop and come to require the skilled services of the readers of this text. For chronic wounds, in particular, the cause of the wound may be difficult to identify from the history. Chapters in this section will address diagnosis and treatment of chronic wounds caused by neuropathy, pressure, and vascular disease. A careful examination of the wound and an understanding of how different causes manifest physically is often required to allow the clinician to identify the cause. The diagnostic process is critical because different etiologies may require very different interventions. Ideally, no two wounds should receive identical interventions nor should any cookbook approach be taken. The characteristics of the wound and the lifestyle of the patient, including home, work, family, and financial resources, should dictate a unique plan of care for each patient.

Chapters 8, 9, and 10 specifically address the characteristics and specific prevention, diagnosis, and intervention strategies for wounds caused by neuropathy, tissue loads, and vascular insufficiency. Chapter 11 addresses how to assess wounds based on the characteristics observed in the wound, regardless of the etiology. However, Chapter 11 also should not be used in isolation. The characteristics of the wound may indicate a particular type of intervention but, as discussed above, other factors must be considered before a plan of care is developed. Development of the plan of care and choosing interventions are described in the next unit.

Acute Wounds

7

OBJECTIVES

- List causes of acute wounds.
- Describe the wounds caused by surgery, including amputations and possible complications such as infection and dehiscence.
- Define the following terms and describe the mechanisms by which these wounds occur: lacerations, incisions, abrasions (road rash), and degloving (avulsion).
- Discuss the complications of puncture wounds and bites.
- Describe the major types of gun shot wounds and contrast the injuries caused by bullets and shot.
- List common causes of toxic ulcerations.
- Discuss the complications involved in fractures; discuss pin care with external fixation.
- List common pathological skin conditions that produce open wounds and describe their etiologies.

Acute wounds are typically managed initially in the emergency department or by the surgeon creating them. Under some circumstances, acute wounds may be seen in other settings as determined by the physician due to the nature of the wound for a more continuous type of intervention, such as debridement and dressing changes. Some of these wounds also carry with them a high risk of complications, requiring prolonged intervention. Acute wounds may be referred to other clinicians in the cases of gross contamination requiring cleansing of the wound before closure, a blistered wound such as a second-degree burn over a large area or a third-degree burn over a small area, infection of an acute wound, the presence of unhealthy tissue within the wound such that primary closure is not feasible, compromised immune system, dehiscence (defined below), and any other reason for tertiary/delayed primary closure.

CLEANLINESS OF ACUTE WOUNDS

The mechanism of injury, age of the wound, cleanliness, and extent of the injury are critical factors in the plan of care for acute wounds. Several terms have been used to describe the cleanliness of a wound. The terms "tidy" and "untidy" indicate a degree of contamination with foreign materials. "Clean," "clean-contaminated," "contaminated," and "dirty" have also been used. A clean or tidy wound has little, if any, foreign material and a low level of bacterial contamination. A kitchen accident with broken glass or a knife would be considered tidy or clean, although some bacteria will be introduced. A dirty or untidy wound is contaminated additionally with foreign materials that are likely to produce inflammation as well as carry large numbers of viable bacteria and spores. Even contaminated wounds are not expected to become infected unless local factors shift the balance in favor of bacterial proliferation. Local factors include necrotic tissue, foreign bodies, hematoma, and dead space. Systemic antibiotics are considered to be of little value in the treatment of acute wounds unless a therapeutic level can be obtained within 4 hours of wounding, and the use of systemic antibiotics after this time may, in some cases, increase infection rate. Wound infection is indicated by either localized purulent drainage or surrounding cellulitis and excessive inflammation. Systemic antibiotics may be used in the case of spreading cellulitis without purulent drainage. Surgically closed wounds with purulence, on the other hand, require opening, irrigation, and drainage. Once bacterial burden is below 100,000 per gram, delayed closure has a 96% success rate.[1]

How clean the wound is can often be inferred from the mechanism of the injury. A wound from farming equipment or a bite is likely to have a much greater degree of contamination than one from a piece of glass or kitchen knife. Also, the possibility of embedded materials and amount of tissue necrosis surrounding the wound can be deduced from the mechanism of injury. The age of a wound is important in deciding whether closure or healing by second intention is preferable. The longer a wound is left untreated, the greater the risk of infection. However, the local blood supply is also a factor in the decision whether to close a wound. A greater blood supply provides a better immune response. Facial injuries are commonly sutured even after 12 hours. In the past, the concept of a "golden period" dictated that closure must be accomplished within 6 to 12 hours, or the wound should be left open to heal by secondary intention. Modern practice with better debridement and antibiotic coverage allows greater latitude on how long a wound may be left open before surgical closure.[2]

CLOSURE OF ACUTE WOUNDS

The viability of tissue surrounding the wound must also be assessed to determine whether to close a wound. Lacerations, in particular, produce flaps of skin that may lose their blood supply. If this is the case, that part of the wound will need to be left open for two important reasons. First, sutures will not hold in devitalized tissue; and second, this devitalized tissue is likely to become infected. The amount of tissue loss in a wound needs to be determined to develop a plan for closure. Some areas of a wound can be sutured and other areas left to heal by secondary intention or to receive a graft where tissue loss occurs. Determining the amount of tissue loss can be difficult to assess where tissue is elastic and taut. Plastic surgeons can often develop a plan to close a wound entirely, even with some tissue loss, by various techniques. The depth of injury also affects the plan of care. A small wound can be allowed to re-epithelialize regardless of the depth of the wound, whereas a large wound with full-thickness injury will need to be grafted.[3,4]

Acute wounds are cleaned before closure. The surrounding skin needs to be carefully prepped, usually with an iodophor such as povidone-iodine. The wound itself is irrigated and debrided. Simple lacerations with minimal tissue injury usually require only irrigation. The more complex the wound and the more extensive the tissue necrosis, the more extensive the irrigation and debridement need to be. The cause of the wound will also determine how extensive the irrigation and debridement need to be. An untidy wound, such as an industrial accident, farming accident, or bite, will need more extensive care. Heavily contaminated wounds can be cleaned with pulsatile lavage or a syringe with an attached catheter. With cleaning of the wound, any embedded material is removed, and a decision of whether debridement is necessary is made. Foreign materials left in the wound will produce inflammation and infection. Long-term consequences include excessive scarring and tattooing. If necrotic tissue or unremovable embedded material remains in the wound, debridement becomes necessary. Debridement needs to be done judiciously to minimize the amount of tissue removed from the wound so that the wound can be closed with minimal scarring.

Local anesthesia for closure is dependent on the extent of the repair. For simple repairs, either 1% or 2% lidocaine is sufficient. For repairs that may require more than 1 hour, a longer-acting drug is needed. Bupivacaine may be used, but it takes longer to achieve anesthesia than lidocaine. Most wounds are infiltrated with epinephrine in combination with lidocaine. Epinephrine acts as a vasoconstrictor, which decreases bleeding during repairs and decreases the vascular washout of lidocaine from the tissue, which increases lidocaine's duration of action.

A variety of suture materials are available, with specific advantages for different situations. Suture material may be either absorbable or nonabsorbable and either monofilament or braided. Absorbable sutures are used subcutaneously or for special conditions in which suture removal is not desired. Polyglycolic acid sutures are braided and degrade by autolytic action rather than phagocytosis, so the risk of tissue reaction is decreased. Nonabsorbable sutures are used for the skin and may be braided or monofilament. The spaces within the braid are a concern for producing tissue reactions or for harboring bacteria. Monofilament sutures, however, are more difficult to tie. Sutures come in different sizes. 6-0 is preferred by many experts for more meticulous work such as the face, whereas 4-0 works well on other parts of the body. Wounds may be approximated with staples, especially skin grafts. Surgical adhesives are also available and wounds may be approximated with tape. Taping reduces the time required for wound closure and the need for local anesthesia but may not produce as precise closure as suturing.

Suturing techniques are critical for a good outcome. Poor technique can lead to excessive scarring or dehiscence. Deep layer approximation becomes necessary when an injury involves subcutaneous tissue. Failure to provide deep layer approximation increases tension on the outer sutures, leading to a poor result. Moreover, this procedure reduces the risk of fluid accumulation and infection below the skin. Suturing the skin can be done in a number of ways. The critical component is to gain closure of the wound with minimal tension. Following closure, swelling will increase the tension on the sutures. Excessive tension produces circulatory compromise of the edges of the wound and can lead to infection, dehiscence, or both. Sutures can generally be removed in 5 days on the face and 7 days on the trunk. Extremity sutures may be allowed to remain longer than 7 days. Formerly, surgeons were concerned about leaving sutures in too long because of inflam-

mation caused by reaction to the suture material. Newer synthetic materials allow a longer time to assure adequate wound strength. In some cases, application of skin tape is performed following suture removal to reduce tension on the immature scar to prevent scar widening or dehiscence. The tape strips are allowed to remain for several days until they loosen and detach on their own.[3,4]

SURGICAL WOUNDS

This type of wound usually presents the least potential for complications. The skin is prepared with an antiseptic such as povidone-iodine and the wound is created under sterile conditions. In addition, areas surrounding the sterile field are draped to avoid contamination. Possible complications may result from contamination released by surgery in the gastrointestinal tract or undetected bleeding, forming a hematoma. The other major complications are related to suturing technique. As discussed above, excessive tension can cause necrosis of the wound margins, leading to infection or dehiscence of the wound. Dehiscence is discussed later in the chapter. In addition, poor nutrition, corticosteroid use, diabetes mellitus, and smoking are among the potential causes of delayed healing and may prevent healing or lead to necrosis of the wound margins or infection. Adequate preparation of the skin is critical to prevent surface flora from being carried into the wound. For this reason, shaving of hair is discouraged. Instead, hair should be trimmed sufficiently to prevent loose hairs from entering the sterile field or hairs becoming entangled in the sutures. Shaving is likely to abrade the skin and may drive surface bacteria into the skin. Preparation of the skin is then done after hairs are trimmed from the area of interest. Circular biopsy punches of the skin may be approximated with sutures to decrease the size of the scar. Alternatively, these wounds could be covered with an occlusive dressing and allowed to heal by secondary intention.

AMPUTATION WOUNDS

Depending on the cause and site, amputation wounds may need to be closed in different ways. In general, a suture line is not desired on a weightbearing surface. To create a suture line on the anterior surface of a residual limb, the sufficient viable skin must be left on the posterior surface of the extremity to be brought over the weightbearing surface and sutured to the anterior surface. If this condition cannot be met because of excessive loss of functional limb length, equal amounts of skin from the posterior and anterior surface of the limb can be sutured across the weightbearing surface. This approach, however, risks damage and possible dehiscence with early weightbearing, which is a common goal of postamputation rehabilitation.

Sufficient soft tissue is needed between the skin and the residual bone to prevent injury to the skin making contact with a prosthesis. Dehiscence of amputation wounds occurs often and these are usually referred for wound management to assist in healing by second or third intention. These wounds are also closed by gradual third intention in which sutures are placed across the wound and tied as the wound becomes clean and sufficiently filled with granulation tissue to minimize tension on the sutures. A dehiscent sternal wound is shown in Figure 7-1.

INFECTION

Infection control is discussed in detail in Chapter 18. Any defect in the skin places an individual at risk of infection; and even with intact skin, exposure to some microbes can cause infection. Basically, one must analyze the combination of which microbes are present, the wound environment, and immune status of the patient. Careful skin preparation before surgery, thorough cleansing/irrigation, and debridement minimize but do not eliminate the risk of infection for a person with normal immunity by reducing bacterial counts in and around the wound. Diminished immunity even under optimal conditions of a clean wound with minimal necrotic tissue represents a much higher risk of infection than a run-of-the-mill contaminated wound in a person with normal immunity.

Wound environment is addressed by debridement and form of wound closure. The presence of necrotic tissue greatly increases the risk of infection by a number of microbes normally contaminating wounds. A high blood flow reduces the risk of infection due to the ability of immune cells to reach the wound and mount an attack against pathogens. Necrotic tissue provides nutrients for microbes and protects the microbes from immune cells. In particular, the formation of a biofilm around fissured, avascular bone fragments can produce intractable osteomyelitis. Occlusion of a wound by primary closure or placement of an occlusive wound dressing on a wound provides a warm, moist environment conducive to growth of pyogenic and other bacteria, and is likely to cause abscesses to form. As the factors determining the risk of infection are analyzed, the decision to suture a wound, leave a wound open, or close part of a wound and leave another part open must be made. A rather untidy wound in a highly vascular area of a person with minimum necrosis is likely to be sutured following thorough irrigation. A wound with substantial necrotic tissue will likely be debrided and allowed to heal by secondary intent. Prophylactic antibiotics may also be administered in cases in which risk of infection is greater than normal. The need for a tetanus booster also needs to be determined at this time.

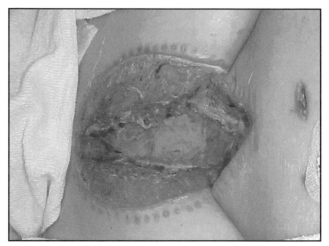

Figure 7-1. Dehiscent sternotomy wound. Note the degree of gapping and inflammation of the suture wounds. (Also shown in Color Atlas following page 274.)

DEHISCENCE

The opening of a surgical wound is termed *dehiscence*. This type of wound is caused by the failure of sutures or staples to maintain primary closure of a surgical wound for a number of reasons. A wound dehisces when the sutures, staples, tape, adhesive, or the skin itself is overcome by pressure or shear. Common causes include excess or improper lifting, necrosis of the wound edges due to vascular compromise or infection, or weakness of the skin caused by corticosteroids or other causes. Sternotomy wounds caused by open heart surgery and other procedures are frequently dehisced by patients who ignore lifting restrictions or are not taught proper transfers and other precautions to reduce sternal stress. These precautions include avoidance of shoulder extension, bilateral abduction, and pushing up in bed from long sitting. Instead, the patient needs to be taught to roll into sidelying and drop the legs off the bed as a counterweight to come to sitting. Some patients may prefer to scoot in prone until the legs are cleared from the bed. Abdominal surgical wounds may dehisce due to lifting but also due to intra-abdominal pressure or bloating. Infection can cause a wound on any part of the body to become dehiscent. In many cases, the dehiscent wound becomes so contaminated or the potential for tissue loss or necrosis is so great that primary closure is not attempted again. In this case, the typical approach is lavage, antibiotics, and delayed primary closure when the wound is clean and stable and sufficient granulation tissue formation has occurred to relieve strain on the apposed edges of delayed primary closure. In other cases, secondary closure is allowed to continue to completion, which may take months for some large abdominal wounds.

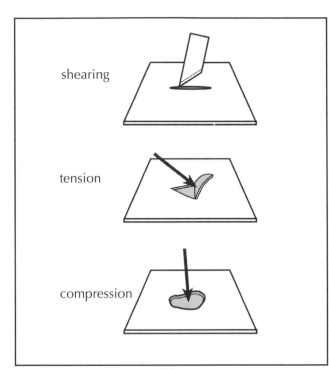

Figure 7-2. Mechanisms of lacerations.

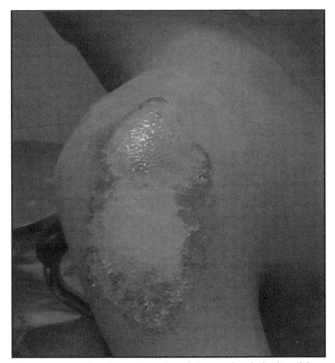

Figure 7-3. Abrasion ("road rash") on the left shoulder. Note the lack of pigmentation of the abraded skin and the darkening of the necrotic epidermis on the edges of the wound. (Also shown in Color Atlas following page 274.)

LACERATIONS

Lacerations are among the most common wounds seen in emergency departments. As occurs with any acute wound, lacerations typically have a high risk of contamination. Frequently, however, they can be cleansed sufficiently to allow primary closure with sutures, glue, staples, or tape. They are caused by three basic mechanisms: shearing, tension, and compression (Figure 7-2). A shearing injury is created by a small amount of energy focused on a small area, basically a sharp edge such as a knife or broken glass. The tissue is divided, but minimal cell injury occurs beyond the sharp edge. These wounds can be cleansed and repaired with primary intention with a thin scar and little risk of infection. Striking the body with a blunt object at an angle with high energy creates a tension injury. A triangular flap is created (partial avulsion). The tissue flap is at risk of ischemic necrosis with the loss of blood supply from the free edges, especially if the flap base is distal rather than proximal. The risk of infection is greater due to the potential for ischemia and greater tissue destruction compared with a shearing force. A compression injury is caused by a high force striking straight on, especially over superficial bone. The wound will have jagged and even shredded edges with much greater cell injury than the other two types. The injury may extend to subcutaneous tissue, including the bone. These wounds are at much greater risk of infection, requiring extensive cleansing, irrigation, and debridement. Primary repair is very extensive and may develop a cosmetically poor scar.

In many cases, primary repair is not achievable because of the extent of cell injury.

INCISIONS

Wounds caused by sharp objects such as scalpels or scissors during surgery are called incisions. Incisions produced with sharp objects by accident or by attack may be categorized with lacerations (above); knives and broken glass are frequent culprits. A deep wound caused by a sharp, narrow object such as an ice pick, nail, or bites by some animals is classified as a puncture wound and is discussed on the next page. Incision wounds are managed in much the same way as lacerations caused by shearing.

ABRASIONS

Abrasions are also common injuries. Their prevalence is difficult to determine because many are self-treated. These wounds are caused by tangential shearing of skin by a rough surface (Figure 7-3). Because they commonly occur along the road surface during cycling or motorcycle accidents to ejected, unrestrained passengers or pedestrians, the term "road rash" is often used to describe this injury. Abrasions are superficial wounds and usually only need cleaning and protection. Thorough cleansing is important to remove contaminants for two reasons: microbes must be removed to prevent infection, and contaminants that are not removed may permanently remain in the skin causing discoloration, called *tattooing*.

DEGLOVING (AVULSION)

A more serious injury in which the skin is pulled from the body is called degloving. This term is particularly descriptive for the upper extremity. It is similar to a tension laceration, but no flap remains; the base of what would be a flap is torn. This type of injury is sometimes called an avulsion. Degloving occurs during motor vehicle or industrial accidents in which skin catches on a sharp edge while the body is moving away from the object (Figure 7-4). This occurs in motor vehicle accidents in which the skin of a driver or passenger becomes caught on torn metal as the person is ejected from the vehicle. The skin is then torn and pulled away from body. Depending on the body part, this injury is covered by either a partial or full-thickness graft. The types of grafts are discussed further in Chapter 19.

PUNCTURE WOUNDS

Long, pointed objects such as ice picks, knives, and animal teeth can produce puncture wounds. The feet may also be punctured by nails and other fasteners by stepping on them. The seriousness of puncture wounds is primarily due to the tremendous risk of contamination deep into the body, particularly bone. To assess the risk of a puncture wound and to guide treatment, a puncture wound scoring system has been developed. The scale consists of four areas of 1 to 3 points and one area with either 0 or 9 points. The items consist of age of the wound, shape of the wound, depth of the wound, footwear at the time of puncture (if in the foot), and radiographic evaluation. The scoring system is given in Table 7-1.

A score of 1 to 4 indicates need for local cleansing; 5 to 8 indicates local cleansing, irrigation, and debridement (I & D), exploration, and placement of a drain. Any score greater than 9 indicates the need for lavage, intravenous (IV) antibiotics, and hospitalization.

ANIMAL BITES

Several vertebrates may inflict humans with bite injuries, ranging from armadillos to zebras. More common are bites from cats, squirrels, mice, rats, guinea pigs, and rabbits; however, of particular importance are dog bites. A wide range of dog sizes leads to a wide range of injury. Most dog bites occur on the lower extremities. In children, however, wounds may also occur on the head, neck, face,

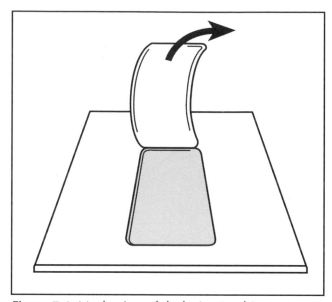

Figure 7-4. Mechanism of degloving (avulsion).

and upper extremities. Wound infections are estimated to occur in 5% to 10% of dog bites and at a greater rate with cat bites. Multiple organisms are likely to be obtained; however, IV antibiotics are not typically used unless a patient is at high risk for infection. Tetanus shots, however, are given as they would for puncture wounds. Several breeds of dogs can create extensive damage during a bite, causing crush injuries in addition to lacerations and punctures. Crush injuries are more likely to cause tissue necrosis and hematomas that increase the risk of wound infection. Multiple bites during an attack may require thorough debridement of the affected area and grafting.[5]

Cat bites are more likely to become infected. These injuries are more likely to cause puncture, rather than crushing or laceration wounds. Inoculation of the puncture wound or lack of medical attention are likely causes of the higher infection rate of cat bites. Small rodents kept as pets are more likely to cause thin lacerations with lower risk of infection than cat or dog bites.

GUN SHOT WOUNDS

Pistols, rifles, and shot guns have the potential to transfer enormous amounts of energy and injury to the body. A tremendous range of projectile velocity exists ranging from BB guns to high-powered rifles. In addition to the soft tissue wounds, gun shots have the potential to cause multiple wounds even with a single projectile. In many cases, the injuries are immediately lethal or lethal in a short time due to direct and indirect injury to the brain (herniation) and tearing of major blood vessels. These wounds may also cause limb amputation. The damage produced by bullets is determined by caliber and type. Several

Table 7-1

Foot Puncture Wound Scoring System

Category	0	1	2	3	9
Age		< 6 hrs	6 to 24 hrs	> 24 hrs	
Classification		Small, sharp, clean edges; superficial	Ragged, irregular margins; moderate depth	Irregular edges, necrotic tissue, foreign body and drainage	
Depth	Presence of concomitant disease = 1 additional point	Only epidermis and dermis	Through dermis with no structural involvement	Through dermis with structural involvement	
Footwear		None	Stockings	Stockings and shoes	
Radiographic Exam	No evidence of osseous involvement				Osseous involvement

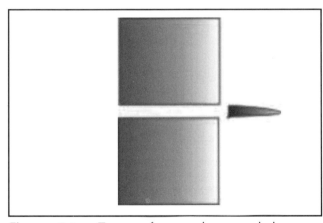

Figure 7-5a. Types of wounds caused by gun shots—high-velocity bullet going through a thin target produces a narrow wound.

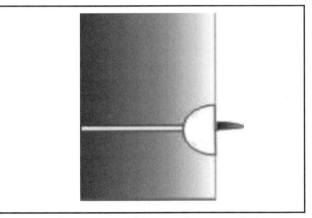

Figure 7-5b. Types of wounds caused by gun shots—high-velocity bullet going through an intermediate target produces cavitation during exit and a large exit wound.

types of bullets have been designed to maximize tissue injury by several mechanisms. Although the bullets or shot may be quite hot as they enter tissues, they also carry clothing and skin into the wound and, therefore, the wound is likely to become infected.

Bullets may be arbitrarily divided into low and high velocity. A low-velocity bullet fired from a typical .22 caliber pistol may travel at a rate of less than 1000 feet per second, whereas a high-powered rifle may propel a bullet greater than 3000 feet per second. In addition, the size of the bullet, the distance from which the gun is fired, and the characteristics of the tissue struck determine the wound produced. The characteristic of the wound produced is determined by the set of physical principles termed *wound ballistics*. Low-velocity bullets and shot may lodge in tissue with an entry wound only, whereas high-velocity bullets produce both an entry and a larger

exit wound, producing devastating cavitation (Figures 7-5a through 7-5d).

The basic types of wounds produced by gun shots include a small linear entry wound and a small or possibly no exit wound with a narrow track of tissue damage. Depending on the depth of the tissue struck, the bullet may produce enormous tissue damage by cavitation with a small exit wound (Figure 7-5a) or an enormous exit wound due to cavitation occurring at the exit (Figure 7-5b). A bullet may also produce a wound with no exit wound but tremendous internal damage produced by cavitation, due to complete dissipation of the bullet's kinetic energy within the tissue (Figure 7-5c). In addition to the damage caused by the tracking of the bullet through tissue, secondary missiles are produced by fragmentation of either the bullet itself or bone struck by the bullet. On occasion,

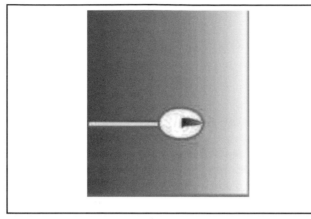

Figure 7-5c. Types of wounds caused by gun shots—high-velocity bullet going through a thick target produces cavitation within the tissue and may become lodged.

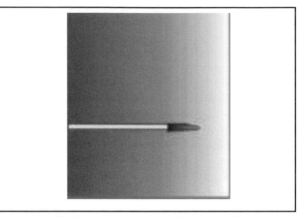

Figure 7-5d. Types of wounds caused by gun shots—low-velocity bullet becoming lodged in a thick target.

the bullet may enter a vein and produce a bullet embolism, typically lodging in the right ventricle.

The amount of damage imparted by a bullet is dependent on the change in kinetic energy ($0.5\ mv^2$) as it passes through tissues. Deformation of a bullet as it passes through tissue causes greater loss of energy and, therefore, more transfer of energy to tissues and tissue damage. As the formula for kinetic energy implies, velocity is more important than caliber in terms of inflicting damage (eg, a .223 caliber M16 rifle produces approximately three times the kinetic energy of a .45 caliber handgun due to the difference in velocity). When a bullet strikes the more dense medium of tissue, its flight becomes unstable; the more unstable it becomes, the more energy it transfers into the tissue. The instability can manifest itself as a tumbling or yawing motion, which increases the surface area of the bullet striking the tissue. Moreover, the irregular movement increases the probability that the bullet may deform or even fragment. For this reason, the transfer of energy from bullets to tissue becomes greater with the velocity of the bullet. With the exception of special handguns, pistols produce low-velocity wounds and most rifles produce high-muzzle velocities. The transfer of energy is directly related to how aerodynamic the bullet is, inversely related to the mass of the bullet, directly related to the caliber, and directly related to the density and tensile strength of the tissue struck.

High-velocity bullets create additional damage due to the process of cavitation. Low-velocity bullets push tissue aside, shearing and damaging tissues in a track approximated by the caliber of the bullet. With high-velocity bullets, cavitation is produced by waves of rapid stretching, compression, and shearing of tissues as a bullet passes through them. Cavitation can create an enormous wound several centimeters wider than the bullet. Tissue in front of the bullet is accelerated forward and laterally, creating a

negative pressure behind the bullet. This wave of tissue expansion and collapse repeats rapidly as the bullet passes through the tissue, creating even greater damage. The size of the defect caused by cavitation is dependent on the combination of depth of tissue and the velocity of the bullet. At higher velocities, the cavity occurs closer to the entrance and the wound will be larger. At a given combination of velocity and tissue thickness, the cavity may occur during exit, causing a large, ragged exit wound. A lower-velocity bullet passing through a smaller depth of tissue may not produce cavitation. On the other hand, a high-velocity bullet passing through a large depth of tissue may produce a small or no exit wound with a large cavity. For this reason, the track of the wound needs to be examined carefully. Cavitation is also dependent on the tensile strength of the tissue. Very soft tissues, such as internal organs, suffer greater cavitation than hard tissues, with skeletal muscle having an intermediate susceptibility to cavitation.

Shot gun shells are available in different sizes and velocities. Shells are classified by their diameter and the number of shot pellets in the shell. Typical shot guns use either 12 or 20 gauge shells with shell diameters of .729 and .614 inches in diameter, respectively. The pellets within the shell are given numerical sizes as well, typically ranging from .08 to .11 inches in diameter. Damage is inflicted by the deceleration of a large number of small lead spheres striking the tissue. At the muzzle, the pellets generally have a velocity of 1000 to 1500 feet per second. However, these small, spherical pellets have poor aerodynamic properties and lose kinetic energy traveling through the air before striking tissue. For this reason, the distance of the body from the shot gun is the chief determinant of the damage inflicted. At very close range, the individual pellets behave as a large single missile. As the pellets diverge, they become singular missiles. Depending on the characteristics of different shells, the damage inflicted at different ranges will vary. At a close range (1 to 2 yards) a large, ragged entrance wound is produced, and depending on the depth of tissue, an exit wound may or may not occur. At greater distances, the size of the entrance wound increases and multiple single shot wounds will surround the central wound. As distance increases to about 20 yards, the spray pattern becomes large (1 to 3 feet across), wounds become singular, and fewer shot pellets will strike the body with low kinetic energy. At greater than 50 yards, the probability of damage diminishes rapidly except for the eye. As discussed above with bullets, shot guns can also produce severe injury and death due to the damage to deeper structures.

Although these missiles achieve great kinetic energy and create tremendous heat on striking tissue, bullets and pellets of shot should be considered contaminated. At one time, it was considered that bullets were sterilized by the heat generated. However, pieces of material from the body surface are carried into the body and several studies have indicated that microbes can be carried into the body by bullets. Gun shot wounds are generally not closed and require thorough irrigation and filling of the tracts with nonocclusive materials such as packing strip, or if large enough, with a bandage roll. Substantial necrosis of tissue surrounding the tracts is expected, and irrigation and debridement may need to be carried out for several days, and the material used to fill the tracts is frequently soaked in topical antibiotic solution such as triple antibiotic.[6]

Psychosocial issues are common with gun shot wounds. The ability of the clinician to handle these issues may influence the patient's adherence to the plan of care. In recent years, strategies for gang-related shooting to minimize risk of punishment by law enforcement have developed specific targets for shootings. Shootings involving the spine became popular to avoid being charged with murder. More recently, the groin has become a popular target with the risk of paralysis of a single lower extremity.

TOXIC ULCERATIONS

Ulcerations caused by chemicals injected by arthropod bites are categorized as toxic ulcerations. Notable among these, particularly in the southern United States, is the venom of the brown recluse spider. The venom spreads rapidly through fatty tissue and can produce ulcers several centimeters wide and deep. One of the author's first wound care experiences was a brown recluse injury that created an ulcer 10 cm x 8 cm x 7 cm deep in the buttocks of a woman bitten while sitting on a wooden latrine seat. These wounds can be cleaned and healed, but may take several weeks to months depending on the size of the wound. As with any wound, the potential for infection exists if the wound is not debrided. With appropriate debridement and dressings, these wounds should heal without complication.

WOUNDS ASSOCIATED WITH FRACTURES

Fractures represent two sets of potential problems related to wound management—wounds created by open fractures and surgical wounds to repair the fracture. The exception would be a closed fracture managed with closed reduction and immobilization. Wounds are created by bone fragments in open fractures and by surgeons for either open reduction or for external fixation. Open fractures are frequently accompanied by skin loss in the area, although some of these lacerations can be surgically repaired. In other cases, severe avulsion or degloving injuries can cause large areas of skin to be torn from the limb. Open reduction wounds will typically be closed surgically and several incisions may be created, depending on the procedure used. In certain types of injuries, fracture blisters may form and cause severe wounds, often associated with infection. Within this section, care for pins used for skeletal traction following a fracture and external fixation used for management of complex fractures or limb-lengthening will be addressed, as well as fracture blisters.

Open Fractures

An open fracture, formerly known as a compound fracture, causes tearing of the soft tissues against the sharp edge of the fractured bone. The risk of open fracture depends on several factors, including the mechanism of the injury, the type and amount of soft tissue surrounding the bone, and the pliability of the bone. Open fractures are more likely to occur with injuries caused by high-energy mechanisms such as car and motorcycle accidents and falls from great heights. Twisting injuries or blows perpendicular to long bones are also more likely to cause open fractures. A bone stabilized by thick, pliable tissues such as the femur of an athlete is less likely to tear through soft tissue than a superficial bone with little support, such as the distal tibia. Finally, brittle bones of the elderly are more likely to tear soft tissue than the highly pliable bones of very young children.

Open fractures present several serious problems. Bone and soft tissue are exposed to the external environment and depending on the circumstances, the contamination can be very extensive (eg, a farm implement accident). Contamination of bone with bacteria increases the risk of osteomyelitis, which can be very difficult to clear. Large amounts of necrotic tissue may be present in the wound due to injury from the sharp bone. In addition, the border between necrotic and healthy tissue may be difficult to determine early. Failure to remove necrotic tissue from the wound increases the risk of infection. Neurovascular compromise is always a threat with an open fracture, especially the radial nerve with midshaft humerus fractures and the peroneal nerve with tibial/fibular fractures, although certainly any peripheral nerve is at risk. Nerve injuries caused by open fractures and in some cases even closed fractures or severe sprains can lead to *complex regional pain syndrome* (CRPS), a condition of persistent pain and autonomic dysfunction requiring protracted physical therapy to manage. CRPS is a term that encompasses the variety of dysfunctions formerly known as reflex sympathetic dystrophy, shoulder-hand syndrome, minor causalgia, major causalgia, and others. These conditions are characterized by mechanical allodynia in which normal mechanical stimulation is perceived as pain and is accompanied by swelling and atrophy of the skin and bone. Sensory re-education and desensitization are performed in physical therapy. Autonomic blockade of sympathetic ganglia with local anesthetic is sometimes used but is not successful for many individuals with CRPS.

Pin Care

Pin care addresses three issues: compromised circulation, pin reaction, and infection. Compromised circulation is caused by excessive skin tension on the pin leading to necrosis of skin around the pin. Pin reaction is described as inflammation due to tissue reaction to the presence of the pin. Signs of inflammation (redness, swelling, tenderness, and discharge) must be present for more than 72 hours to be considered a reaction, and clear drainage alone is not considered to be pin reaction. Excessive movement of the pin and blockage of drainage increase the risk of pin reaction.

Minor pin reaction refers to a situation in which redness, swelling, tenderness, or clear drainage is present and improves with lancing of the skin. A major pin reaction or infection is defined as a condition that does not improve with lancing and results in the need to remove pins due to the risk of osteomyelitis and the difficulty of managing it. Problems include the development of an abscess around the pin, presence of necrotic tissue around the pin promoting infection, and excessive motion, which increases the risk of infection. Six issues related to pin care include the frequency of pin care, cleansing solutions, use of ointments at the pin-skin interface, management of crusts on the pins, when to use sterile technique, and the use of dressings.[7]

It is widely held that keeping the pins clean and allowing a slow drainage from the tissue onto the pins is the best strategy for avoiding infection. Thus, recommendations are aimed at promoting free flow of drainage, avoiding disturbance of the normal balance of skin flora, and avoiding skin and subcutaneous tissue irritation. Frequency of pin care needs to be individualized. Too frequent pin care causes inflammation, whereas infrequent observation can lead to serious problems. A simple guideline is for pin site care every 8 hours in the presence of drainage and daily with no drainage. Although many individuals commonly use hydrogen peroxide and/or povidone iodine, recommendations are for the use of normal saline only. Normal saline dilutes the bacteria present on the pins, whereas disinfectants have been associated with a higher, not lower, rate of infection. The recommendation is to clean only the pin with alcohol, whereas skin cleansing should only be done as needed and with normal saline. Cleansing also needs to be performed by sweeping away from the skin and avoiding moving contaminants toward the open wound.

Ointments are not recommended, as they can occlude the pin hole and allow infection to occur. For the same reason, the recommendation is to remove crusts from the pin-skin interface to allow drainage to occur. Some authors have suggested that with pins used for skeletal traction placed in areas with little soft tissue, crust removal is not necessary; but with external fixators, crusts should be removed. Gauze dressings are recommended for covering the pin sites to reduce surface contamination and to absorb drainage. Dressings should not hold moisture against the skin nor should they be cut before placing them over the wounds, as frayed ends may irritate the wound. Sterile technique has only been recommended during hospitalization due to the presence of multi-resistant organisms and potentially reduced resistance.[8]

Fracture Blisters

These wounds occur in a small percentage of fractures in general but are much more likely to occur in areas of superficial bone with tight skin (5% in these areas). They may also occur in other injuries that do not produce fractures, such as severe ankle sprains, and to areas such as the elbow, foot, and distal tibia. In these areas, tissue injury can cause edema between the dermal and epidermal layers of skin. Because of the proximity of the involved bone or ligaments and the lack of skin mobility in these areas, separation of the epidermis from the dermis with subsequent necrosis of the epidermis results. Fracture blisters are four times more likely to occur if surgical stabilization is delayed more than 24 hours. Wound infections, delayed fracture treatment, fracture nonunion, increased hospital stay, and increased costs of care may result from these blisters. The presence of a fracture blister causes surgical incisions to be placed in areas that may not be optimal for the surgical procedure due to the risk of spreading infection from the blister. Compression may not be useful for prevention of fracture blisters because veins are more superficial in the areas where blisters tend to occur, and compression is likely to impede venous flow; whereas compression tends to aid deeper venous return. Useful prevention is aimed at early immobilization, elevation, and surgical repair of twisting injuries of the foot, ankle, elbow, and distal tibia. Rupture of the blister is not recommended; rather a dry, absorbent dressing to protect the blister is recommended. Occlusive dressings such as hydrocolloids are recommended once the blister ruptures, if the wound is clean. Topical antibiotics are not recommended unless the wound is infected and not healing. Systemic antibiotics are recommended if infection occurs. In this case, occlusive dressings should not be used. Re-epithelialization of fracture blisters is expected in 4 to 21 days depending on individual factors.[9]

Irrigation and Debridement

Acute wounds are also deliberately formed to treat infections, particularly those of the diabetic foot. When deep infection is suspected, irrigation and debridement may be indicated. This procedure is also used for infected surgical wounds, osteomyelitis, puncture wounds, tunneling, or sinus tracts. The procedure is often followed by placement of a drain, packing, and delayed primary closure. Packing of the wound with saline-moistened gauze is done to prevent the wound from filling with granulation tissue. When the wound is clean and stable, tertiary closure is used.

SKIN DISEASES

Blistering diseases, in particular, may produce acute wounds. Blisters may be formed either by the separation of the epidermis from the dermis or dermis from the basement membrane. In either case, the disease process results in the loss of the barrier to infection and fluid loss. *Epidermolysis bullosa* is a genetic disease characterized by defective desmosomes. *Pemphigus* is an autoimmune disease affecting desmosomes, allowing separation within the dermis, and is life threatening. *Pemphigoid* is a disease that superficially resembles pemphigus, but the separation occurs between the epidermal and dermal layers. Blistering may also be toxin-mediated. The condition popularly known as *Staphylococcal scalded skin syndrome* (SSSS) is caused in neonates by an epidermolytic toxin of a particular strain of *Staphylococcus aureus*. The skin may come off in sheets and patients must be handled very delicately to prevent further damage. Hypersensitivity reactions may also cause blistering. In particular, Stevens-Johnson syndrome produces blistering of the skin and mucosa. A number of pharmaceuticals, especially antibiotics and sulfonamides, have been linked to this syndrome. Treatment is generally performed by protecting the skin with silver sulfadiazine ointment, although this compound has also been linked to Stevens-Johnson syndrome. Once the skin is at low risk for infection, daily application of sterile hydrogel sheets can be performed. They are soothing, retain fluid and heat, and do not adhere to the wound, making dressing changes less painful for the patient. The patient can also avoid the discomfort of the agitation necessary to remove silver sulfadiazine.

OPERATIVE REPAIR

Operative repair of ulcers represents surgical management and, as such, is performed only by a qualified and licensed surgeon. Possible techniques for operative repair include direct closure with sutures, staples, or adhesives. Another common means, especially for full-thickness burns, is skin grafting, in which a portion of tissue is removed completely from the body and transplanted to another site, where it is revascularized. A third type is the flap in which the transplanted tissue is transferred with its own blood supply. In some cases, the transplanted tissue is not completely excised and may have a number of different tissue types within it.

In certain cases, healing by first, second, or third intent is not adequate for wound closure. Operative repair is addressed in the Agency for Health Care Policy and Research (AHCPR) pressure ulcer treatment guidelines (see Appendix). At the time of publication, the recommendation was for operative repair for clean stage III or IV pressure ulcers not responding to optimal care, although it was stated that more research was needed to identify criteria clearly. Operative repair should not be undertaken until a wound is clean, stable, and free of necrotic tissue. In the case of large wounds, conventional treatment, including debridement and dressing changes, may be carried out for several weeks followed by grafting. Operative repair is recommended only for patients who are medically stable, adequately nourished, and otherwise able to tolerate surgery. In some cases, especially terminal illness, wound closure is not a feasible goal; simple protection of the wound may be sufficient.

For the operative repair candidate, a number of factors may improve operative outcome. Preoperatively, the clinician should address smoking cessation, treatment for spasticity, wound colonization, urinary and fecal incontinence, and urinary tract infection.

Common procedures include direct closure (third or delayed primary intent), skin grafting, skin flaps, musculocutaneous flaps, and free flaps. The advantages and disadvantages of postoperative care are also discussed in this chapter. Because the ischial tuberosities are a leading cause of pressure ulcers in chairbound individuals, a school of thought was once to perform prophylactic ischiectomy. This procedure is not recommended by the AHCPR guidelines.

Postoperative follow-up care for operative repair of ulcers includes using an appropriate support surface. An air-fluidized bed, low air loss bed, or Stryker frame is recommended for up to 2 weeks postop, depending on multiple factors, especially the patient's ability to remain off the operative surface and the risk for development of new ulcers. Tissue viability in the operative site should be monitored carefully with a slow increase in the time that the patient is positioned on the flap or graft. Monitoring flaps or grafts for pallor or redness that persist after 10 minutes of pressure is recommended. In addition, shear forces, including excessive stretching of the operative site, should be avoided.[10]

Direct Closure

If possible, direct closure of an acute wound is preferable to prevent contamination and chronic inflammation. Indications for direct closure include lacerations with minimal tissue loss, surgical wounds, and other incisions. Regardless of the cause of the wound, for direct closure to be the method of choice, the wound must be clean and likely to heal. Prior to direct closure, the site must be irrigated and debrided of any foreign material or necrotic tissue. A surgeon may choose delayed primary closure (tertiary closure) if significant undermining or contamination is present. Should direct closure be chosen, deep sutures are placed in the depth of the wound to decrease stress on skin. Surgical staples or adhesives (glue) may be used in the place of sutures.

Skin Grafts

Skin grafts are indicated for wounds that are not expected to close spontaneously in a reasonable time in patients with available donor sites and sufficient blood flow to the area to be grafted to revascularize the graft. Either split-thickness or full-thickness grafts may be used, depending on the area to be covered. The advantage of a split-thickness skin graft is its ability to cover a larger area due to meshing, which allows a surface area approximately three times as large to be covered as the donor area and the ability to reharvest the same donor site. However, the drawbacks of cosmetic problems and function on flexor surfaces may require a full-thickness graft. The stretching of the meshed graft has the important effect of converting a single large defect in the skin into multiple small wounds that can heal by re-epithelialization. As the donor site heals by re-epithelialization, it can be reharvested after 10 to 14 days to provide a graft for another area of the body.

Full-thickness grafts have sufficient strength to function on flexor surfaces such as the anterior elbow, axilla, and posterior knee, and are much more cosmetically acceptable than the residual diamond effect left in a healed split-thickness skin graft. However, full-thickness skin grafts can only cover a third of the area that a split-thickness graft can, and the available surface area for taking full-thickness grafts may be limited.

Cultured skin is another way of covering a wound. A small piece of skin is harvested from the patient and grown under optimal conditions in a laboratory setting. After several weeks, a piece of skin originally only a few cm^2 may reach a size approaching a square meter. Precautions following successful grafting include the risk of infection, protecting the graft from the effect of shear for 7 to 14 days, and the need for lubrication.

Flaps

In certain cases, flaps are preferable to grafts. Benefits of using a flap rather than a graft include better-quality skin cover, sensation is more likely to remain intact with a flap, the provision of padding, the ability to cover exposed anatomical structures and prostheses, the ability to maintain blood supply and cosmesis, and the possibility of functional restoration.

Flaps are classified based on the type of tissue grafted and the anatomical relationship between the donor and graft site of the flap. Tissue type may include skin and subcutaneous tissue, muscle with or without overlying skin, or bone with or without original overlying tissue. The anatomical relationship between the donor and graft sites may be classified as *local*, in which the tissue harvested is adjacent to the defect to be filled; *distant*, in which the harvested tissue is attached temporarily to its original site until vascularization occurs at the new location; and a *free flap*, which has been removed from its donor site but blood vessels anastomosed to blood vessels in the new location.

Skin Flaps

Although the purpose of using a skin flap rather than a skin graft is the presence of intact blood vessels, blood supply to the skin flap can be unpredictable. If blood vessels are identifiable within the flap, the preference is for a flap with an axial arterial supply running the length of the flap. An axial supply can provide a larger flap than one with horizontal blood supply.

Muscle Flap

This type of flap can be created without overlying skin but then must be covered with a split-thickness skin graft. As with the skin flap, an axial blood supply is preferred with perforating blood vessels to revascularize skin. In contrast to skin flaps, muscle flaps provide padding. Good blood supply decreases risk of infection or failure of the graft to take.

Free Flap

To perform a free flap, the surgeon must be able to identify vessels to anastomose in both the flap and the recipient site. If this vessel anastomosis can be done, the free flap provides well-vascularized tissue to a site that does not have a good local site. In addition, a skilled surgeon may be able to anastomose a nerve. Other specialized flaps exist, and the reader is directed to texts covering these flaps.[10]

SUMMARY

Acute wounds are typically managed in the emergency room or operating room, but complications may involve other clinicians. The purpose of this chapter is to understand the mechanisms of these wounds and what may lead to the referral to clinicians reading this material. Common causes of acute wounds include burns, discussed in Chapter 19, dehiscence of surgical wounds, amputation wounds, lacerations, incisions, gun shot wounds, and open fractures. A brief discussion of operative repair is also included in this chapter.

STUDY QUESTIONS

1. Why is a gun shot wound likely to become infected even if the bullet reaches a high temperature?

2. What are the advantages and disadvantages of placing an amputation wound at the distal end of the residual limb?

3. What are the relative risks of poor outcomes from the three basic types of lacerations? Which is generally better, a triangular flap with its apex distal or proximal?

4. What are the potential problems created by an open fracture and the use of external fixation?

5. Why is a clean wound, that is free of infection, required for operative repair?

REFERENCES

1. Robson MC, Shaw RC, Heggers JP. The reclosure of post-operative incisional abscesses based on bacterial quantification of the wound. *Ann Surg.* 1970;171:279-282.

2. Robson MC. Wound infection. A failure of wound healing caused by an imbalance of bacteria. *Surg Clin North Am.* 1997;77:637-650.

3. Finley JM, McConnell. *Emergency Wound Repair.* Baltimore, Md: University Park Press; 1984.

4. Kaplan EN, Hentz VR. *Emergency Management of Skin and Soft Tissue Wounds. An Illustrated Guide.* Boston, Mass: Little, Brown, and Company; 1984.

5. Driscoll JA. Integumentary management of the patient with multiple traumatic injuries. *Acute Care Perspectives.* 1999;7(3):1-18.

6. Swan KG, Swan RC. *Gunshot wounds. Pathophysiology and management.* Chicago: Year Book Medical Publishers; 1989.

7. McKenzie LL. In search of a standard for pin site care. *Orthopaedic Nursing.* 1999,18:73-78.

8. Ward P. Care of skeletal pins: a literature review. *Nursing Standard.* 1998 12: 34-38.

9. Varela CD, Vaughan TK, Carr JB, et al. Fracture blisters:Clinical and pathological aspects. *J Orthop Trauma.* 1993, 7:417-427.

10. Peacock EE. *Wound Repair.* Philadelphia, Pa: WB Saunders; 1984.

Neuropathic Ulcers

OBJECTIVES

- Assess risk factors for neuropathic ulcers.
- Discuss control of diabetes mellitus.
- Discuss American Diabetes Association recommendations.
- List causes of Charcot's foot and describe interventions to minimize its effects.
- Discuss how other complications of diabetes mellitus affect mobility.
- Describe the etiologies and treatments of other neuropathies.
- Perform a foot screening.
- Discuss appropriate footwear for individuals with neuropathy.
- Discuss strategies for prevention of neuropathic ulcers.

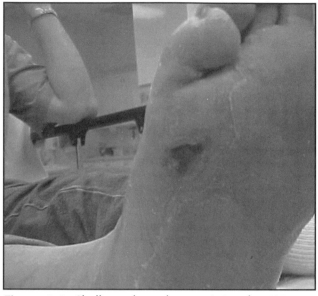

Figure 8-1. Shallow ulcer characteristic of a Wagner grade 1 ulcer. Note the dryness and callus formation over the entire plantar surface.

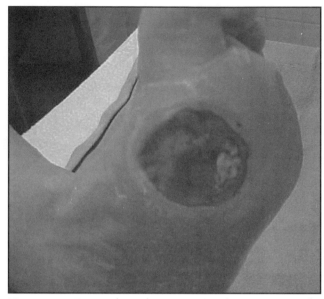

Figure 8-2. Deep ulcer characteristic of a Wagner grade 2 ulcer. Note the thick rim of callus around the wound. Also note the presence of hammer toes, which increase the shearing forces under the metatarsal heads during gait. (Also shown in Color Atlas following page 274.)

BACKGROUND

Discussion of neuropathic ulcers is commonly directed toward plantar ulcers of the diabetic foot. In Western countries, diabetes mellitus represents the major cause of peripheral neuropathy; as such, ulcers caused by the lack of neural function are observed most commonly in the feet of individuals with diabetes mellitus. Other causes include spinal cord injury, tumors, stroke, spina bifida, syringomyelia, other sensory neuropathies, and leprosy (Hansen's disease).

Although diabetes may also cause peripheral vascular disease, neuropathic ulcers are caused by mechanical factors, not vascular. A person may have both arterial insufficiency and neuropathy due to diabetes. However, the wounds caused by these two etiologies are generally easy to distinguish (Table 8-1). Arterial insufficiency is painful, occurs on the distal part of the foot, the affected extremity has a low ankle-brachial index (ABI), and the wound has an irregular shape and pale wound base. Neuropathic ulcers occur on areas of weightbearing and shearing, especially under metatarsal heads and sites of bony abnormalities (Figures 8-1 and 8-2). The wounds are round and not painful. It is clear, however, that arterial insufficiency may exacerbate neuropathic ulcers, and neuropathy may exacerbate arterial insufficiency ulcers. Although the lack of sensation is commonly believed to be the root cause of plantar ulcers in diabetic feet, this type of ulcer is generally due to neuropathy of all three systems—sensory, motor, and autonomic.

Sensory neuropathy results in the loss of protective sensation. Motor neuropathy produces weakness of intrinsic foot muscles and changes in the shape of the foot with altered biomechanics and risk of injury. Thirdly, autonomic neuropathy causes the loss of sweating to protect the skin against drying. As a result of damage to all three neural systems, damage is allowed to go undetected, altered biomechanics of the foot cause pressure and shear in typical locations, and dry, hyperkeratotic skin and callus increase pressure and shear on skin with the result of round/elliptical wounds occurring under bony prominences.

It is estimated that 15% of all individuals with diabetes mellitus will develop foot ulcers. Moreover, 20% of all hospital admissions of those with diabetes mellitus are due to foot ulcers. People with diabetes mellitus average one hospital admission per year for foot ulcers after 65 years of age. The most common sites of diabetic foot ulcers include the plantar great toe, 30%; the head of first metatarsal, 22%; the dorsum of digits, 13%; the plantar aspect of the other toes, 10%; the fifth metatarsal head, 9%; the second metatarsal head, 6%; the arch, 4%; the third metatarsal head, 2%; the fourth metatarsal head, 2%; and the heel, 1%.

PATHWAYS TO DIABETIC LIMB AMPUTATION

In addition to neuropathic ulcers, diabetes mellitus frequently leads to amputation.[1] The reasons for amputation of diabetic limbs are multiple and many pathways lead to

Table 8-1

DIFFERENTIAL DIAGNOSIS OF ULCERS CAUSED BY NEUROPATHY AND ARTERIAL INSUFFICIENCY

	Neuropathic	*Ischemic (Arterial Insufficiency)*
Appearance	Round or elliptical, dry surrounding skin	Irregular, wet or dry gangrene, atrophy of skin, thickened nail, loss of hair, rubor of dependency
Location	Sites of pressure or shear during weight-bearing and ambulation	Distal, especially toes and heels, but may occur anywhere arterial vessels occlude
Pain	None, but may have dysesthesia	Painful
Tests	Sensory testing shows loss of protective sensation, loss of vibration, position sense, reflexes	Low ankle-brachial index; low transcutaneous oxygen; claudication during treadmill test

Table 8-2

CAUSAL PATHWAYS TO AMPUTATION WITH DIABETIC NEUROPATHY

1. Neuropathy
2. Minor trauma
3. Ulceration
4. Faulty healing
5. Gangrene
6. Amputation

amputation. The usual pathway (72%) consists of minor trauma, cutaneous ulceration, and wound-healing failure.[2] Factors cited as indications for lower extremity amputation are as follows: ischemia, 46%; infection, 59%; neuropathy, 61%; faulty wound healing, 81%; ulceration, 84%; and gangrene, 55%. Initial minor trauma was cited in 81% of cases of lower extremity amputation in persons with diabetes mellitus (Table 8-2). Because statistically identifiable and potentially preventable events appear to precede most amputations, the federal government has instituted a program through the National Institutes of Health called the LEAP program (Lower Extremity Amputation Prevention).[3] It consists of educational material for both individuals with diabetes and clinicians caring for them. A number of the principles come directly from these materials. These include screening and proper fitting of footwear. As discussed earlier, all patients need to be evaluated and treatment needs to be developed based on individual needs. This is particularly true for patients with diabetes mellitus. Multiple systems are affected by this disease, particularly with lack of glycemic control. Of particular importance in this discussion are neuropathy; athero-

sclerosis, which leads to peripheral vascular disease and ischemic heart disease and stroke; renal disease; retinopathy; and glycolysation of proteins. Glycolysation has been suggested to cause reduced elasticity of skin, tendons, and ligaments. The triple threat of neuropathy needs to be carefully addressed by evaluating sensory, motor, and autonomic function. Sensory neuropathy leads to glove and stocking sensory loss, which is characterized by loss of sensation occurring distally and progressing proximally. Glove and stocking sensory loss results from the greater probability of damage to longer neurons, and as disease progresses, shorter neurons become involved. Therefore, sensory loss is most likely to occur first in the foot and progress centrally. Sensory loss may also progress to the hand, usually about the time that sensory loss occurs near the knee. Sensory loss is also manifested as bizarre, brief burning sensations, termed *dysesthesia*, and chronic discomfort of the feet. Treatment of diabetic foot pain is addressed at the end of this chapter.

Motor neurons are also affected based on the probability of longer neurons being affected preferentially. The muscles most affected are those located within the foot itself; however, several muscles attached to the foot are innervated by much shorter neurons. Frequently, the peripheral neuropathy results in a combination of weak intrinsic flexors and normal extrinsic extensors, which produce foot deformities and may contribute to limited joint mobility. Anatomical changes, in turn, lead to biomechanical abnormalities resulting in pressure and shearing under metatarsal heads, shearing under other bony prominences, and a condition known as tip-top-toe syndrome, in which the tips and tops of toes are damaged by friction against the inside of the patient's footwear.

Autonomic involvement causes loss of sweating, which results in dry skin and loss of control of blood vessels within the foot. Increased blood flow to the foot has been implicated in resorption of bone in the foot, leading to the deformity known as Charcot's foot. Charcot's foot carries with it an increased risk of fracture of osteopenic bone and subsequently an increased risk of other shear/pressure points on the foot. As a result of triple neuropathy, individuals with poor glycemic control experience a number of factors, which left unmanaged are nearly certain to result in a downward spiral of the person's health. These conditions include dry, flaky skin prone to hyperkeratosis and cracking, which can provide a portal for bacterial entry, especially if the patient soaks the feet. Deformities of the foot produce abnormal pressure and shear points manifested initially as callus, erythema, and hemorrhage under callus. Callus itself is a risk factor for ulceration because callus formation increases load on the tissue by 30%.[4] A simple demonstration of the effect of callus can be performed by having a person with normal sensation walk with a coin taped in the bottom of the shoe. Moreover, the lack of sensation decreases voluntary reduction of tissue load on the foot. Whereas a person with normal sensation and an injury to the foot will reduce gait-induced stresses on the foot, the person lacking pain is likely to forget to alter the gait pattern.

FACTORS LEADING TO FOOT WOUNDS

A single factor is unlikely to alone cause plantar ulcers. Generally, several factors interact to cause the wound and, therefore, several factors must be addressed in the treatment plan. Among these problems are altered biomechanics, an insensate foot, arterial insufficiency, the inability to monitor the feet, competition for time and resources with other pathologies, bad information received from others, and denial. Denial is particularly easy with an insensate foot competing with more immediate life-threatening problems such as end-stage renal failure, lack of feeling in the damaged foot, and poor mobility and vision limiting the ability to inspect one's feet.

Treatment of neuropathic ulcers is very different from ulcers caused by arterial insufficiency (ischemia). Arterial insufficiency must be referred to a vascular surgeon for appropriate treatment. Differential diagnosis is based on the location, appearance, and special tests. Differential diagnosis is also important because both are associated with diabetes mellitus. Some individuals with diabetes mellitus will predominantly or solely have neuropathy, whereas other individuals may have severe atherosclerosis, yet no neuropathy. The usual case seems to be neuropathy appearing prior to ischemia, although often both are present.

WAGNER GRADES FOR NEUROPATHIC ULCERS

The Wagner scale is used for prognosis and intervention decisions regarding neuropathic ulcers. The scale does not represent a progression of a given wound, rather it represents an increase in the severity and invasiveness required for treatment of the wound. As the descriptions detail, neuropathy, infection, and ischemia are progressively involved. The scale ranges from grade 0 to grade 5. A grade 0 ulcer represents damage to the foot, but the skin remains intact. Severe subcutaneous tissue injury may be present and, as such, minor trauma to the foot may lead to a serious infection of the necrotic tissue within the foot. Grade 1 describes a partial-thickness or superficial ulcer (see Figure 8-1). A full-thickness wound with subcutaneous involvement is classified as a grade 2 neuropathic ulcer (see Figure 8-2). Note that only two grades are used to denote the depth of the ulcer. A wound is classified as a grade 3 ulcer when infection is present, manifested as either an abscess or osteomyelitis (Figure 8-3). Progression to forefoot gangrene is documented as a grade 4 ulcer, and grade 5 represents gangrene of most of the foot. Treatment of neuropathic ulcers according to Wagner grade is described later.

Interventions for neuropathic ulcers include local wound care and periodic foot screening for deformities, callus formation, sensation, reflexes, strength, and range of motion. Decreased range of motion of the articulations of the foot are predictive of future ulceration. Inspection of footwear and either off-loading or protecting the foot may become necessary. Of all possible interventions, metabolic control is the most important factor for long-term health. Patients must be reinforced and rewarded by all members of the health care team to maintain blood glucose as close to normal (about 100 mg/dL) as possible. With multiple demands on the patient's life, blood glucose control is often difficult prior to ulceration but only becomes more difficult with infection. In fact, rising blood glucose is suggestive of infection.[5]

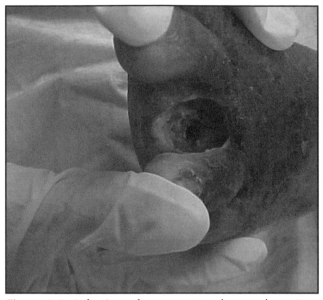

Figure 8-3. Infection of an amputated second ray (toe and metatarsal). Infection is characteristic of Wagner grade 3 ulcers.

PROTECTING THE FOOT

Several means are available for protecting the foot. These include bed rest, crutch walking, total contact casting, walking splints, cut-out sandals, diabetic shoes, and custom shoes. Bed rest is largely impractical due to the potential for severe cardiopulmonary decline and exacerbation of blood glucose control. For many individuals, especially older patients with multiple health problems, crutch walking is also impractical. Diminishing balance due to loss of proprioception and vision creates safety concerns. Moreover, the tremendous prevalence of obesity in type 2 diabetes mellitus and the potential for cardiovascular disease with increased energy demands of crutch walking compared with unaided gait may increase the risks associated with ambulation with crutches.[6] More detailed discussion of protecting the foot is discussed later in the chapter.

WOUND CARE

Appropriate local wound care consists of debridement, selection and application of appropriate dressings, application of topical agents and modalities, and protection of surrounding skin. The American Diabetes Association recommends aggressive debridement to viable tissue due to the high risk of infection of open wounds with necrotic tissue and frequent immunosuppression. Trimming callus should be done as needed. Callus is formed by abnormal shearing forces on the skin. Even with removal of the abnormal shear, callus often returns and must be debrided by either peeling or by shaving the tissue tangentially with a sharp scalpel.

Dry gangrene should never be debrided. As a general rule, necrotic tissue is removed from a wound to allow healing from viable edges of the wound toward the center. In the case of dry gangrene, no healthy tissues exist under the necrotic surface. Debridement exposes necrotic tissue to the outside environment. This, combined with the frequent immunosuppression of individuals with poor glycemic control, creates tremendous risk for a rapidly progressing infection of the extremity. Stated simply, no good comes from debriding dry gangrene, and tremendous risk is associated with removal of the covering of the moist necrotic tissue below.

When cleansing a neuropathic ulcer, avoid using a whirlpool or any type of soaking. Soaking increases the risk of maceration and potential for skin cracking, providing a portal of entry for bacteria. When selecting a dressing, the clinician must first consider the high risk of infection. An appropriate dressing allows frequent observation and avoids occlusion. A cavity requires loose filling to promote healing from the center of the wound toward the periphery. Available fillers include alginates and hydrofibers, amorphous gels, and various gauze products such as 4 x 4 gauze sponges. However, gauze promotes inflammation, which in turn leads to continual use of gauze due to drainage caused by the inflammatory response to gauze products. One particular study demonstrated that collagen-alginate filler increases healing compared with gauze, but at a higher cost per dressing change. On the other hand, the ease of dressing removal and comfort of the alginate or hydrofiber dressings produces greater patient satisfaction.

Topical agents shown to be effective for wound healing include the growth factors that are now commercially available. Two types have been approved by the Food and Drug Administration (FDA). These include Regranex (Ortho-McNeil Pharmaceutical, Inc., Raritan, NJ) and Procuren (Curative Health Services, Inc., Hauppauge, NY). Procuren is only available at specific wound care centers run by the individuals who prepare Procuren from the patient's own blood. Growth factors are separated and amplified from a blood sample. The process is extremely expensive. Regranex is recombinant platelet-derived growth factor. Both of these are discussed in more detail in Chapter 17. Topical antiseptics and antibiotics are not recommended due to cytotoxicity. The American Diabetes Association (ADA) instead recommends oral or parenteral antibiotics. Chemical debriders are not recommended by the ADA due to the risk of infection in these wounds. Sharp debridement down to healthy tissue is recommended instead.

PROTECTION OF SURROUNDING SKIN

In addition to glycemic control and off-loading of the foot, protection of the skin is vitally important. Compromise of skin integrity in a foot with diminished immunity and possibly necrotic tissue represents a tremendous risk for infection and movement toward limb amputation. Management of drainage needs to be considered carefully. The presence of moisture on surrounding skin is likely to cause maceration and cracking of the skin, providing a portal for infection. In addition, excessive dryness of skin can cause cracking. Cracking can be prevented by moisturizing the skin of the foot other than the web spaces. Web spaces tend to accumulate moisture. Use of cotton batting or lamb's wool between toes will wick moisture away from the web spaces to protect this area.

WOUND MANAGEMENT BY WAGNER GRADE

A grade 0 ulcer has intact skin and must be protected by off-loading the foot by total contact casting or other methods described below, including orthotics or special shoes. The foot needs to be inspected for the presence of subcutaneous necrosis and potential breach of the skin. An analogy to a volcano is often drawn. Subcutaneous necrosis below intact skin frequently produces a greenish hue to a circumscribed region beneath at-risk skin. Management of grade 1 and 2 ulcers includes local wound care as described later, management of edema, protection from maceration, and protection of the foot by total contact casting or another method. Total contact casting (described on page 85) both off-loads and controls edema. The control of edema, however, presents two serious challenges to clinicians: resolution of edema may compromise the fit of the total contact cast, causing damage to the skin under the cast; on the other hand, increased swelling within the cast may cause severe ischemic injury. Patients must be taught to monitor the cast carefully and seek immediate care if swelling causes vascular compromise within the cast. They must return for recasting if it becomes too loose.

Grade 3 ulcers require referral to an orthopedic surgeon who may perform resection of bone or bony prominence, and incision and drainage of the abscess or bone with osteomyelitis. The surgeon may decide that selective removal of foot bones may be required to rid the foot of infection. If an incision and drainage approach is taken, the incision and drainage wound used to gain access to the interior of the foot requires packing the open wound to prevent filling with granulation tissue. Instead, the surgeon will repair the incision with tertiary (delayed primary) closure. Therefore, generation of granulation tissue will increase the size of the foot and may exacerbate any deformities. Oral or parenteral antibiotics, not topical, are recommended by the ADA. Total contact casting is contraindicated for Wagner grades 3 to 5. Wounds should be cleaned by sharp debridement and selective cleansing, such as pulsatile lavage with concurrent suction rather than whirlpools and wet-to-dry dressings.

Grades 4 and 5 neuropathic feet with dry gangrene require referral to a vascular surgeon with possible revascularization or amputation of the limb.

AMERICAN DIABETES ASSOCIATION CLINICAL PRACTICE RECOMMENDATIONS

Every year, the ADA publishes clinical practice recommendations in its journal *Diabetes Care* and also makes this information available on its website (*www. diabetes.org*). According to the ADA, the first step is to identify risk factors for foot ulcers/amputations. The most important risk factors include having diabetes mellitus for more than 10 years; being male; poor glucose control; the presence of cardiovascular, retinal, or renal complications; peripheral vascular disease; and a history of ulcers or amputation. In addition, several direct foot-related risk factors for amputation have also been identified: peripheral neuropathy; altered biomechanics; evidence of increased pressure manifested as callus, erythema, hemorrhage under a callus; limited joint mobility; bony deformity; or severe nail pathology (Table 8-3).

The ADA recommends an annual foot examination for all individuals with diabetes mellitus to identify risk conditions, including assessment of protective sensation, foot structure, biomechanics, vascular status, and skin integrity. Based on the results of the yearly foot examination, more attention should be paid to certain individuals. Those identified with one or more risk factors should be evaluated more frequently for development of additional risk factors. Secondly, people with neuropathy are recommended to have visual inspection of their feet at every visit to their regular health care providers. Elements of a foot examination of a person with low risk are listed in Table 8-4.

SENSORY TESTING ON THE FOOT

In addition to other tools used to determine sensory integrity, diabetic foot screening commonly uses Semmes-Weinstein monofilaments to assess risk of plantar ulceration in ambulatory, sensory-impaired individuals. These special monofilaments are designed to bend at a calibrated force. Starting with the thinnest monofilament in the set, each monofilament is touched to skin for a total of 1.5 seconds: bending for half a second, left bent for half a second, and removed for half a second (Figures 8-4a through 8-4e). A person with normal sensation should feel a 10-g monofilament bend. Excessive callus on the foot will, however, decrease the sensitivity of even normal feet. Once a person is able to feel a given monofilament, the clinician stops and records the value. In some cases, a clinician may wish to perform a more thorough test and actually map the entire foot. For a screening procedure, a sin-

Table 8-3

ADA RISK FACTORS FOR FOOT ULCERATION AND AMPUTATION

1. Diabetes mellitus for more than 10 years
2. Male
3. Poor glucose control
4. Presence of cardiovascular, retinal, or renal complications
5. Peripheral vascular disease
6. History of ulcers or amputation
7. Peripheral neuropathy
8. Altered biomechanics
9. Evidence of increased pressure manifested as callus, erythema, and hemorrhage under a callus
10. Limited joint mobility
11. Bony deformity
12. Severe nail pathology

Table 8-4

ELEMENTS OF FOOT EXAMINATION FOR A LOW-RISK PERSON WITH DIABETES MELLITUS

1. Use of Semmes-Weinstein monofilament or vibration to detect loss of protective sensation
2. Taking a history for claudication or examination for pedal pulses
3. Examination of skin integrity, expecially between toes and under metatarsal heads
4. Examination for erythema, warmth, and callus on soles of feet
5. Examination for bony deformities of the foot
6. Evaluation for limited joint mobility
7. Evaluation of gait and balance

gle 10-g monofilament may be used for a prescribed number of standardized sites. In addition, the clinician should check the foot for deformities and decreased strength, which may alter weightbearing pattern and gait, and visually inspect the skin on each foot. Further sensory testing should be done to distinguish between small and large sensory neuron loss. Reflexes and vibrations are carried by large neurons. Loss of these functions indicates a greater degree of neuropathy because loss of neurons generally occurs first in small neurons, progressing to large neurons. Sensations such as temperature and pinprick are carried by smaller, more susceptible neurons. Loss of large neurons is particularly critical. Motor neurons and position sense are carried by large neurons. Loss of the position senses, proprioception, and kinesthesia are likely to exacerbate the problems caused by sensory neuropathy. A typical gait for a person with diminished proprioception includes short, slapping steps and abnormal progression from heel-strike to toe-off.

Limited range of motion of the foot and ankle are particularly devastating. A normal foot relaxes and splays to absorb shock as contact is made with the floor. As weight moves from the hind foot to the forefoot, the foot becomes more rigid to allow transfer of force to propel the body forward. Limited range of motion not only causes more energy to enter the plantar surface of the foot as the rigid foot hits the floor, but limited dorsiflexion and first toe extension limit the ability to transfer pressure from the metatarsal head region to the toes.[6] This, in turn, creates a shearing force on the metatarsal heads, especially the first. As a minimum, these biomechanical abnormalities need to be addressed with appropriate footwear from an orthotist or pedorthist.

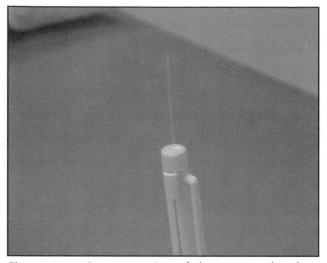

Figure 8-4a. Sensory testing of the neuropathic foot using a 10 g monofilament. This figure shows a typical monofilament used for testing.

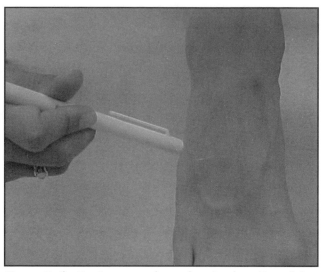

Figure 8-4b. Testing procedure, showing bending of the monofilament on the dorsal foot testing location.

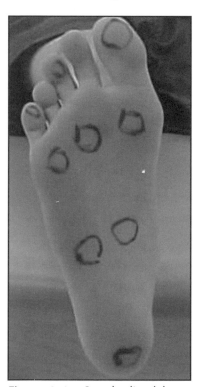

Figure 8-4c. Standardized locations drawn on the plantar surface of the foot.

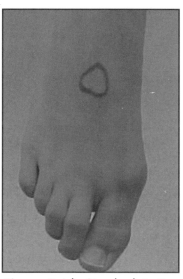

Figure 8-4d. Standard testing location on the dorsum of the foot.

Prevention of high-risk conditions is also recommended. Those at high risk include individuals with distal symmetric polyneuropathy and autonomic neuropathy. Two major recommendations for these individuals are tight control of blood glucose and smoking cessation. In addition, specific recommendations for management include wearing well-cushioned walking or athletic shoes, education on implications of sensory loss and self-monitoring, footwear to distribute pressure if signs of high pressure are evident, debridement of callus to decrease pressure caused by walking on the relatively nondeformable callus, and a vascular evaluation if claudication is determined by history or an exercise test. Extra wide or deep shoes are recommended if bony deformities such as hammer toes (Figure 8-5) and bunions are present. Referral to a qualified pedor-

Footwear must be checked for proper size and construction. Shoes assembled with nails must be discarded; rubberized or crepe soles are more practical than hard, leather soles because of their ability to dissipate mechanical stresses on the foot. A tracing of the bare foot should be made and compared to the shoe. An orthotist or pedorthist can select a shoe with an appropriately shaped last to match the shape of the patient's foot.

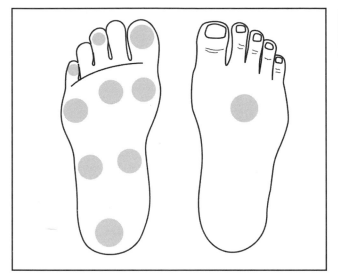

Figure 8-4e. Testing locations for the plantar foot on the left and dorsal foot on the right.

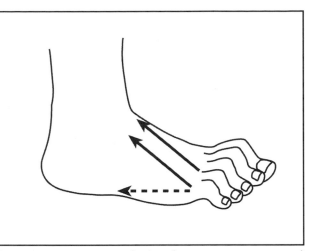

Figure 8-5. Forces producing hammer toes—normal strength of the long extensors of the toes combined with weakness of the intrinsic toe flexors.

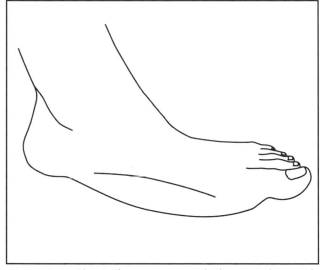

Figure 8-6. Classical appearance of Charcot's foot with boat-shaped plantar surface.

thist or orthotist for custom-molded shoes should be done if severe deformities, including Charcot's foot (Figure 8-6), are present (Charcot's foot is described further in the next section). Individuals with milder foot deformities may need to perform foot tracing before buying shoes to make a comparison of the shape of the foot to the last of the prospective shoe (Figures 8-7a and 8-7b). Screening for pressure points on the foot may be performed with a foot imprinter. This device consists of an inked mat with a grid system on the underside. Pressure on the imprinter mat causes the inked grid to contact the paper below. The grid system is designed such that low pressures only create a wide grid on the paper, whereas higher pressure creates finer grid lines. Note the high pressures under the first metatarsal head in Figures 8-8a through 8-8h. More

sophisticated means of pressure mapping are available but are quite expensive.

Patient education efforts need to be directed at risk factors and appropriate management, implications of loss of protective sensation, self-monitoring for changes in the foot, foot and nail care, selection of appropriate footwear, and smoking cessation. Learning ability should be assessed individually and the program should be tailored to the patient's preferred learning style. Excellent videotapes are available from the National Hansen's Disease Programs in Baton Rouge, La. These tapes are available to be copied and returned to the center so that clinicians can provide patient education. Certain segments are available in both English and Spanish. Some very useful demonstrations for important interventions are also available on the videotape.

CHARCOT'S FOOT

A particularly devastating complication of neuropathy is the complex of sensory, motor, and autonomic changes that lead to structural and vascular changes known as Charcot's foot. An acutely swollen foot with no significant radiographic changes may represent the early stage of Charcot's foot, requiring careful observation, rest, elevation, immobilization, and referral to a specialist who is experienced in treating Charcot's foot. Charcot's foot is most common with diabetes mellitus but may occur with other diseases. Up to 13% of those seen in high-risk diabetes mellitus clinics have this condition. In general, Charcot arthropathy refers to skeletal damage secondary to neuropathy and may be defined as neuropathic osteoarthropathy. In the diabetic foot, the term Charcot's foot is used to describe a progressive condition of multiple osteoarthropathy characterized by joint dislocation,

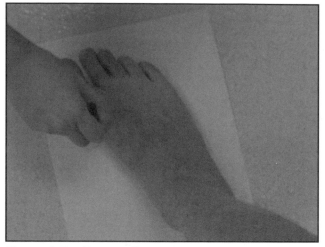

Figure 8-7a. Foot outline to compare to prospective shoes. This figure shows tracing of the foot.

Figure 8-7b. The completed tracing of the foot. This tracing is cut from the sheet of paper and placed inside shoes to determine if the shape of the shoe is suitable.

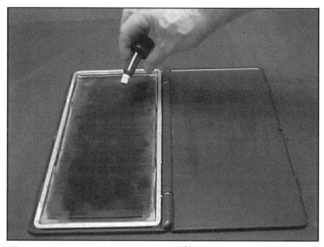

Figure 8-8a. Foot imprinter. A low-cost screening tool for rapid determination of excess forces on the foot. This figure shows that the grid on the underside of the rubber mat is inked.

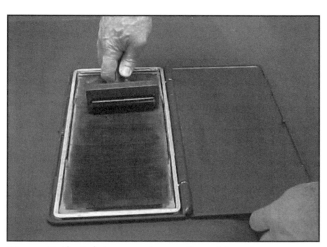

Figure 8-8b. Ink is spread over the grid surface.

pathologic fractures, and deformities. The most common deformity is a boat-shaped foot in which the concavity of the arch of the foot is not only lost, but the bottom of the foot becomes convex (see Figure 8-6). The toes frequently lose contact with the support surface of the foot, and tremendous shear forces are exerted at the metatarsal heads. Pathological fractures of the diabetic foot and deformities must be considered high-risk factors.

Charcot arthropathy was named for a prominent French neurologist and was first described as a consequence of syphilis. It was originally believed to be due to lack of sensation and accumulated trauma, but was later shown to have a neurovascular component. This includes an increased blood flow due to denervation accompanied by demineralization of the bones of the foot. Osteopenia combined with the loss of sensation leads to fractures of the foot. Moreover, motor denervation and resultant muscle imbalance lead to a very high risk of ulceration of the plantar surface as well as dorsal surfaces of hammer toes.

Diagnosis of Charcot's Foot

Unilateral swelling, elevated temperature, and erythema are early signs of Charcot's foot development. These events are associated with the increased blood flow caused by denervation of blood vessels of the lower extremities. Further examination may reveal joint effusion, bone resorption by imaging techniques, an insensate foot, and usually some degree of pain. Approximately 40% of those with Charcot's foot have already experienced ulceration. Because of the swelling, heat, erythema, and pain of Charcot arthropathy, this condition may be confused with osteomyelitis. Differential diagnosis can be performed with a bone scan, blood work (especially white blood cell count), and bone biopsy.

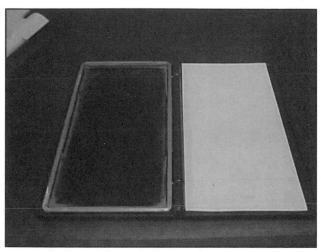

Figure 8-8c. Paper is placed in the tray located under the rubber grid.

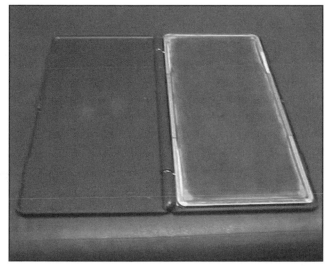

Figure 8-8d. The rubber grid is rotated into its tray with the smooth side up and inked, grid side down.

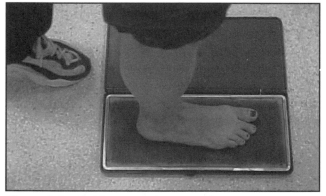

Figure 8-8e. Subject stepping onto the mat.

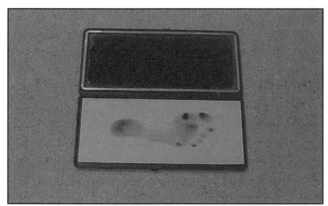

Figure 8-8f. High-pressure areas are indicated by more densely marked portions of paper. Higher pressures are necessary for the progressively closer portions of the grid to come in contact with the paper below it. Note high pressures on the head of the first metatarsal and proximal, lateral portion of the first toe.

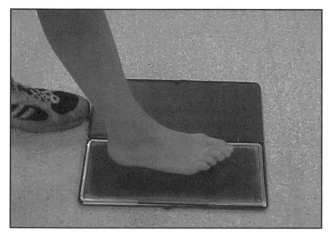

Figure 8-8g. Second subject stepping on the mat.

For convenience of discussion, Charcot's foot has been described as having four stages. The first stage is characterized by a hot, red, swollen foot with bounding pulses. During stage 1, resorption of bone produces severe osteopenia. For diagnosis, an increase of 2°C is considered necessary. During the second stage, dissolution, fragmentation, and fracture of bone occurs as osteopenia weakens bones too much to support the biomechanics of the foot. A patient is considered to be in stage 3 with development of a rocker bottom foot deformity. Stage 4 consists of plantar ulceration with possible progression to infection, gangrene, and amputation. Interventions to prevent progression of Charcot's foot during stage 1 are nonweight-bearing of the affected extremity and, if appropriate, the use of total contact casting until skin temperature is normal. If the disease progresses to stage 3, the patient will need molded shoes or special Charcot shoes with molded inserts and possible surgery to repair deformities to prevent progression to stage 4. Unfortunately, the process may progress to stage 4, and damage to the foot may become so severe as to require amputation.

Another classification of Charcot arthropathy is based on radiographic, thermometric, and clinical signs into either the acute phase or postacute phase. Acute Charcot arthropathy may be treated with immobilization and reduction of stress, including decreased weightbearing with crutches. Unfortunately, unloading one foot overloads the contralateral foot. With the likelihood of bilateral disease, the other foot is placed at greater risk of fracture. Other options that do not overload the contralateral extremity include using a total contact cast for 5 to 6 months, arthrodesis, open reduction, and internal fixation of the fractures.

Long-term solutions can be instituted during the postacute phase. The classification of the postacute phase may be given after temperature of the affected foot is within 1°C of the contralateral foot. At this time, the patient may be fitted for orthotic shoes using a removable cast walker until a custom shoe is ready. In about 25% of cases, reconstructive foot surgery is performed.

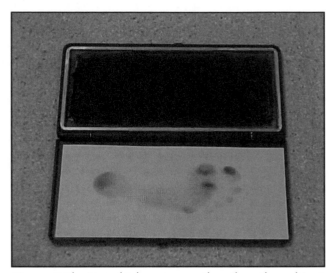

Figure 8-8h. Note high pressures (less than the subject in Figure 8-8f) under the first and second metatarsal heads and first toe.

AMERICAN DIABETES ASSOCIATION POSITION STATEMENT ON FOOT CARE

This position statement addresses management of neuropathic foot ulcers in an attempt to publicize what the ADA believes to be optimal care.[7] Also, the predisposing factors and possible complications relevant to diabetes mellitus should be taken into account rather than simply addressing the open wound. The first priority of the clinician should be determining the ulcer's etiology. Once known, the interventions directed toward cause of the ulcer can be addressed, as well as prevention of further ulcers and potential complications that might delay healing. Next, the ulcer's size, depth, and involvement of deep structures should be established. The clinician should examine the wound for purulent exudate, necrosis, sinus tracts, and odor. The surrounding skin should then be assessed for signs of edema, cellulitis, abscess, and fluctuation as well as ruling out systemic infection. The ADA also states that the physical exam should include a vascular exam. The ability to gently probe through the ulcer to bone highly predicts osteomyelitis. A radiological exam should be done by the physician to exclude subcutaneous gas, presence of foreign body, osteomyelitis, and Charcot's foot. Distinguishing between Charcot's foot and osteomyelitis may be difficult in some cases. According to the ADA's position statement, plain radiographs showing periosteal resorption and osteolysis are consistent with, but not diagnostic of, osteomyelitis. Rather, a bone scan, white blood cell count imaging, magnetic resonance imaging, or bone biopsy may be necessary to distinguish between osteomyelitis and Charcot's foot.

Bacterial cultures and antibiotics are also addressed in the position statement. Because bacterial infections of foot lesions tend to be polymicrobial, broad-spectrum antibiotics should be used immediately but should be modified based on culture results and patient response to treatment. As discussed more thoroughly in Chapter 18, swab cultures are not sufficient for management decisions. Deep specimens obtained by curettage at the base of the wound should be used instead. In terms of debridement of neuropathic ulcers, the ADA's position is that abscessed infections should be incised and drained with debridement down to viable tissue. The ADA does not specifically endorse the use of topical agents. Rather, it states that the use of topical agents is controversial and no adequate evidence exists for their use. Contrary to popular practice of soaking ulcers, the ADA states specifically that prolonged immersion of feet in water is not recommended.

With regard to mechanical stress, the ADA recommends minimizing weightbearing on ulcers by bedrest, or when ambulatory, by crutches. Also recommended is heel and ankle protection and daily inspection of both lower extremities. Other suggested protection includes the use of total contact casts for protecting healing ulcers, and either shoe inserts or special shoes for those with foot deformities. Candidates for vascular reconstruction include those with slow or inadequate healing, decreased pulses, and decreased pressure by Doppler exam and avoiding vasoconstrictor drugs.

Metabolic control is probably the greatest predictor of long-term health in persons with diabetes mellitus and perhaps even more so in individuals with neuropathic ulcers. Open wounds can make management of blood sugar more complex. Infection and inflammation can cause wide fluctuations in blood sugar. Surgical or medical treat-

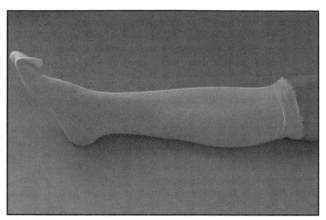

Figure 8-9a. Total contact casting. Stockinette applied from the knee, beyond the toes, and folded onto the dorsal surface.

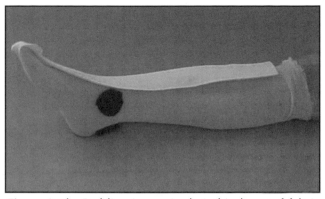

Figure 8-9b. Padding is required. A thin layer of felt is placed over the crest of the tibia, and foam is placed over both malleoli and the insertion of the heel cord.

ment of the neuropathic ulcer can help control blood sugar. Moreover, poor glucose control hinders healing, and overall nutritional status should be monitored by an appropriate clinician.

Post-healing management needs to continue to address potential complications. Anyone with neuropathic ulcers is at high risk of future ulceration and requires an education program that emphasizes daily inspection, possible job modification, prescribed footwear, walking or athletic shoes, soft insoles, extra-depth shoes, custom-molded inlays, and custom-molded therapeutic shoes.

OFF-LOADING TECHNIQUES

Removing the causes of neuropathic wounds is not practical. The optimal outcome is to alleviate the mechanical forces causing the wounds on a temporary basis in order to allow healing. Following healing, more definitive measures can be undertaken to minimize future ulceration. The two most important aspects are patient education and adherence to the plan of care. To prevent lower extremity amputation, the clinician must evaluate the patient's understanding of the plan of care and willingness to adhere to the plan. Based on this information, the clinician can select the most appropriate off-loading techniques. The available techniques differ in the clinician's skill level in applying them, the perceived adherence of the patient, and the patient's or caregiver's skill level to follow up at home. Techniques discussed below include total contact casting, walking splints, the Charcot restraint orthotic walker (CROW), DH pressure relief walker, healing sandal, and OrthoWedge healing shoe.[8,9]

Total Contact Casting

This technique was developed primarily in Carville, La at the National Hansen's Disease Programs. Total contact casting is used for diabetes mellitus and other chronic sensory neuropathies, such as Hansen's disease (leprosy). This technique is based on the concept of protecting the foot against repetitive stress on insensate feet. Total contact casting is the preferred method of temporary off-loading of the foot for Wagner grades 0, 1, and 2 provided no contraindications exist. Contraindications include grades 3 to 5 wounds, fragile skin, and poor adherence to the care of the total contact cast. Poor adherence and failure to follow up as directed may cost the patient's limb or worse.

Total contact casting reduces excessive plantar pressure by redistributing pressure and immobilizing the foot and ankle to correct biomechanical problems and minimize shearing. The cast also controls edema and protects the foot from trauma. Statistically, healing occurs 73% to 100% of the time over 37 to 65 days, with an average of 43 days. In addition, those who have used total contact casting for neuropathic ulcers experience fewer hospitalizations for infection or amputation. However, total contact casting does have the potential for some problems. One study reported that 43% of those using total contact cast reported minor complications. Those listed included abrasions from suboptimal fit and fungal infections treated topically. Other possible risks include undetected osteomyelitis or deep infection, sepsis, amputation, or death. However, these complications can be minimized by careful application and frequent follow-up.[10]

Total contact casts are constructed of plaster bandages used for other types of orthopedic casts (Figures 8-9a through 8-9f). One significant difference is in the amount of padding used. In a total contact cast, a minimum of padding is used. First, the web spaces are protected by cotton batting or lamb's wool. A length of stockinette is applied to the leg and foot. The distal end of the stockinette is brought to the top of toes to prevent pressure on toes caused by a seam in the stockinette. The proximal end should extend to the knee. Padding is placed over the malleoli, around the toes, and along the crest of the tibia.

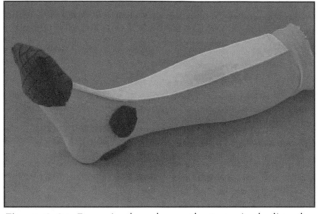

Figure 8-9c. Foam is placed over the toes, including the metatarsals, with beveling of the edge under the metatarsal head to improve foot biomechanics.

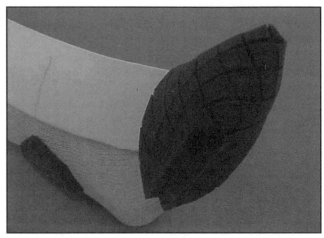

Figure 8-9d. Close-up view of foam over the forefoot.

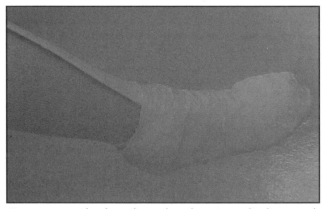

Figure 8-9e. The first plaster bandage is applied. Several turns around the ankle are necessary to maintain rigidity.

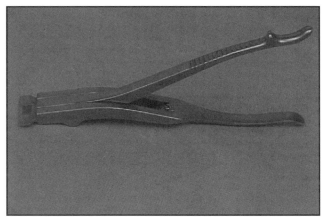

Figure 8-9f. Cast spreaders used to remove a cast.

Quick-set plaster bandage is applied distally to cover the toes and applied with overlapping spirals proximally up the leg. Typically two to three plaster bandages are needed to cover a leg. The surface of the plaster is smoothed with water as the bandages dry. Extra care is needed to reinforce the cast at the ankle. The cast is only allowed to come to about a finger's width below the head of the fibula. A shorter cast is more susceptible to torque, and a longer cast will interfere with knee range of motion. The cast should end about one inch below the head of the fibula to avoid damage to the peroneal nerve. The cast may then be reinforced by a layer of fiberglass casting tape. The use of layered plaster allows visualization of drainage from the wound into the cast. Fiberglass improves the durability of the cast but compromises visualization of drainage. The fiberglass roll must be wet with cold water and applied quickly to prevent premature hardening.

The initial cast is generally worn for 1 week, and subsequent casts are worn up to 2 weeks. The clinician must be confident in the patient's ability to follow directions and monitor the fit of the cast, and seek emergency care for the cast when needed. Some individuals place a rubber heel on the cast to allow ambulation. Others fit the patient for a postoperative sandal to wear on the bottom of the cast to protect it. Casts may be worn in the shower if care is taken to protect them from water. A plastic trash bag can be secured over the cast and towels may be wrapped over the top of the cast and attached with rubber bands to absorb any leakage into the plastic bag.

Walking Splint

An alternative to total contact casting is the walking splint. It is similar to a cast but made of more durable materials and is cut along both sides to allow it to be taken off. It is secured with velcro straps or elasticized bandage rolls. Like the total contact cast, the foot and ankle are immobilized, pressure is distributed more evenly on the plantar surface, and edema is prevented. A walking cast has the advantage of allowing frequent inspection of the foot, but the disadvantage is that the patient may fail to wear the device. With this device and the next two described below, off-loading of an infected ulcer may be performed. Because of the inability to monitor the wound, infection is an absolute contraindication for total contact casting.

Charcot Restraint Orthotic Walker

The CROW has features in common with the walking splint. The orthosis is a rigid polypropylene boot walker with a rocker sole. The anterior half of the shell is removable with velcro straps and shares the advantages and disadvantages of the walking splint. The device is not custom-made and, as such, may allow more movement and provide less edema control than a total contact cast or walking splint, both of which are customized. The rocker sole built into the orthosis allows pressure and shearing forces to be minimized. A custom-molded insert is used to accommodate the shape of the foot.

DH Pressure Relief Walker

Similar to the CROW, the DH pressure relief walker is an extended foot-ankle orthosis, covering the leg to just below the head of the fibula. It is similar to the boots used for lower extremity fractures and features a rocker sole bottom and customizable insole. The insole consists of an array of hexagonal plugs attached with velcro. Individual plugs are easily removed and can be reconfigured as needed to determine the optimal pressure relief for the patient's foot. The advantages and disadvantages are similar to the CROW and walking splint, with the exception of edema control. The DH pressure relief walker is not rigid and may allow swelling to occur. The convenience of pressure relief without custom molding may be considered an advantage but is also a disadvantage because the insole will not conform carefully to the plantar surface of the foot. One published study, however, indicates that this orthosis is as effective as total contact casting for reducing forefoot pressure.[11]

OrthoWedge Healing Shoe

The OrthoWedge healing shoe, as the name implies, has a wedge-shaped sole, providing 10 degrees of dorsiflexion and suspends the forefoot, as the wedged bottom part of the sole extends only to the metatarsal head. The design limits motion of the ankle and foot, similar to the orthoses described above, but removes weightbearing nearly completely from the forefoot. The patient will also ambulate with a shorter stride, similar to the other orthoses described. Because the device only covers the foot, edema control is not provided. The orthosis is readily removed for inspection of the foot and, of course, can be left off by the patient. An awkward gait may lead to noncompliance by some patients.

Healing Sandal

Another device to assist in healing of neuropathic ulcers that is less invasive but probably less effective and, therefore, recommended for individuals at lower risk of not healing is the healing (cut-out) sandal. A sandal is molded to the shape of the foot with thermoplastic with a relief area cut into the sandal. The bottom of the foot requiring relief is marked with ink, betadine, benzoin, or other suitable marking substance and the individual is asked to stand on the thermoplastic material. The inked thermoplastic is cut out. This process may require several trials to create the proper shape. When the material is cut out properly, the thermoplastic is cemented to an orthopedic sandal. These sandals may, however, cause pressure around the ulcer. Use of this option necessitates meticulous callus removal. Callus formation on the edges of the cutout may generate unacceptable pressure around the wound. A similar procedure can be performed with either felt or foam padding cut to fit around the ulcer to relieve pressure on the site. Like the walking splint, the healing sandal has the disadvantage that the patient may choose to walk without the device. Other disadvantages are the lack of ankle immobilization and edema control. Only total contact casting guarantees that the patient will wear the device at all times during ambulation. Of particular concern is that the patient will remove an orthosis when retiring for the night and if getting up in the middle of the night, will ambulate at what he or she can rationalize as an insignificant distance.

SHOES

Following complete healing of the wound, definitive treatment to minimize risk of recurrence or new ulcerations is to fit the patient for appropriate shoes. The risk of recurrence of plantar ulcers has been reported to be 26% for those wearing special shoes, compared with 83% who wore their own shoes. Either off-the-shelf or custom shoes may be needed for long-term use. Custom-fit shoes designed for the individual require a mold of the foot, analysis of normal and abnormal forces on the foot, and modifications to relieve abnormal pressures. A patient may be referred to an orthotist or pedorthist for proper fitting or molding of custom shoes. In the case of lost range of motion of the foot or fixed deformities, a steel shank rocker bottom can be used to off-load the metatarsal heads. Constructed properly, special shoes can off-load a foot to nearly normal amounts of pressure and shear. Medicare Part B will supply a maximum of one pair of custom shoes per year. The patient must use the shoes prudently. Some have advocated that the patient purchase a new pair every year and rotate through different shoes. If this strategy is undertaken, the clinician must ensure that the older shoes are still effectively off-loading the foot.

WALKING PATTERNS

A number of ambulation strategies have been proposed to reduce peak plantar pressure. Shortening and slowing step length has been shown to reduce pressure, presumably by decreasing push-off forces. Mueller has proposed what he terms a "hip strategy" to reduce plantar pressure.[12] In this strategy, ground-reaction forces are reduced by using hip flexion to advance the swinging extremity, rather than plantar flexion and strong toe-off of the fixed extremity. The patient is also instructed to shorten step length but not walking speed. Another proposed strategy is the step-to gait pattern. By decreasing the length of the step on the uninvolved extremity by stepping to the involved foot, forefoot pressure is reduced by 53%. Many patients naturally adopt these walking strategies when placed in off-loading footwear. Just as compliance is an issue with footwear, it is even more critical if gait pattern is the major preventative strategy. In particular, patients may not wish to be seen ambulating in public with an unusual gait pattern.

ULCER RECURRENCE AND FAILURE TO HEAL

By definition, the term *ulcer recurrence* can apply after 6 months of closure. Recurrence has been shown to happen in 34%, 61%, and 70% of cases after 1, 2, and 3 years respectively. Recurrence after total contact casting has been reported to be between 32% and 57%. Failure to heal is reported to occur in 10% to 22% of cases. Reasons reported for failure to heal include undiagnosed infection and failure of the patient to adhere to the treatment plan. Failure to heal is also reported to be correlated with presence and degree of autonomic neuropathy.

Total contact casting is reported to be cost-effective. A typical 8-week course of treatment includes six to eight casts, costing in the range of $810 to $1050. On the other hand, a short stay in an acute care hospital (3 to 5 days) costs more than $2000, not including physician fees, diagnostic work-ups, and procedures or medications. Other options are less costly than total contact casting and are suitable alternatives for patients who can be trusted to use the orthoses as instructed.[13]

DIABETIC NEUROPATHY

Diabetic polyneuropathy has a prevalence of 7.5% in newly diagnosed diabetes mellitus, which increases with the duration of diabetes mellitus. Diabetic polyneuropathy is estimated to be present in 50% of individuals after 25 years of diabetes mellitus with an overall 30% prevalence, which is similar in types 1 and 2. This condition is manifested in more than one way, and one person may have two or more types of peripheral neuropathy at once. The types are classified by their anatomical distribution into diffuse neuropathy and focal neuropathy. Diffuse neuropathy may present as distal symmetric sensorimotor polyneuropathy, autonomic neuropathy, or symmetric proximal lower limb motor neuropathy. Focal neuropathy may be superimposed on diffuse neuropathy and present as a complex clinical picture of one or more very specific neurological deficits with no systematic anatomical basis, autonomical dysfunction, and homogenous distal neurological deficits.

Distal symmetric polyneuropathy is the most common type of neuropathy seen with diabetes mellitus. Its distal nature is based strictly on probability; the longer the neuron, the more likely it is to be affected. Because this form of peripheral neuropathy is based on neuron length, its risk is increased with height. Both small- and large-diameter neurons are involved. However, the earliest manifestations occur in small-diameter neurons, leading first to loss of normal pain and temperature sensation. Derangement of nociceptive neurons frequently leads to neuropathic pain, which may be described as burning, sharp, shooting, or deep aching. As the neuropathy advances, signs and symptoms of large neuron involvement become evident. These include the loss of vibratory sensation and proprioception, and absent or reduced deep tendon reflexes, especially the ankle jerk and slow nerve conduction velocity in advanced disease. Numbness, tingling, and a sensation of tightness may also be reported in advanced disease. Because motor neurons are the largest type by diameter, motor symptoms occur later and distally. The loss of strength of distal lower extremity muscles leads to deformities of the foot, altered biomechanics, and high risk of ulceration.

Autonomic neuropathy is present in 40% of individuals with type 2 diabetes mellitus at the time of diagnosis. Typical manifestations of autonomic neuropathy include sexual dysfunction, gastroparesis (diminished motility of the stomach and gastrointestinal tract), diabetic diarrhea, bladder atony, loss of sweating in the feet, and cardiovascular abnormalities such as postural hypotension, loss of normal heart rate variability, and arrhythmias leading to sudden death. The pathophysiology of peripheral neuropathy includes damage caused by sorbitol accumulation, ischemia of neurons due to atherosclerosis, and diminished expression of nerve growth factor. Excessive blood glucose is converted to sorbitol, which, in turn, accumulates in tissues. Sorbitol accumulation causes decreased production of myoinositol and taurine, which leads to decreased Na/K ATPase and slowed nerve conduction velocity. Researchers have attempted to correct nerve injury secondary to sorbitol accumulation with aldose reductase inhibitors, but have yet to be successful in restoring neuronal function.

Pharmacological Treatment of Neuropathic Pain

Neuropathic pain can be severe and debilitating. It is frequently cited by patients/clients as a reason for not participating in exercise programs. Complaints of sudden burning, shooting pains (dysesthesia), and pins and needles (paresthesia) are common. Patients/clients often report a greater intensity and frequency of neuropathic pain in affected limbs during weightbearing and exercise. Recently, however, several drugs have been shown to be very effective to certain individuals in reducing neuropathic pain. These include tricyclic antidepressants such as amitryptyline; the anticonvulsant drug gabapentin, which stimulates inhibitory central neurons; and capsaicin, which is used as a topical analgesic for arthritis and musculoskeletal pain. Capsaicin, the active ingredient of chili peppers, is believed to work by depletion of substance P, thereby preventing the transmission of pain information to the spinal cord.

Summary

Neuropathic ulcers are formed by a chain of events including loss of sensory, motor, and autonomic innervation of the foot, leading to loss of protective sensation, altered biomechanics of the foot, and dryness of the foot. Foot screening is performed at regular intervals and more frequently in patients with established high risk. The Wagner scale evaluates a series of progressively worse conditions, rather than a continuum of wound severity. The Wagner scale begins with neuropathic ulcers but continues into the realm of arterial insufficiency. A noninfected foot without arterial insufficiency needs to be protected from further injury by off-loading, including total contact casting. Total contact casting may not be appropriate for all individuals. Infection (stage 3) needs to be cleared before casting. Stages 4 and 5 require referral and further evaluation by a vascular surgeon. Other options for off-loading are less effective but allow better inspection of the affected foot.

Study Questions

1. Trace the sequence of events leading to lower extremity amputation.
2. Distinguish between diabetic ulcers caused by arterial insufficiency and by mechanical forces on the foot.
3. Discuss the roles of motor and autonomic neuropathy in causing neuropathic ulcers.
4. What is the basis for the Wagner scale? Does it represent increased severity of a given condition?
5. What is the value of testing for pain, vibration, reflexes, and muscle strength in the diabetic foot?
6. Why is bedrest frequently a poor option for off-loading a diabetic foot?
7. Describe indications for different types of off-loading devices for aiding neuropathic ulcer healing.

References

1. Nelson RG, Gohdes DM, Everhart JE, et al. Lower extremity amputations in NIDDM: 12-year follow-up study in Pima Indians. *Diabetes Care.* 1988;11:8-16.
2. Pecoraro RE, Reiber GE, Burgess EM. Pathways to diabetic limb amputation. Basis for prevention. *Diabetes Care.* 1990;13:513-521.
3. Bureau of Primary Health Care. LEAP program. Available at: http://www.bphc.hrsa.dhhs.gov/leap/. Accessed 2001.
4. Young MJ, Cavanaugh PR, Thomas G, et al. The effect of callus removal on dynamic plantar foot pressures in diabetic patients. *Diabetes Med.* 1992;9:55-57.
5. Edmonds ME, Blundell MP, Morris ME, et al. Improved survival of the diabetic foot: the role of a specialized foot clinic. *Q J Med.* 1986;232:763-771.
6. Sims DS, Cavanaugh PR, Ulbrecht JS. Risk factors in the diabetic foot. Recognition and management. *Phys Ther.* 1988;68:1887-1902.
7. American Diabetes Association Position Statement. Preventive Foot Care in People with Diabetes. *Diabetes Care.* 2000; 25:S69-S70.
8. Cotanzariti AR, Haverstock BD, Grossman JP, Mendicino RW. Off-loading techniques in the treatment of diabetic plantar neuropathic foot ulceration. *Adv Wound Care.* 1999;12:452-458.
9. Mueller MJ. Off-loading techniques for neuropathic plantar wounds. *Advances in Wound Care.* 1999;12:270-271.
10. Sinacore DR. Total contact casting for diabetic neuropathic ulcers. *Phys Ther.* 1996;76:296-301.
11. Lavery L, Vela SA, Lavery DC, Quebedeaux TL. Reducing dynamic foot pressure in high-risk diabetic subjects with foot ulcerations. *Diabetes Care.* 1996;19:818-821.
12. Brown HE, Mueller MJ. A step-to gait pattern decreases pressures on the forefoot. *J Orthop Sports Phys Ther.* 1998;28:139-145.
13. Helm PA, Walker SC, Pulliam GF. Recurrence of neuropathic ulceration following healing in a total contact cast. *Arch Phys Med Rehab.* 1991;72:967-970.

Pressure Ulcers

9

- Describe the components of tissue loads that place a person at risk for ulcer development: pressure, shear, friction, heat, and humidity.
- Describe the physiological effects of tissue loading.
- List at-risk sites for development of pressure ulcers.
- List and discuss the relative efficacy of pressure relief/reduction devices.
- Discuss methods for off-loading body segments.
- Demonstrate use of available tools for quantifying risk.

BACKGROUND

Pressure ulcers are among the most costly preventable injuries, and as such, various agencies including the National Pressure Ulcer Advisory Panel (NPUAP)[1] and the Agency for Health Care Policy and Research (AHCPR)[2] have published materials to develop a common language and guidelines for prevention and treatment of pressure ulcers (see Appendix). The scope and mission of the AHCPR has since changed. The name was also changed to the Agency for Healthcare Research and Quality (AHRQ) to indicate these changes.

Pressure ulcers have a high prevalence and incidence in acute- and long-term care. Certain conditions are associated with a very high prevalence and incidence: quadriplegia (60% prevalence), femoral fractures (66% incidence), critical care (33% incidence, 41% prevalence), and a total cost of $1.3 billion. For 1992, a study performed for the AHCPR estimated an average of $21,000 per ulcer in hospital charges and $2900 in physician charges and additional charges by hospitals of $10,986 and $1200 in physician charges, for hip fractures due to pressure ulcers.[2]

TISSUE LOAD

Although this chapter deals with the topic of pressure ulcers, factors other than pressure are also to blame for the necrosis of tissue between a support surface and a bony prominence. The term *tissue load* is more inclusive than pressure, although the term *pressure ulcer* and its predecessor *decubitus* are unlikely to be replaced by the term *tissue load ulcer*. Tissue loading is caused by pressure, friction, and shear, and is exacerbated by moisture and temperature (Figure 9-1). In many cases, shear is more of a problem than pressure, particularly in the individual left in a head up, reclining position greater than 30 degrees. Friction and shear are related phenomena. Friction is always present when shear is present. Friction relates to the injury caused directly by moving one surface across another. The coefficient of friction determines the amount of energy transferred into a surface as another is dragged across it. Shear refers to a tangential force applied to a surface as two surfaces are moved in opposite directions. For example, friction occurs as a patient is passively moved across the surface of a sheet. Friction may then denude skin. Shear presents the same detrimental effects as friction on the skin. In addition, blood vessels are distorted, potentially causing ischemia in the sheared skin. Therefore, shear is a greater risk factor for tissue injury than friction alone. Shear commonly occurs in an individual sitting or lying in a position with the head elevated more than 30° degrees for a prolonged time.

Prevention of pressure ulcers is accomplished by managing tissue loads by decreasing pressure, friction, and shear; optimizing moisture and temperature, using proper

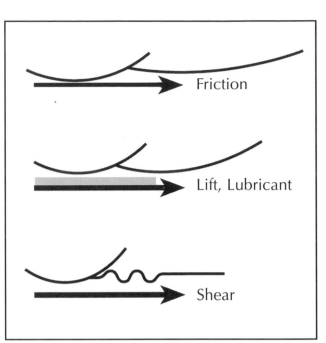

Figure 9-1. Tissue loads other than pressure, placing skin at risk.

positioning techniques; and using appropriate support surfaces. Different considerations are made for the patient in bed and the patient in a chair.

DEFINITIONS

The NPUAP defines a pressure ulcer as any lesion caused by unrelieved pressure resulting in damage of underlying tissue. These usually occur over bony prominences and are staged to classify the degree of tissue damage observed. Definitions are given for four stages of ulcers. The staging system refers to the depth of injury observed and does not necessarily correspond to an observable progression of tissue injury. In extreme cases, a wound may not be observable at all until an ulcer exposing subcutaneous tissue appears.

A stage I ulcer was initially defined as an area of a non-blanchable erythema of intact skin. This definition, however, proved inadequate for heavily pigmented skin. Recently, the definition has been expanded to include increased warmth or altered coloration of skin (redness of caucasian skin or purplish tint of more heavily pigmented skin).

A stage II pressure ulcer is defined as a partial-thickness wound involving epidermis, dermis, or both, but does not extend through the entire depth of the dermis (Figure 9-2). Once a wound does extend into subcutaneous tissue, but not through the fascia, it is classified as a stage III ulcer. Any wound that extends through the fascia and deeper is classified as stage IV. These full-thickness wounds may damage muscle, bone, ligaments, or tendons. Fascia is usually easily identifiable as a clear, smooth, shiny

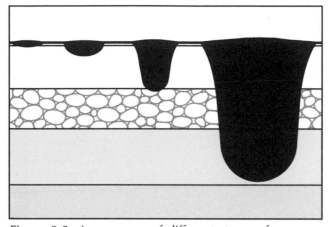

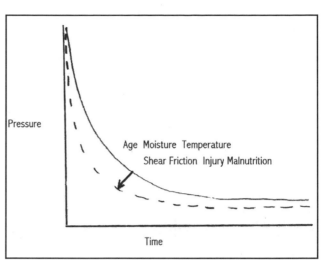

Figure 9-2. Appearance of different stages of pressure ulcers. Stage I is characterized by nonblanchable erythema, which can be difficult to distinguish in heavily pigmented skin. Stage II is characterized by ulceration of the epidermis and may extend into, but not through, the dermis. Stage III ulcers may extend through the dermis, up to but not deeper than the fascia. Stage IV ulcers extend more deeply than fascia and may involve subcutaneous tissues such as muscle, bone, tendons, and ligaments.

Figure 9-3. Theoretical effects of pressure and time on tissue viability. Note the hyperbolic relationship between time and pressure in that either a high pressure for a short time or a lower pressure for a long time may lead to tissue necrosis. Also note the theoretical shifting of the curve based on nutrition, mobility, and skin condition.

layer, making distinction of stage II versus III and III versus IV fairly simple once the base of the wound is visible. For this reason, staging of pressure ulcers should not be done before the base of the wound is visible.

Although the definitions are straightforward, some limitations need to be kept in mind. First, detection of stage I ulcers can be very difficult in darkly pigmented skin. Very careful observation needs to be performed, including detecting either an increase in temperature or a violescence (eggplant-like purple) compared with surrounding skin. When eschar is present, accurate staging is not possible. Many clinicians may be tempted to guess at the extent of an ulcer. However, good practice dictates that staging not be done until eschar has been removed. Moreover, ulcers under casts, orthotic devices, and support stockings are difficult to assess and require extra work to remove the device to examine the skin on a regular basis. The assignment of numbers to classify extent of the wound does not necessarily imply progression in ulcer severity. For example, a stage I ulcer may have very little tissue damage or it may have extensive necrosis beneath intact skin. A related problem is the insistence of certain agencies to "reverse stage" a wound as a means of documenting healing of a wound. The NPUAP has issued a position statement advising against this practice. As discussed in Chapter 2, a wound with subcutaneous involvement fills with granulation tissue and contracts; it does not fill with the same tissue that was originally in the wound. Therefore, once a wound is classified as a stage IV ulcer, it cannot be logically classified as a stage III, II, or I, because

the tissue markers on which the definitions are based do not exist. Instead, an appropriate description includes the original stage and the measurable depth of the current state of the wound. As an alternative to back staging a pressure ulcer, the National Pressure Ulcer Advisory Panel has developed the Pressure Ulcer Scale for Healing tool (PUSH tool). The tool and instructions are given at the end of this chapter. This tool allows the clinician to document progress toward healing by identifying positive changes in the pressure ulcer.

RISK FACTORS

A number of factors may be responsible for the development of pressure ulcers (Table 9-1).

Typically, a combination of lack of mobility, lack of cognition/motivation to move, and exacerbating factors of nutrition and incontinence are at fault. In particular, individuals with spinal cord injuries, diabetes mellitus, hip replacement surgery, femoral fractures, ICU patients with hypotension, and elderly patients with multiple diseases are at risk. Sites of wound development are generally located in underlying tissues between bony prominences and support surfaces, thereby developing a wound that is either round or elliptical.[3]

Although many individuals tend to dwell on the pressure aspect of risk for pressure ulcers, pressure alone does not cause ulceration; tissue necrosis is a function of both time and pressure. A graph of the combination of the two produces a hyperbolic curve, implying that the product of pressure and time is a constant (Figure 9-3). Classically,

---
Table 9-1

RISK FACTORS FOR PRESSURE ULCERS

Physical Causes of Immobility

• Altered neuromuscular integrity
  Diminished strength
  Altered muscle tone (spasticity, rigidity, dystonia, athetosis, flaccidity, etc)
• Altered musculoskeletal integrity
  Decreased range of motion
  Traumatic injury
  Muscle disease, other
• Devices (splints, casts, orthoses, restraints)

Cognitive Causes of Immobility

• Altered state of consciousness, stupor, coma
• Prolonged anesthesia
• Diminished motivation to self-reposition
• Pain

Diminished Sensation

• Spinal cord injury
• Spina bifida
• Head injuries
• Peripheral neuropathy
• Other

Excessive Moisture

• Use of moisture-resistant support surface
• Urinary incontinence

Fecal Incontinence

Emaciation

Malnutrition

Management

• Inappropriate turning/repositioning schedule
• Inappropriate support surface
• Neglect of immobility issues
• Failure to clean following episodes of incontinence
• Harsh cleaning procedures
• Failure to moisturize/protect dry skin

---

the risk has been defined as an unrelieved 70 mmHg of pressure for 2 hours to produce irreversible injury. However, a greater pressure takes less time and a lower pressure for greater than 2 hours can cause tissue necrosis. For example, a very high pressure can be developed by allowing a lower extremity to hang over a bed rail. Without relief, necrosis of tissue between a bony prominence and a bed rail can occur in less than 1 hour. Conversely, a pressure of 40 mmHg left unrelieved for several hours may produce injury.

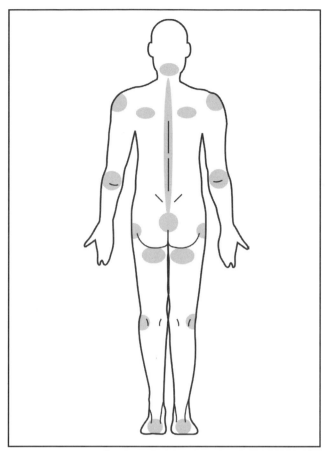

Figure 9-4. At-risk areas for skin breakdown.

Another problem is that the assumption that a pressure of 70 mmHg will develop between a support surface and a bony prominence for every individual is unrealistic. For example, the pressure at a bony prominence of an obese person may be much lower than 70 mmHg, whereas the same position for an emaciated person may be much higher than 70 mmHg. Therefore, a turning schedule should be individualized, taking into account all factors relevant to the individual: lack of weight shifting, lack of soft tissue over bony prominences, poor nutrition, excess moisture, shearing stresses, prolonged reclined sitting in either a bed or a chair, shearing skin over the sacrum, dragging the patient across sheets, wrinkles in sheets, incontinence, and the use of moisture-resistant mattresses.

At-risk areas that need particular attention include: heels, greater trochanters, sacrum, occiput, epicondyles of the elbow in the person lying in bed, the sacrum in a person reclining in either a bed or chair, and the ischial tuberosities in a person sitting erect (Figure 9-4). The occiput is easily neglected in a person with a neurologic injury. Too often necrosis of the skin over the occiput is not discovered in time to prevent injury in a person whose head is not repositioned due to risk of injury to the head or spine. For anyone with limitations of mobility, heel pro-

tection using pillows, splints, or heel lifts must be used. However, pressure ulcers can develop in a number of other locations with bony prominences including the face; vertebral processes; ribs; spine of the scapulae; acromion processes; along the iliac crests; posterior superior iliac spine; anterior superior iliac spine; the anterior, lateral, and medial surfaces of the knee; the tibial crest; malleoli; first and fifth metatarsals, and toes. Results of an ongoing survey of acute care hospitals, with most recent results reported in November 1995 show a consistent prevalence of pressure ulcers, sites of the ulcers, characteristics of the patients, and depth of the ulcers.[4] The ongoing study consistently shows the sacrum and heels to be the most common locations (36% to 39% and 19% to 30%, respectively) over the four surveys. The greatest number occurred in the age group of 71 to 80 in all four surveys, with a slightly lower number in 81 to 90 and somewhat less in the age group 61 to 70. Areas at risk and other characteristics of patients are likely to be different for different populations. One might surmise that a population that is primarily chair-bound, rather than bed-bound, would show fewer heel ulcers and more ischial ulcers, and individuals unable to turn their heads would be at greater risk for occipital ulcers. Therefore, the clinician must be aware of particular areas at risk dependent on the circumstances of individual patients.

Knowledge of risk factors allows the clinician and caregivers of those at risk to reduce the risk of developing pressure ulcers. Key among the risk factors is immobility or the lack of volition to move. In the clinical situation, rather than simply assessing the risk factors informally, several tools have been developed in an attempt to quantify risk. Quantification allows clinicians and caregivers to speak a common language in terms of risk factors and also provides the clinician with an objective means of decision-making. The goals of the tools described in this chapter are to both identify individuals in need of prevention measures and address specific factors that put them at risk. Interventions may then follow directly from addressing the factors. Physical therapy may be prescribed to improve mobility and instruct the patient in the use of assistive and adaptive devices. Specialized support surfaces and orthoses may be ordered. In addition, issues with incontinence may be addressed.

The AHCPR recommends that bed- and chair-bound individuals and anyone with an impaired ability to reposition be systematically evaluated for risk factors. In addition to immobility, risk factors include incontinence, malnutrition, and altered mental status. Mental status includes both the level of consciousness and any psychological impairments that would decrease the person's awareness of the need to reposition. Furthermore, the AHCPR recommends that individuals be assessed on admission to acute care and rehabilitation hospitals, nursing homes, home

---

Table 9-2

SCORING BASED ON THE NORTON SCALE

	4	*3*	*2*	*1*
Physical condition	good	fair	poor	very bad
Mental condition	alert	apathetic	confused	stupor
Activity	ambulant	walk/help	chair-bound	stupor
Mobility	full	slightly limited	very limited	immobile
Incontinent	not	occasional	usually/urine	doubly

Adapted from AHCPR guidelines.

care programs, and other health care facilities, and should be reassessed at periodic intervals. As recommended by the AHCPR, all assessments of risk should be documented. This not only provides legal protection for the clinician and facility, but also allows changes in the patient's status to be evaluated easily. Three major instruments described below are the Norton scale, the Braden scale, and the Gosnell scale.

The Norton scale (Table 9-2) is a sum of ordinal scale values for overall physical condition, mental condition, activity level, bed mobility, and continence. Each item is scored between 1 and 4, and the five item scores are added. Risk is then determined by the sum. The lowest possible score is 5 and the highest is 20. A score of 14 or less indicates risk for developing pressure ulcers, and a score of 12 or less indicates high risk. Based on the risk, prevention and intervention strategies may be undertaken. Although some of the items require judgment of the clinician, the reliability of the scale is sufficient for most needs. As with any instrument using ordinal scales, the numerical differences cannot be treated mathematically. For example, a score of 7 does not necessarily represent 30% more risk than a score of 10.

The Braden scale (Table 9-3) uses some similar indicators of risk. It has six items, also on an ordinal scale of 1 to 4. With this scale, risk also increases with a lower score. This scale uses sensory perception rather than mental condition and moisture rather than incontinence. It, similar to the Norton scale, uses mobility and activity level. The Braden scale scores two additional items. Risk of friction and shear (which are somewhat related to bed mobility) and nutrition are addressed in this scale, but not in the Norton scale. The Braden scale does not give a score to the clinician's overall impression of physical condition. The scale gives a maximum score of 23; one item (friction and shear) only scores between 1 and 3. For this scale, a person with a score of 16 or below is generally considered to be at risk, although for certain populations a score of 17 to 18 is considered to be at risk for development of pressure ulcers.

The Gosnell scale is an adaptation of the Norton scale. One major difference is the reversal of the scores such that a high number represents a greater risk. With this adaptation, 5 is the lowest possible score, indicating the least risk, and a score of 20 represents the greatest risk. Other differences between the Gosnell scale and Norton scale is the replacement of "physical condition" with nutrition. Other items appear on the tool but are not directly used in the scoring. In addition, very detailed instructions are included on the tool.

SKIN CARE AND EARLY TREATMENT

Those identified as having risk factors need interventions, including education of patient, family, and caregivers, to maintain and improve tissue tolerance to pressure in order to prevent injury. The AHCPR recommends that all individuals at risk should have a systematic skin inspection at least once a day, paying particular attention to the bony prominences; the results of the skin inspection should be documented. Historically, a process of trying to toughen the skin has been proposed as a means of increasing tolerance to tissue load. To the contrary, this practice has been shown to cause damage, rather than prevent injury. AHCPR guidelines state clearly that the practice of massaging over bony prominences should not be used.

Incontinence presents two problems. First is the presence of excessive moisture on the skin; second is the physical composition of urine and feces. Both are generally acidic. Urine pH can range from 6 to 3 and feces can contain a large quantity of bile acids. Because incontinence is such an important risk factor, skin cleansing should occur at the time of soiling and at routine intervals. Hot water and harsh detergents should not be used. Instead, many mild cleansing agents are available that can both minimize irritation and maintain appropriate moisture of the skin. Although removal of acidic urine and feces is important, minimizing force and friction applied to the skin is equally important to prevent skin injury. On the other hand, drying of the skin can also lead to injury. Prevention of injury must also include minimizing low humidity (<40%)

Table 9-3

SCORING BASED ON THE BRADEN SCALE

	1	*2*	*3*	*4*
Sensory perception	completely limited	very limited	slightly	no impairment
Moisture	constantly moist	moist	occasionally	rarely
Activity	bed-bound	chair-bound	walks occasionally	walks frequently
Mobility	completely immobile	very limited	slightly	no limitations
Nutrition	very poor	probably inadequate	adequate	excellent
Friction and shear	problem	potential problem	no apparent problem	

Adapted from AHCPR guidelines.

and exposure to cold. Moreover, dry skin should be treated with appropriate moisturizers. Various moisturizers are available. These moisturizers vary in their concentration of solids. Watery lotions with a low concentration of solids are not as effective as emollients with a higher concentration of oil and solids. An effective moisturizer will retain fluid within the skin while protecting the skin from excessive external sources of moisture such as incontinence, perspiration, or wound drainage. On occasion, these sources of moisture may not be controllable. Various absorptive pads or garments may be necessary under these conditions. However, all underpads and briefs are not suitable for this purpose. Only those made of materials that absorb moisture and wick it away from the skin should be used. General-purpose underpads may be suitable for those at low risk for a few days, for example individuals at low risk for pressure ulcers after surgery with copious drainage from surgical wounds. Moisture barriers should be used for the individual who frequently has moisture on the skin. See Chapter 17 for more information on skin care products.

For the person at risk, extra care, including referral to physical therapy, becomes necessary to prevent skin injury due to friction and shear forces. The patient, family, or caregivers should be instructed in proper positioning and transferring techniques. One may wish to use lubricants, (eg, corn starch), protective dressing materials (eg, transparent film), or hydrocolloid dressings, skin sealants, or protective padding. Because lack of mobility is the most important cause of pressure ulcers, referral to physical therapy to improve mobility should be made if potential for improvement exists and improved mobility is in accordance with patient and family goals. In some cases, maintaining current activity level, mobility, and range of motion is an appropriate goal, which may also require a course of physical therapy.

SUPPORT SURFACES

The terms *pressure relief* and *pressure reducing* have specific meanings. A pressure-relieving surface provides an interface pressure measurement below 25 mmHg. Pressure-reducing devices provide an interface pressure of 26 to 32 mmHg. Interface pressure refers to the pressure measured between a support surface and bony prominences such as greater trochanters. The purpose of definitions based on 32 mm is to avoid pressures greater than the accepted standard for capillary closing pressure. This number is based on the assumption that an interface pressure greater than 32 mmHg deforms capillaries sufficiently to cut off blood supply to the tissue between the support surface and the bony prominence. This number is based on a 1930 study of healthy younger men and may vary tremendously between men, women, and with age and cardiovascular status.[5]

A number of terms are used to evaluate support surfaces. Indentation load deflection is tested with specific equipment using specific testing procedures. A standard test of 25% indentation load deflection examines the load necessary to compress a surface to 75% of its original height. This load is expected to be within the range of 25 and 35 pounds. The 65% deflection is determined similarly. The ratio of the load necessary to compress the surface to 35% of its original height to the load necessary to compress the surface to 75% of its original height is termed the *support factor.* A high ratio indicates a surface that initially gives to provide comfort but maintains firm support. Density of foam refers to the weight in pounds of a cubic foot of foam. Density should be greater than 1.8 lb/ft^3 to prevent bottoming out and premature fatigue of the foam.[6]

In addition, several terms are used to describe the performance of support surfaces. *Immersion* allows bony prominences to sink into the support surface so that pressure can be borne by tissues surrounding the bony prominences (Figure 9-5). A support surface with low immersion places more pressure against a bony prominence as the surrounding tissues make little contact with the support surface. The term *envelopment* refers to the ability of the support surface to deform around any irregularities. Superficially, these two terms seem similar. Both are related to the property of deformation. Immersion refers more specifically to the "give" of the surface, whereas envelopment refers to the contouring of the surface to what is placed on it. A surface may have both good immersion and envelopment or may be good in just one property.

Postural stability refers to the ability of the patient to be held in place by the surface. A high immersion may provide good postural stability. However, a support surface with good envelopment provided by allowing material in the support surface to flow beneath the cover may produce poor postural stability. Many support surfaces may be constructed of combinations of materials to optimize these three characteristics. In addition, seat cushions may be precontoured. The covers used on the support surface influence the overall performance of the support surface. A tight cover reduces both immersion and envelopment. A cover designed to lower friction and shear may reduce postural stability. Moisture and temperature control may also be important considerations. Certain materials have a low heat transfer rate, which allows retention of heat by the skin surface, whereas others may have a high heat transfer rate, which reduces the skin/body temperature. The process of "draining" heat from the body is known as *heat sink. Moisture vapor transmission rate* refers to the movement of moisture through the surface. Again, certain materials may cause accumulation of moisture.[7]

Choice of support surface may become an exercise in compromise, as a support surface with one good characteristic may become less useful because of a poor characteristic. For example, some materials used in fluid-filled cushions can provide excellent envelopment but provide poor postural stability and cause retention of heat and moisture.[8]

Pressure-Reducing Devices

A number of classifications of pressure-reducing devices (PRDs) have been described in the literature. One sensible classification categorizes surfaces as alternating pressure

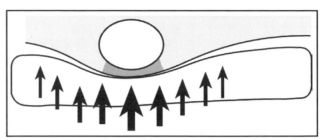

Figure 9-5. Effect of cushion on pressure exerted on bony prominences.

pads, beds, mattress overlays, mattress replacements, and enhanced overlays and mattresses.

Alternating pressure pads consist of a pump that periodically directs air to one set of cells while simultaneously allowing air to be released from another set, resulting in the alternation of pressure points over a given time. To be effective, these devices must be at least 2.5 inches in depth. Beds, by definition, are integrated systems including a frame and any control devices for the support surface. These may be further categorized as air-fluidized beds, low-air-loss beds and low-air-loss beds with adjuvant features. Air-fluidized beds consist of a tank filled with silicone microspheres that are circulated with an air pump and a sheet to contain the microspheres. The features of this support surface are described in greater detail below. Low-air-loss beds are also described below. They consist of interconnected air cells that are monitored for pressure and allow air to be lost as pressure increases within a cell. An air pump replaces air as needed when weight is shifted from a cell. These have a minimum depth of 5 inches and may require a stool to allow patient mobility. Low-air-loss beds with adjuvant features are basically the same type of support surface but include features such as vibration or periodic movement of a patient across the surface in an effort to reposition the patient to maintain airway clearance.

Mattress overlays fit over a standard mattress. These include air, foam, gel, or water. These types are described below. Air overlays should be at least 3 inches in depth. Foam features include a density of 1.35 to 1.8 lb/ft^3 and a 25% indentation load deflection of 25 to 35 lbs. A waterproof and friction-reducing cover should be part of the overlay. A minimum depth of 2 inches is recommended for gel overlays and 3 inches for water.

Mattress replacements, as the name implies, are meant to fit into standard bed frames and to replace the mattress, as opposed to an overlay or dedicated bed. These, like overlays, may be air, foam, gel, or water. Because they replace a mattress, the recommended thickness is greater. For air it is 3 inches, foam is 5 inches and includes the features also mentioned for the overlay. Recommended gel depth is 5 inches, as is that of water mattress replacements.

Table 9-4

CLASSES OF SUPPORT SURFACES

Alternating Pressure Pads

Bed
- Air-fluidized beds
- Low-air-loss beds
- Low-air-loss beds with adjuvant features

Mattress Overlays
- Air
- Foam
- Gel
- Water

Mattress Replacements
- Air
- Foam
- Gel
- Water

Enhanced Overlays and Mattresses

Alternating Pressure Mattresses

Low-Air-Loss Overlays

Nonpowered Adjustable Zone Overlays

Low-Air-Loss Mattresses

Low-Air-Loss Mattresses with Adjuvant Features

At this time, enhanced overlays and mattresses include alternating pressure mattresses, low-air-loss overlays, nonpowered adjustable zone overlays, low-air-loss mattresses, and low-air-loss mattresses with adjuvant features (Table 9-4).

Support surfaces may also be categorized by the materials used in them. Elastic foam is designed to deform to accommodate a load placed upon the support surface and may consist of a series of layers, may be contoured, or may be combined with another material such as gel or air-filled chambers. A combination of foam and either gel or air chambers allows postural stability because of properties of immersion and envelopment. Foam alone loses its resilience and bottoms out as the foam degrades with time ("impression set"), and foam has a limited ability to envelope and allow immersion. The stiffness of foam must strike a compromise between envelopment of soft foams and bottoming out. Precontouring a foam support surface provides immersion and envelopment as well as postural stability. Foam, however, can also retain heat and moisture against the skin and requires a porous cover and construction with open cell foam to allow moisture to move through the surface.

Viscoelastic foam is constructed of open cell foam and is temperature sensitive. The foam nearest the skin becomes softer due to the increased temperature of the foam. The viscoelastic nature helps the foam conform to the body surface and reduce interface pressure. Solid gel support surface functions in the same way as viscoelastic foam. Gel also has the disadvantage of retaining heat if the surface is used for more than 2 hours and retaining moisture on the skin.

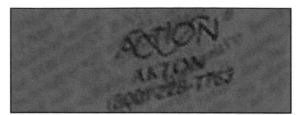

Figure 9-6a. Gel mattress overlay. (Also shown in Color Atlas following page 274.)

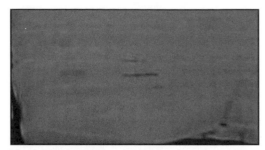

Figure 9-6b. Static air overlay.

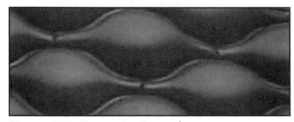

Figure 9-6c. Dynamic air overlay.

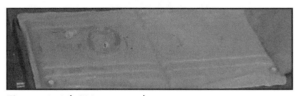

Figure 9-6d. Water overlay.

A fluid-filled support surface may be filled with air, water, or viscous fluid materials and have interconnected chambers. Pressure is accommodated by the flow of the fluid between chambers, permitting envelopment and immersion. Air-filled cushions must be inflated optimally to prevent bottoming out with underinflation and excessive pressures with overinflation. In addition, gel-filled surfaces may periodically require adjustment of the gel through the surface to prevent bottoming out. Fluid-filled support surfaces have the advantage of being deformable without the large restoring force of surfaces such as foams. This property allows very low interface pressures to occur if the surface is maintained properly.

Any individual assessed to be at risk for developing pressure ulcers should be placed, when lying in bed, on a pressure-reducing device. Foam, static air, alternating air, gel, and water mattresses are discussed below. In addition, anyone determined to be at risk for developing pressure ulcers should avoid uninterrupted sitting in a chair or wheelchair. Appropriate cushions or chair bottoms should be supplied commensurate with risk. For the individual with musculoskeletal injuries of the lower extremities but otherwise able to reposition, a simple wheelchair with a sling seat may be sufficient. At the other extreme, a person with quadriplegia who is unable to reposition and lacks sensation should have a specialized pressure-reducing cushion. In addition to reducing pressure, seating arrangements must also take into consideration postural alignment, distribution of weight, balance, and stability. The AHCPR guidelines recommend that an individual should be repositioned, shifting the points under pressure at least every hour or be put back in bed if consistent with overall patient management goals. However, allowing a person to remain in bed also carries the risk of pressure ulcers. Moreover, lying in bed presents a tremendous risk to gen-eral health, including risk of thromboembolism, pneumonia, gastrointestinal disease, renal disease, and bone demineralization. Individuals who are able should be taught to shift weight every 15 minutes, and a written plan for the use of positioning devices should be supplied and reviewed with each individual. A patient who has a pressure ulcer on a sitting surface should avoid sitting. If pressure on the ulcer can be relieved, limited sitting may be allowed.

Pressure-reducing devices can be divided into cushions, bed overlays that fit onto an existing support surface, and specialty beds (Figures 9-6a through 9-6d). Foam in the form of a cushion or mattress overlay is inexpensive, but has limited use for an individual at risk. Foam is a good insulator and is very absorbent; therefore, it increases temperature, retains moisture, and is easily contaminated. Foam cushions and mattress overlays are useful only for comfort in patients at low risk of developing ulcers. They should never be used for a patient with any ulcers present. Water flotation devices are designed to disperse weight more evenly than standard mattresses. This effect only exists with proper filling; over- or underfilling negates their effectiveness. Moreover, their effectiveness for sufficient pressure reduction at the greater trochanters and heels is questionable. They tend to bottom-out easily and may become cold or leak. Like foam, water flotation is useful for lower risk and only if the ulcer is not on the heel or greater trochanter. As a rule of thumb, they should only be used for patients who are independent in mobility and weight-shifting, although many healthy individuals enjoy this technology in everyday beds and pillows.

Gel overlays and seat cushions are more useful than foam and water flotation. In particular, these overlays are capable of dispersing both pressure and shearing forces (Figures 9-7b and 9-7c). However, these overlays and cushions are costly and heavy, and they allow moisture to

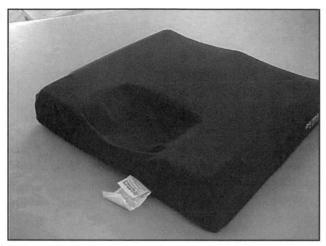

Figure 9-7a. Support surface for a chair: Isch-dish (Span-America Medical Systems, Inc. Greenville, SC).

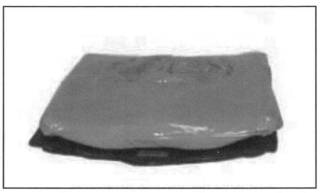

Figure 9-7b. Support surface for a chair: Jay J2 gel cushion (Sunrise Medical, Longmont, Colo).

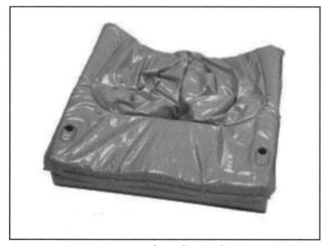

Figure 9-7c. Support surface for a chair: Jay J2 Deep Contour gel cushion (Sunrise Medical, Longmont, Colo).

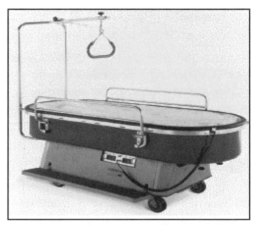

Figure 9-8a. Clinitron II air-fluidized therapy unit (2001 Hill-Rom Services, Inc., Batesville, Ind., Reprinted with permission, all rights reserved).

accumulate. Gel overlays are useful for minimal- to moderate-risk patients and patients with manageable ulcers and independent mobility. They are frequently used on operating tables for prevention during long procedures that carry risk of pressure ulcers. Gel seat cushions (Figures 9-7b and 9-7c) can be very expensive but effective for the person with a spinal cord injury or other loss of sensation below the waist.

The next most effective type of PRD is static air. These devices allow movement of air among channels to redistribute pressure and, to some extent, shear. Drawbacks include the potential for over- or underfilling, which decrease effectiveness, the potential for seams to fatigue and leak, and accidental puncture. Static air cushions and overlays can be useful for minimal- to moderate-risk patients and patients with manageable ulcers and independent mobility. Static air is also very effective for wheel-chair cushions. They are easy to clean and transport, as opposed to water flotation and gel PRDs.

Dynamic air systems consist of adjacent compartments that alternately inflate and deflate, reducing the time that any area is exposed to a high pressure. These can be very useful for moderate-risk, mobility-dependent patients and those with manageable ulcers. Dynamic air systems may take the form of a specialty bed or an overlay system placed upon a standard bed.

Specialty beds consist of either low-air-loss, air-fluidized, or combination units (Figures 9-8a through 9-8c). These beds or overlays are recommended for stage III or IV ulcers on multiple turning surfaces. Because of the expense of providing support surfaces, most facilities have developed specific criteria for determining medical necessity, such as a specific score on one of the risk assessment tools or the guidelines described in the AHCPR publication. Low-air-loss devices are now available in overlays as well as traditional beds. In either case, the unit consists of compartments inflated separately with sensors and a pump to maintain proper pressure in each segment as air is lost

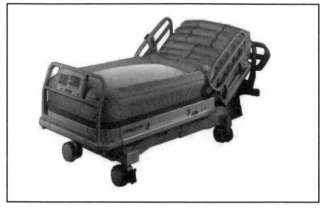

Figure 9-8b. Clinitron Rite-Hite air-fluidized therapy unit (2001 Hill-Rom Services, Inc., Batesville, Ind., Reprinted with permission, all rights reserved).

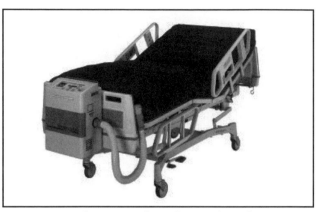

Figure 9-8c. Flexicare Eclipse low-air-loss therapy unit (2001 Hill-Rom Services, Inc., Batesville, Ind., Reprinted with permission, all rights reserved).

slowly through the compartments to dissipate pressure. The cover is water vapor permeable; therefore, clinical decisions for managing wound drainage must take into account the greater evaporation of moisture from the wound. Pressure and airflow may be adjustable for individual compartments. Some higher-end units provide airway clearance by either vibrating or rotating through an arc of movement to reduce time any given lung segment is left in a dependent position. Low-air-loss beds are very expensive; large hospitals may own a small number or they may be rented for hospital or home use. These devices are particularly useful for mobility-dependent, moderate- to maximal-risk patients, and patients with difficult to manage ulcers. The compressibility of the air segments would make mobility and cardiopulmonary resuscitation difficult without the safety mechanisms built into the units. Air can be let out rapidly in emergency situations by use of a "CPR" switch. Deflating the bed can be useful for transfers into and out of the bed, depending on the patient's height. Mobility can be improved by temporarily increasing the pressure within the segments by using a "maximum inflation" or equivalent function. Deflation of the bed is generally more useful for shorter patients and maximum inflation for taller patients.

Pressure-Relief Devices

Air-fluidized beds are the only true pressure-relief devices. These bed pumps drive air through ceramic silicon-coated soda lime beads, which are 1½ times as dense as water. The density of the floating beads causes the patient to float with a vapor-transmitting sheet in between. The bed consists of a tank filled with microspheres, controls, a heater, and blowers beneath. The bed is also designed to minimize friction, shear, and maceration. Body fluids drain into the tank, clumping the beads, which then settle out and can be removed. Moreover, drainage causes sodium ion release from the beads, ren-

dering the medium bacteriostatic. In addition, the temperature of the microspheres is controllable. Appropriate dressings need to be placed on the wound to avoid desiccation, in contrast to beds with vapor-impermeable sheets. Because these beds support the patient with the least pressure, they are indicated for patients with the greatest risk of developing pressure ulcers or for pressure ulcers to heal. As with low-air-loss beds, air flow can be turned off for emergency situations, such as administration of CPR. In one type of bed, the head of the bed cannot be directly elevated; this is accomplished by placing a wedge in the bed while the bed is turned off and then re-inflating it. It is very difficult for patients to transfer from these beds; however, patients placed in these beds generally are not capable of transferring from a bed. A combination of air-fluidized and low-air-loss bed is also available exclusively from Hill-Rom. The upper section uses low-air-loss and the lower section uses an air-fluidized tank. Unlike the standard Clinitron bed, this bed allows the head to be elevated. The upper section protects the upper body from pressure, while the lower section provides optimum pressure relief where most pressure ulcers are most likely to develop. Air-fluidized beds may also be used for patients with extensive burns to promote healing of burned posterior regions and graft donor sites, Stevens-Johnson syndrome, necrotizing fasciitis, and other skin conditions, and may be used for end-stage cancer.

Selection of Pressure-Reducing Devices

The performance characteristics suggested by the AHCPR for decisions on support surfaces included providing an increased support area, low moisture retention, reduced heat accumulation, shear reduction, and pressure reduction properties. Other properties for consideration are the dynamic versus static properties and cost per day.

The panel recommended that clinicians assess all patients with existing pressure ulcers to determine their risk for developing additional pressure ulcers. If the patient remains at risk, a pressure-reducing surface should be used.

Static support surfaces are recommended for patients who are able to assume a variety of positions, can stay off the ulcer, and those who do not cause the device to bottom out. Bottoming out is defined as a distance of less than 1 inch between the surface below the specialized support surface and bony prominences. This is established by placing a hand under the device to feel if the support surface is greater than 1 inch thick. More sophisticated computer-aided devices are capable of mapping areas of increased pressure more precisely.

Dynamic support surfaces are recommended for patients who are unable to assume a variety of positions, who cannot stay off the ulcer, or who cause a static support surface to bottom out. Another indication for a dynamic support surface is a wound that does not show evidence of healing. Air-fluidized beds are indicated for patients at high risk for developing pressure ulcers and patients with ulcers that are difficult to manage. Low-air-loss beds are indicated for moderate-risk patients and those with manageable ulcers. Overlay-type PRDs are indicated for patients at minimum to moderate risk and ulcers that do not require pressure relief to heal. At the time the AHCPR guidelines were written, panel members could not find any compelling evidence that one support surface for beds performed better under all circumstances.

In the original guidelines, kinetic therapy beds were not addressed. These beds take two basic forms. One type (no longer available from the manufacturer) mechanically rotates the support surface, thereby rotating the patient's area of support from supine to prone. The other type rocks from side-to-side. Newer specialty beds accomplish the same rocking motion by rhythmically inflating and deflating air chambers across the bed from side-to-side. In addition, these newer beds can provide airway clearance by vibrating the support surface. The use of this type of bed, however, does not eliminate the need for a turning schedule.

Sitting offers a different set of problems. Positioning considerations in sitting include an assessment of postural alignment and interventions such as instruction, orthoses, or cushions to provide postural alignment. Positioning should be used to ensure optimal distribution of weight, balance, stability, and continuous pressure relief. Although more favorable from a cardiopulmonary standpoint, sitting—even in a well-cushioned chair—causes very high interface pressures. Recommendations from the AHCPR guidelines include avoiding sitting if an ulcer develops on a sitting surface such as the sacrum or ischial tuberosities. Bear in mind, however, that these guidelines were created prior to the development of newer seating cushions. One type in particular, the Isch-dish (see Figure 9-7a), takes

weight completely off the ischial tuberosities and sacrum, and redistributes weight to the posterior thighs. If pressure can be totally relieved, the guidelines recommend that the patient may sit a limited time. As with the bed-bound individual, he or she should have an individualized written plan. In addition, each person should have an individually prescribed cushion, be repositioned every hour, and should shift weight every 15 minutes, if possible.

Medicare Part B Support Surface Guidelines

Policies for reimbursement for support surfaces are divided into groups I, II, and III. Criteria for group I devices are complete immobility, limited mobility, or any stage ulcer on the trunk or pelvis and at least one of the following contributing factors: impaired nutritional status, fecal or urinary incontinence, altered sensory perception, and compromised circulatory status. The need for a pressure-reducing device needs to be included in a plan of care established by the patient's physician or home care nurse, documented in the medical records including education of the patient or caregiver on prevention or management of pressure ulcers, regular assessment by a health care practitioner, appropriate turning and positioning, appropriate wound care, appropriate management of moisture (incontinence), nutritional assessment, intervention consistent with the overall plan of care, and a written order must be provided by the physician. Devices in group I include alternating air pressure mattresses and overlays, gel mattress or overlay, and water pressure mattresses and overlays.

Group II products include low-air-loss beds noted as "powered air flotation beds," powered pressure-reducing air mattress, nonpowered advanced pressure-reducing overlay for mattress, powered air overlay for mattress, and nonpowered advanced pressure-reducing mattress. Requirements for a group II product include the following: multiple stage II pressure ulcers located on the trunk or pelvis and the patient has been using a group I support surface as part of a comprehensive treatment program with worsening or no improvement over the past month, or large or multiple stage III or IV pressure ulcers on the trunk or recent myocutaneous flap or skin graft for a pressure ulcer on the trunk or pelvis with surgery within the past 60 days. The patient must also be on a group II or III support surface immediately prior to discharge. Coverage is limited to 60 days for operative repair of ulcers. Again, a written order and a comprehensive plan as described above for group I surfaces are required. Use of the group II surface is allowed until the ulcer is healed or documentation in the medical record shows that other aspects of the plan of care are being modified to promote healing, or that the group II surface is medically necessary for wound management.

Group III only includes air-fluidized beds, such as the Clinitron. Requirements include the presence of a stage III or IV pressure ulcer, the patient is bed- or chair-bound due to severely limited mobility, the patient would require institutionalization without the air-fluidized bed, and failure of more conservative treatment. A comprehensive plan of care including the air-fluidized bed is required as described under group I devices. In general, a more conservative plan of care should have been in effect for at least 1 month prior to use of an air-fluidized bed with failure to improve. Other limitations also need to be addressed, including presence of coexisting pulmonary disease, lack of a caregiver willing and able to provide care required by a patient on an air-fluidized bed, and inadequate structural support (these beds are extremely heavy) and electrical system.

TURNING SCHEDULES

The purpose of support surfaces is to protect against the adverse effects of tissue loads, whether pressure, friction, or shear. Any bed-bound individual with compromised mobility or other risk factors should be repositioned according to an individualized schedule that should be written, posted, and carried out by the patient's caregivers. Historically, a recommendation of turning at least every 2 hours has been made. For individuals at high risk, especially those who are emaciated and malnourished, 2 hours may be too long. Moreover, blindly repositioning without regard to neurological deficits, musculoskeletal injuries, or particular areas of skin at high risk is a disservice to the patient. When the sidelying position is used in bed, pillows or wedges should be used to avoid positioning a patient directly on the greater trochanter. Some turning schedules call for a rotation between prone, sidelying to one side, supine, and sidelying to the other side. Rather than positioning a patient directly sidelying, a 30-degree turn from supine can relieve pressure without placing pressure directly over either greater trochanter. Moreover, a patient should never be positioned directly over an ulcer if possible; and if not possible, the patient should be on a pressure-reducing surface.

To prevent injury caused by bony prominences contacting each other, pillows, foam wedges, or other devices should be used to keep the knees or ankles apart. Anyone with impaired mobility who is bed-bound should have a device that totally relieves pressure on the heels, usually by raising the heels off the bed. This may consist of simply placing pillows under the legs or may include more complex devices such as Multipodus boots (Figure 9-9). Donut devices should never be used on anyone at risk for pressure ulcers. These devices are designed only for temporary comfort in individuals not at risk for pressure ulcers.

In addition to pressure, shear must be minimized. Shear results from forces applied tangentially to the skin. Shear stresses increase directly in proportion to the incline of a bed or chair. In the case of reclining, shear is placed on the skin over the sacrum when skin adheres to the support surface as body weight pulls downward. These forces also occur during transfers, turning, and bed mobility. To minimize injury due to shear, the clinician should maintain the head of the bed at the lowest degree of elevation consistent with medical conditions and other restrictions such as increased intracranial pressure, pulmonary edema, congestive heart failure, and gastroesophageal reflux. The use of a trapeze or draw sheets to lift and avoid dragging individuals in bed who cannot assist during transfers and position changes is recommended.

NUTRITIONAL ASSESSMENT

The stage of pressure ulcers has been correlated with nutrition. Particular risk factors cited include low dietary protein and hypoalbuminemia. Moreover, a clear association between malnutrition and new ulcer development has been observed. The AHCPR guidelines recommend an evaluation of nutritional status using a nutrition screening manual. Preferably, a clinical dietician would be available to perform a thorough nutritional assessment. The AHCPR also recommends that a reassessment be made every 3 months.

Nutritional risk factors addressed in the guidelines include inability to take food by mouth, a history of involuntary weight loss, immobility, altered mental status, and educational deficit. The guidelines recommend encouraging dietary intake and supplementation of the diet if the person is malnourished, including nutritional support by tube feeding or other means if necessary. An intake of 30 to 35 kcal per kilogram of body mass each day with 1.25 to 1.50g of protein per kilograms per day.

PAIN ASSESSMENT

Pain management is discussed in Chapter 18. Routine assessment of pain is recommended by the AHCPR, although they also recommended further research into this topic. Specifically addressed is the potential for intensified pain during dressing changes and debridement. They suggest that pain should be managed by eliminating or controlling its source and providing analgesia during painful procedures such as debridement. All patients should be assessed for pain related to the pressure ulcer or its treatment. Controlling the source of pain may include covering wounds, adjusting support surfaces, or repositioning.

PSYCHOSOCIAL ASSESSMENT

In many situations, the health care professionals cannot provide all of the care; the patient or other caregiver must take a major role. Even in the acute care hospital, psychosocial issues may promote or impair the efficacy of provided services. Issues that need to be addressed include whether the patient comprehends the plan of care and if the patient is motivated to adhere to the plan. The clinician needs to understand values, lifestyle, psychosocial needs, and goals of not only the patient but also the family, or if different, the caregiver. The AHCPR guidelines specifically mention mental status, learning ability, depression, social support, polypharmacy or overmedication, alcohol and/or drug abuse, goals, values, lifestyle, sexuality, culture, ethnicity, and stressors.

With these issues in mind, the clinician, patient, family and other caregivers should set treatment goals collaboratively. In addition, when developing a home plan of care, the clinician needs to determine whether the patient and family have the resources available to be treated at home. These resources are not only financial, but also include the ability to understand and the skills to follow through on the treatment plan. Periodic reassessment is also recommended by the AHCPR, and follow-up should be planned in cooperation with the individual and caregiver.

SUMMARY

Pressure ulcers are caused by a number of factors, including pressure, shear, friction, excess moisture, heat or skin dryness, and a lack of nutrition. Both time and pressure on a body surface must be considered in assessing risk of skin injury. Staging of pressure ulcers is based on the tissue involved and, therefore, reverse staging cannot be done logically. With regard to positioning and pressure, the patient's body composition, mental status, and support surface must be considered. Guidelines for appropriate support surfaces are discussed, as is the need for adequate nutritional and psychosocial assessment. Methods to enhance healing of pressure ulcers are discussed in subsequent chapters.

STUDY QUESTIONS

1. Why is body composition important in the risk for developing pressure ulcers?
2. Why are the occiput and lateral condyles of the elbows at such high risk for skin breakdown?
3. Why is reclining such an important risk factor in sacral ulcers?
4. For what reasons would a person require a specialty bed?
5. What options are available for reducing risk of pressure ulcers in a person during sitting?

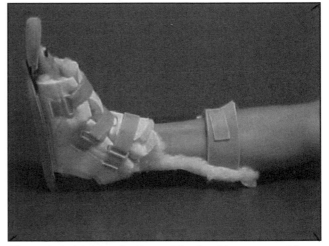

Figure 9-9. Multipodus boot. The heel is protected from the weight of the patient, and loss of dorsiflexion produced by constant weight of sheets and blankets on the foot is minimized.

6. Why are psychosocial factors important in preventing pressure ulcers?

REFERENCES

1. NPUAP. Statement on Pressure Ulcer Prevention 1992. Available at: *http://www.npuap.org/positn1.htm.* Accessed 2001.
2. Panel on the Prediction and Prevention of Pressure Ulcers in Adults. Pressure Ulcers in Adults: Prediction and Prevention. Clinical Practice Guideline, No. 3 AHCPR Publication No. 92-0047. Rockville, MD: Agency for Health Care Policy and Research; May 1992.
3. Calianno C. Assessing and preventing pressure ulcers. *Advances in Skin and Wound Care.* 2000;13:244-246.
4. Barczak CA, Barnett RI, Jarczynski Childs E, Bosley LM. Fourth National Pressure Ulcer Prevalence Study. *Advances in Wound Care.* 1997;10:18-26.
5. Landis EM. Microinjection studies of capillary blood pressure in human skin. *Heart* 1930;15: 209-228.
6. Brienza DM, Geyer MJ. Understanding support surface technologies. *Advances in Skin and Wound Care.* 2000;13:237-244.
7. Brienza DM, Karg PE. Seat cushion optimization: a comparison of interface pressure and tissue stiffness characteristics for spinal cord injured and elderly patients. *Arch Phys Med Rehabil.* 1998;79:388-394.
8. Wells J, Karr D. Interface pressure, wound healing and satisfaction in the evaluation of a non-powered fluid mattress. *Ostomy and Wound Management.* 1998;44:38-54.

PUSH Tool 3.0

Patient Name_____ Patient ID#_____

Ulcer Location_____ Date_____

Directions: Observe and measure the pressure ulcer. Categorize the ulcer with respect to surface area, exudate, and type of wound tissue. Record a sub-score for each of these ulcer characteristics. Add the sub-scores to obtain the total score. A comparison of total scores measured over time provides an indication of the improvement or deterioration in pressure ulcer healing.

Length cm^2	*0* 0	*1* < 0.3	*2* 0.3-0.6	*3* 0.7-1.0	*4* 1.1-2.0	*5* 2.1-3.0	
Width cm^2		*6* 3.1-4.0	*7* 4.1-8.0	*8* 8.1-12.0	*9* 12.1-24.0	*10* >24.0	*Sub-score*
Exudate *Amount*	*0* None	*1* Light	*2* Moderate	*3* Heavy			*Sub-score*
Tissue *Type*	*0* Closed	*1* Epithelial Tissue	*2* Granulation Tissue	*3* Slough	*4* Necrotic Tissue		*Sub-score*
							Total Score

Length x Width: Measure the greatest length (head to toe) and the greatest width (side to side) using a centimeter ruler. Multiply these two measurements (length x width) to obtain an estimate of surface area in square centimeters (cm^2). Caveat: Do not guess! Always use a centimeter ruler and always use the same method each time the ulcer is measured.

Exudate Amount: Estimate the amount of exudate (drainage) present after removal of the dressing and before applying any topical agent to the ulcer. Estimate the exudate (drainage) as none, light, moderate, or heavy.

Tissue Type: This refers to the types of tissue that are present in the wound (ulcer) bed. Score as a "4" if there is any necrotic tissue present. Score as a "3" if there is any amount of slough present and necrotic tissue is absent. Score as a "2" if the wound is clean and contains granulation tissue. A superficial wound that is reepithelializing is scored as a "1". When the wound is closed, score as a "0".

4—Necrotic Tissue (Eschar): black, brown, or tan tissue that adheres firmly to the wound bed or ulcer edges and may be either firmer or softer than surrounding skin.

3—Slough: yellow or white tissue that adheres to the ulcer bed in strings or thick clumps, or is mucinous.

2—Granulation Tissue: pink or beefy red tissue with a shiny, moist, granular appearance.

1—Epithelial Tissue: for superficial ulcers, new pink or shiny tissue (skin) that grows in from the edges or as islands on the ulcer surface.

0—Closed/Resurfaced: the wound is completely covered with epithelium (new skin).

PRESSURE ULCER HEALING CHART

(To Monitor Trends in PUSH Scores Over Time)

Patient Name_____ Patient ID#_____

Ulcer Location_____ Date_____

Directions: Observe and measure pressure ulcers at regular intervals using the PUSH Tool. Date and record PUSH Sub-scale and Total Scores on the Pressure Ulcer Healing Record below.

PRESSURE ULCER HEALING RECORD

Date																
Length x Width																
Exudate Amount																
Tissue Type																
Total Score																

Graph the PUSH total score on the Pressure Ulcer Healing Graph below.

PUSH Total Score	*PRESSURE ULCER HEALING GRAPH*										
12											
11											
10											
9											
8											
7											
6											
5											
4											
3											
2											
1											
Healed 0											
Date											

(Used with permission from the National Pressure Ulcer Advisory Panel, Reston, Virginia)

INSTRUCTIONS FOR USING THE PUSH TOOL

To use the PUSH Tool, the pressure ulcer is assessed and scored on the three elements in the tool:

- Length x Width --> scored from 0 to 10
- Exudate Amount --> scored from 0 (none) to 3 (heavy)
- Tissue Type --> scored from 0 (closed) to 4 (necrotic tissue)

In order to insure consistency in applying the tool to monitor wound healing, definitions for each element are supplied at the bottom of the tool.

Step 1: Using the definition for length x width, a centimeter ruler measurement is made of the greatest head to toe diameter. A second measurement is made of the greatest width (left to right). Multiple these two measurements to get square centimeters and then select the corresponding category for size on the scale and record the score.

Step 2: Estimate the amount of exudate after removal of the dressing and before applying any topical agents. Select the corresponding category for amount & record the score.

Step 3: Identify the type of tissue. Note: if there is **any** necrotic tissue, it is scored a 4. Or, if there is **any** slough, it is scored a 3, even though most of the wound is covered with granulation tissue.

Step 4: Sum the scores on the three elements of the tool to derive a total PUSH Score.

Step 5: Transfer the total score to the Pressure Ulcer Healing Graph. Changes in the score over time provide an indication of the changing status of the ulcer. If the score goes down, the wound is healing. If it gets larger, the wound is deteriorating.

(Used with permission from the National Pressure Ulcer Advisory Panel, Reston, Virginia)

Vascular Insufficiency

OBJECTIVES

- Identify risk factors for wounds caused by vascular insufficiency.
- Perform a differential diagnosis of wounds caused by vascular insufficiency.
- Devise a plan of care including direct interventions and patient education for a patient with vascular insufficiency.

The most common causes of chronic wounds include neuropathy (see Chapter 8), tissue loads (see Chapter 9), and venous insufficiency (venous hypertension) of the lower extremities. Occasionally, wounds may be seen due to arterial insufficiency. The ability to perform a good differential diagnosis between arterial and venous insufficiency becomes critical because the major interventions for correcting venous hypertension are contraindicated in the presence of arterial insufficiency, and untreated arterial insufficiency of a lower extremity may become an emergent condition requiring surgery to prevent limb loss.

ARTERIAL INSUFFICIENCY

Arterial insufficiency ulcers represent necrosis secondary to ischemia of a limb and are usually secondary to atherosclerosis. As described in Chapter 5, measurement of ankle brachial index (ABI) can be performed to assess for arterial insufficiency. This test is a simple ratio of systolic pressure in the ankle from either the dorsalis pedis or the posterior tibial artery to the systolic pressure of the brachial artery. Normally, the ratio of ankle to brachial systolic pressure is 1.1 to 1.0. A value below 0.8 to 0.7 is indicative of arterial disease. In a patient with arterial insufficiency and ABI below 0.45, healing is unlikely.

In a minority of cases, arterial insufficiency may be caused by other arterial diseases such as Buerger's disease (thromboangiitis obliterans). In the most common case of atherosclerosis of the lower extremity, tissues at greatest risk of necrosis are the most distal structures. Normally, blood pressure dissipates little along blood vessels of the lower extremity. However, with obstruction of arterial vessels due to atherosclerotic plaque and thrombosis, necrosis occurs in tissues distal to obstruction, usually on the foot, especially the toes. These wounds tend to be deep wounds with irregular borders outlining the arterial distribution involved. The outward appearance of advanced arterial disease is blackened, dry gangrene on the toes and sometimes more proximal structures. Dry gangrene should not be debrided, because it acts as dressing to protect the tissue beneath it. Debridement of dry gangrene is discouraged because debridement exposes necrotic tissue that can quickly support pathogenic organisms and allow disseminated infection. Severe ischemia may require surgical amputation. In some cases, autoamputation occurs, in which the necrotic tissue, often a toe, withers and falls off the limb.

Conservative treatment for arterial insufficiency consists of local wound care, but dry gangrene should not be debrided as discussed earlier. Reduction of risk factors include smoking, diabetes mellitus, hypertension, hyperlipidemia, and limb protection. Seemingly trivial mechanical trauma may produce ulcers. Padding, lotions, absorp-

tion of excess moisture, and the use of assistive and adaptive devices may help protect limbs at risk for developing infection or injury.

Pharmacological treatment for arterial insufficiency includes thrombolytic drugs, anticoagulants, vasodilators, and pentoxifilline (Trental, Aventis Pharmaceuticals Inc., Bridgewater, NJ). Surgical treatment provided by vascular surgeons includes bypass surgery, endarterectomy, and percutaneous transluminal angioplasty.

VENOUS INSUFFICIENCY

These wounds have a prevalence estimated to be as high as 500,000 to 800,000 in the United States. Venous insufficiency ulcers have also been called venous stasis ulcers due to a lack of understanding of their pathophysiology; they are not caused by lack of venous flow but a diminished diffusion of nutrients through the interstitial space from capillaries. The root cause of venous insufficiency ulcers is venous hypertension and the consequences of capillary hypertension.[1,2] Through a sequence of events described below, venous hypertension leads to malnutrition of the skin and a limited depth of subcutaneous tissue. In many cases, patients will identify trauma to the affected leg as the cause of the wound. In these cases, however, the patient has traumatized necrotic tissue that likely would open into a wound on its own.

Venous hypertension results in elevated capillary pressure to the extent that capillaries begin to leak fluid, macromolecules, and red blood cells into the interstitial space. As a result, edema of the affected extremity occurs, along with hardening of the skin and the presence of hemosiderin staining. The brawniness of the extremity appears to be due to the leakage of protein into the interstitial space with resultant fibrosis. Leakage of red cells and their breakdown leads to the formation of bilirubin, biliverdin, and hemosiderin (a storage form of iron) in the skin with an obvious brownish-yellow discoloration. The appearance of venous insufficiency ulcers is shown in Figures 10-1a through 10-1c. Several theories of how venous hypertension results in malnutrition have been proposed. Three particular theories with merit are pericapillary fibrin cuffs, leukocyte trapping, and microangiopathy (Figure 10-2).

Pericapillary Fibrin Cuffs

The theory of Burnand and Browse[3] is based on the concept of macromolecular leakage due to high capillary hydrostatic pressure. Fibrinogen leaking from capillaries polymerizes into fibrin, creating a diffusion barrier between the capillary and tissues supplied by them. This theory enjoys substantial experimental support but is inadequate to explain tissue PO_2.

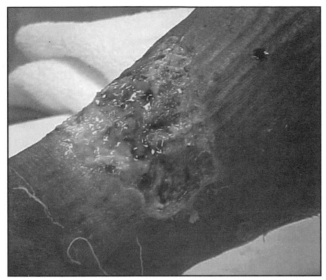

Figure 10-1a. Appearance of venous insufficiency ulcers. Note the irregular borders, location, copious drainage, and red granulation tissue. (Also shown in Color Atlas following page 274.)

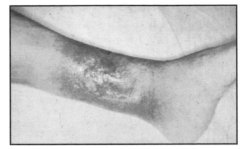

Figure 10-1b. Hemosiderin staining of the lower extremity, characteristic of venous insufficiency. Note, however, that hemosiderin localized to the margins of a wound may occur with wounds caused by mechanical trauma such as pressure ulcers and neuropathic ulcers. Courtesy of Little Rock Veteran's Administration Hospital. (Also shown in Color Atlas following page 274.)

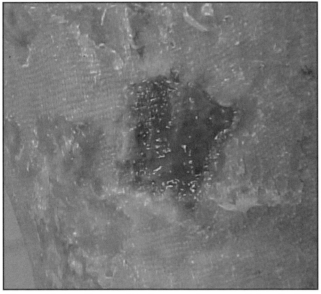

Figure 10-1c. Dermatitis, frequently termed "stasis dermatitis," characteristic of venous insufficiency. Note indentations of skin caused by the weave of the compression bandage. (Also shown in Color Atlas following page 274.)

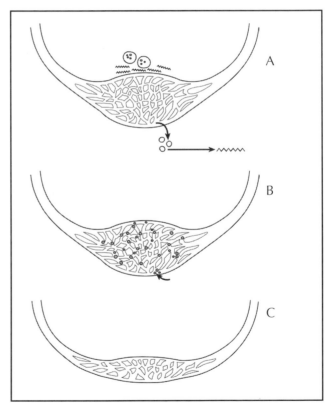

Figure 10-2. Pathophysiology of venous insufficiency. (A) Leakage of proteins from capillaries. (B) Inflammation caused by trapped leukocytes. (C) Rarefaction of capillaries secondary to hypertension.

Leukocyte Trapping

The low pressure gradient across capillaries due to venous hypertension is believed to produce sluggish capillary blood flow and enhance the probability of leukocyte adherence to the capillary endothelium, with increased expression of leukocyte adhesion molecules. Leukocyte adhesion then leads to production of chemical mediators of inflammation and tissue injury.[4]

Microangiopathy

Elevated venous pressure due to calf-pump failure causes elevated pressure and distension of capillaries. Capillary distention can be observed before the tissue injury charac-

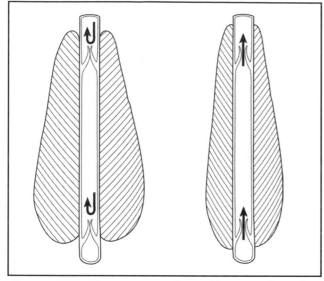

Figure 10-3. Components of a calf pump. Pumping requires the presence of unobstructed vessels, valves to ensure unidirectional flow, and a source of energy (muscle contraction).

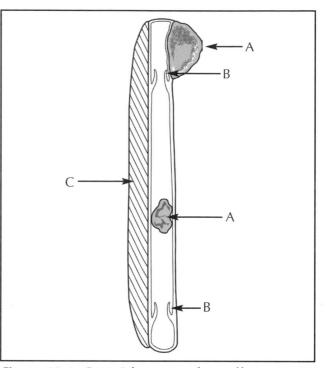

Figure 10-4. Potential causes of a calf pump. (A) Obstruction of the venous vessels from within or outside. (B) Incompetent venous valves. (C) Loss of muscle contraction due to injury or disease.

teristic of venous hypertension can be observed, and the severity of skin damage and capillary injury are highly correlated. A severe reduction in the number of capillaries can be observed within the ulcer itself, and at the edge of the ulcer a large number of damaged capillaries characterized by dilation, elongation, tortuosity, stasis, and thrombosis can be observed. Thus, avascular areas develop, resulting in tissue injury and progressing to tissue death and ulceration. Wound healing would also be expected to be slow or absent given the lack of nutritive circulation. A correlation between loss of capillaries and transcutaneous oxygen $tcPO_2$ has been demonstrated in a series of patients with chronic venous insufficiency. During healing, capillary density improved in all cases in both the ulcer and surrounding skin on the ulcer's edge. A greater increase in capillary density was observed in patients with relatively rapid healing compared with patients with relatively slow healing. In addition, $tcPO_2$ increased rapidly in the fast healers and was initially decreased in the slow healers. Healing was accompanied by an increased $tcPO_2$ in both groups but was higher in the fast healers. Although healing occurred in these patients, the deranged capillary morphology remained. This, in part, may explain the high recurrence of ulceration in patients simply receiving treatment for ulcerations but not for venous hypertension.[5]

Causes of venous hypertension represent calf-pump failure. The calf pump uses contraction of leg muscles to pump blood from the dependent lower extremities by taking advantage of one-way valves present in the veins. Without the calf pump, blood pressure in the foot may increase an additional 100 mmHg for an individual

approximately 6 feet in height when moving from supine to standing. To lower venous and capillary pressure to manageable levels, pumping of blood caused by intermittent contraction of leg muscles must be functional. This pump, similar to any other pump, requires a force to drive flow, patent conduits, and a one-way valving system. The force to drive flow is derived from calf muscle contraction—the veins are the conduits, and the venous valves ensure unidirectional flow from the lower extremities. The components of the calf pump are illustrated in Figure 10-3.

Given the parts of the calf pump, possible causes of calf-pump failure become easily identified. The causes can be categorized as outflow obstruction, valve insufficiency, or loss of muscle pumping action (Figure 10-4). Venous outflow obstruction may occur from within the venous vessels or external compression. Typically, internal obstruction results from deep venous thrombosis or clotting. External compression may result from a tumor, such as an enlarged lymph node in the groin, pregnancy, obesity, or inappropriate application of elasticized garments. Insufficient valves may occur in the deep veins running alongside arteries, superficial veins, or the communicating veins that allow the superficial veins to drain into the deep veins. Many individuals appear to be genetically predisposed to venous valve weakness. Once venous valves

---

Table 10-1

CAUSES OF VENOUS HYPERTENSION

Insufficient Valves

- Insufficient valves of deep veins
- Insufficient valves of communicating veins
- Insufficient valves of superficial veins (varicose veins)

Obstruction of Lower Extremity Veins

- Pregnancy
- Obesity
- Tumor
- Clotting/thrombosis of veins

Insufficient Calf Muscle Activity

- Prolonged standing
- Neuromuscular disease affecting the leg muscles
- Musculoskeletal injury or disease affecting the leg muscles
- Immobilization of the lower extremity

---

begin to fail, a chain reaction of valve failure results. As a valve fails, pressure rises in the veins until inflow becomes equal to outflow. The lack of outflow results in venous hypertension, dilation, and tortuosity. When dilation of superficial veins is evident, the term *varicose veins* is used. The failure of the leaflets of a venous valve to support the column of blood above it increases the height of the column of blood on the valve below it. This, in turn, predisposes that valve to fail until all of the valves below the initially insufficient valve also fail, producing a positive feedback of insufficiency and dilation. Loss of muscle pumping action may occur following neuromuscular or musculoskeletal disease or injury (Table 10-1).

Microcirculatory changes result from venous hypertension. As pressure increases in veins, the outflow pressure of capillaries increases, decreasing flow out of capillaries until pressure within the capillaries exceeds pressure within the draining veins. Edema results from both high hydrostatic pressure and the high concentration of protein in the interstitial space. Elevated capillary pressure drives fluids and macromolecules out of the affected capillaries. Normal loss of plasma proteins can be handled by lymphatic drainage; however, with venous hypertension, proteins leak out faster into the interstitial space than they can be taken up, resulting in an accumulation of interstitial plasma proteins. Edema alone increases the diffusion distance for nutrients. In addition, the presence of proteins, particularly fibrinogen, has been blamed for tissue injury. Interstitial fibrinogen may be converted to the insoluble protein fibrin, which is the major component of thrombi. Excessive water and protein combined with decreased

numbers of capillaries diminish diffusion of oxygen and nutrients required for the health of tissue surrounding the vein. These wounds are usually full-thickness with irregular edges but without subcutaneous involvement. Often, the wound bed appears very healthy with a red, shiny appearance due to good arterial circulation. Unfortunately, many of the wounds do not heal well unless the underlying condition of venous hypertension is corrected. Many individuals have suffered for years through a series of venous insufficiency ulcers because treatment has been directed toward the wound instead of the venous hypertension.

DIFFERENTIAL DIAGNOSIS OF ARTERIAL AND VENOUS ULCERS

The ability to distinguish between arterial and venous insufficiency as causes of ulcers is generally simple with a systematic investigation of the following characteristics: pain, the effect of elevation, the distribution and appearance of the wounds, and special tests described in Chapter 5. Arterial ulcers can be very painful, increasing with exercise and elevation. Venous insufficiency ulcers are relatively pain-free with some discomfort or bursting sensation, which is relieved with elevation. As discussed above, arterial insufficiency produces ulcers on the most distal areas of the body, especially the toes and heels, whereas venous insufficiency creates wounds almost always on the distal leg superior to the malleoli, with approximately two-thirds occurrence on the medial side compared with the

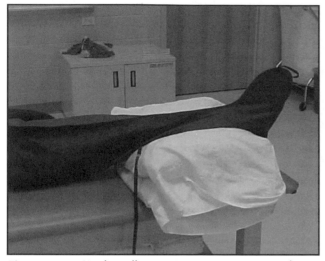

Figure 10-5. Single-cell compression pump. A single air bladder is alternately inflated and deflated. An on-time and off-time must be set, as well as the pressure.

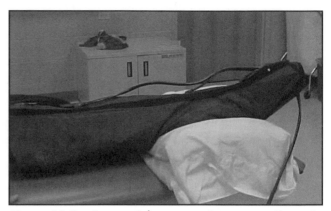

Figure 10-6a. Sequential compression pump. Four air bladders are sequentially inflated in the distal-to-proximal direction. For this model, only the pressure exerted by the pump is adjustable. All four bladders are deflated.

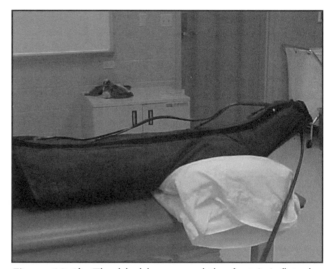

Figure 10-6b. The bladder around the foot is inflated.

lateral side. Arterial insufficiency creates deeper, well demarcated wounds without the presence of granulation tissue. During healing, granulation tissue has more of a pink color, rather than the beefy red color of granulation tissue in wounds with adequate blood flow. By the time arterial insufficiency ulcers begin to appear, the patient usually has pain even at rest. Dry gangrene of severe disease is characterized by depressed, "punched out" blackened areas. Round or elliptical wounds are generally the result of tissue loading caused by either unrelieved pressure over bony prominences or neuropathy of the foot. Moreover, the skin surrounding the arterial insufficiency wound displays signs of ischemia such as pallor or mottling of the skin (variegated coloration of the skin).

The appearance of venous insufficiency ulcers is usually very stereotypical—hemosiderin staining and induration of the surrounding skin with a granulating wound base that looks ready to heal. In a minority of cases, some aspects of the appearance of venous insufficiency ulcers may be overlooked. A history of varicose veins, a job requiring the person to stand still throughout the day, and special tests may then be necessary to confirm the cause as venous insufficiency. Special tests for the vascular system are described in Chapter 5. These tests include the arterial tests of using a Doppler to determine the presence of distal arterial flow, ABI (indicates occlusion if ankle blood pressure is significantly less than the blood pressure in the arm), and pneumoplethysmography waveforms indicating the ratio of blood flow during diastole compared with blood flow during systole. Venous tests include the percussion test, Trendelenberg test, venous filling test, and venous plethysmography (refilling time faster with incompetent valves).

COMPRESSION THERAPY FOR VENOUS ULCERS

Definitive treatment for venous insufficiency ulcers involves compression therapy to ameliorate the underlying cause of venous hypertension.[6,7] Gentle cleansing of wounds should be done with each dressing change. Using typical whirlpool therapy actually creates more problems with venous insufficiency. Typical whirlpool temperatures increase arterial inflow and the dependent position with the thigh compressed over the edge of the whirlpool tank exacerbate venous insufficiency. Compression may be performed with a clinical or home compression pump. Some older compression pumps are single cell units in which a single sleeve inflates and deflates rhythmically (Figure 10-5). Most newer devices are sequential and multicell, in which three or four cells inflate sequentially from distal

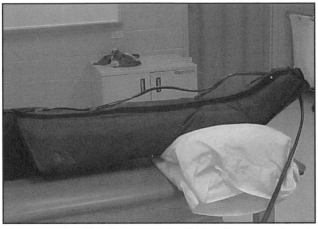

Figure 10-6c. The three proximal bladders are inflated.

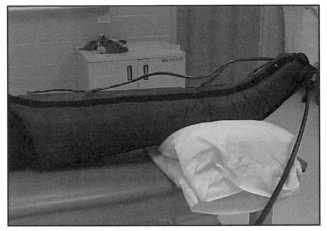

Figure 10-6d. All four bladders are inflated.

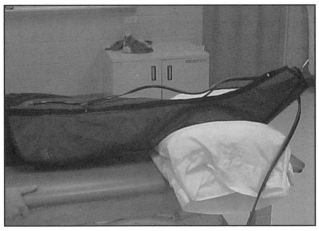

Figure 10-6e. All four bladders are deflated.

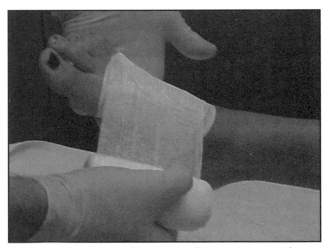

Figure 10-7a. Application of an Unna's boot. Application begins around the metatarsal heads with the bandage applied in a figure-of-eight fashion proximally.

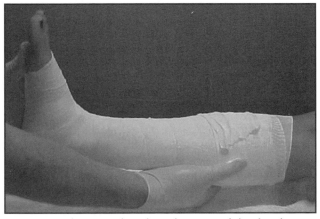

Figure 10-7b. Completed application of the first layer.

(over the foot) toward the knee, then deflate and begin inflation distally toward proximally again (Figures 10-6a through 10-6e). Any wounds should be covered with an appropriate dressing and a plastic bag to prevent soiling the compression sleeve. The bagged extremity is then placed into the compression sleeve and the affected extremity is elevated slightly. Pumping is done for 1 hour with pressure at 50 mmHg, but less than diastolic pressure. Pressure higher than 50 mmHg is believed to compress lymphatic vessels, and pressure less than diastolic ensures some circulation into the extremity for the entire cardiac cycle. If using a single-cell sleeve, 90 seconds on, 30 seconds off is commonly used. A sequential pump is simply allowed to run continuously as described above. If the patient needs to be seen in a clinic, treatment may be done two to three times per week. A more cost-effective strategy is a rental or home unit for more frequent treatments up to twice per day. Compression must be maintained between treatments. Several options are now available. The old standby of the Unna's boot is being replaced. Unna's boot is messy to apply, difficult to regulate the pressure within it (Figures 10-7a through 10-7e) and is typically only useful in ambulatory patients in whom the

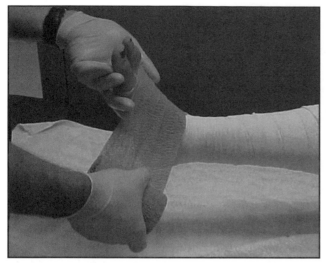

Figure 10-7c. Second layer of cohesive bandaging, also applied in a figure-of-eight. This layer prevents soiling of clothing by the material on the Unna's boot bandage and prevents unraveling.

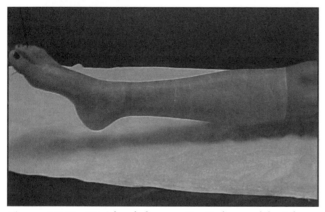

Figure 10-7e. Residue left on patient's leg and foot from the Unna's boot.

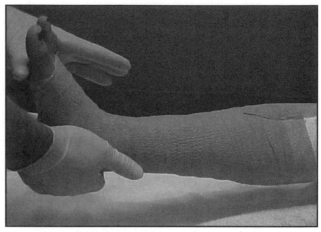

Figure 10-7d. Competed Unna's boot.

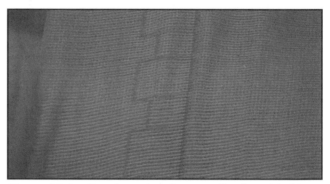

Figure 10-8a. Two-layer bandage application. Markings on the elasticized bandage indicate pressure generated by the bandage when applied in a half-overlapping spiral technique. Short quadrangles are stretched into squares to produce approximately 30 mmHg pressure.

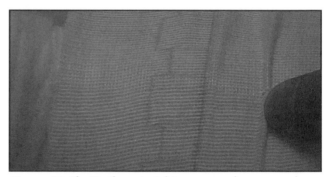

Figure 10-8b. Further stretching causes larger quadrangles to form squares and produce approximately 50 mmHg pressure on the leg.

semirigid dressing aids the calf pump mechanism. In addition, the Unna's boot loses effectiveness as volume of the leg decreases. The bandage material cannot absorb much drainage and maceration of the periwound skin may occur unless other steps are used to manage drainage from the wound. In many cases, compression is achieved solely with bandaging, rather than use of compression pumps.[8]

Multilayer bandaging systems consisting of either two (Figures 10-8a through 10-8g), three, or four layers (Figures 10-9a through 10-9i) can be applied much faster than an Unna's boot. The pressure can be applied easily, the bandages can be removed easily, and the multilayer system creates a more uniform pressure and provides a layer for absorption of drainage. Still unclear at this time is whether short-stretch, long-stretch, or nonstretch bandages are superior in performance. Regardless of the type, the clinician must ensure that the bandaging does not create

excessive pressure and must provide the patient with emergency information on how and under what conditions to remove the compression bandaging. A simple test is to check capillary refill (Figures 10-10a and 10-10b). Compression pumps and bandages should be used until the clinician is certain that edema has been removed as

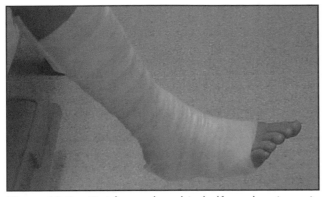

Figure 10-8c. First layer placed in half-overlapping spiral. This layer absorbs drainage and fills in irregularities on the foot and leg.

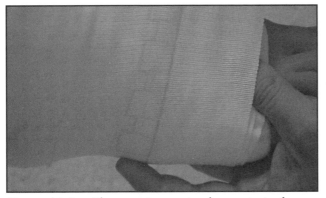

Figure 10-8e. Close-up image to demonstrate formation of squares on the bandage.

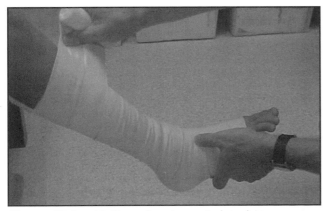

Figure 10-8g. Half-overlapping spiral technique completed.

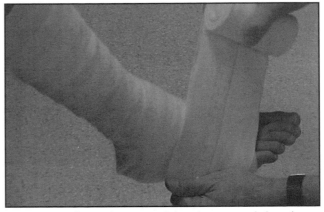

Figure 10-8d. Application of the short-stretch bandage, beginning at the metatarsal heads.

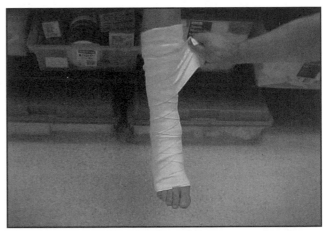

Figure 10-8f. Figure-of-eight technique completed.

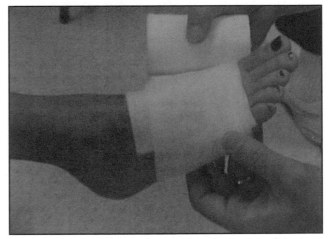

Figure 10-9a. Four-layer bandage application. Beginning of first (absorbent) layer, which serves the same function as described for the two-layer technique.

much as possible. This is determined most objectively by serial measurement with a foot volumeter. At this time, the patient should be fitted for custom compression stockings (Figure 10-11). The clinician must check the other leg to determine if venous insufficiency is also present in that extremity.

In multilayer bandaging systems, the first layer is generally an absorbent layer of cotton batting. This layer also

fills irregular areas such as those around the malleolus where pressure may be low without appropriate padding. Another layer generally found is a short-stretch bandage. A short-stretch bandage applies adequate pressure with lit-

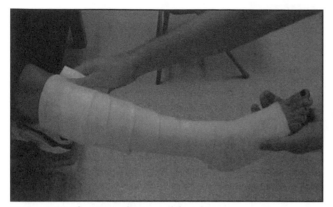

Figure 10-9b. Completion of first layer.

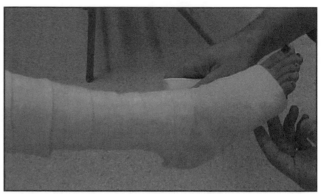

Figure 10-9c. Beginning of half-overlapping spiral technique with longer stretch bandage.

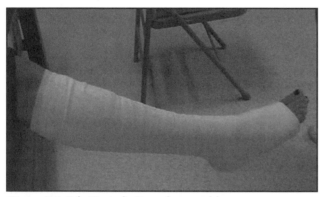

Figure 10-9d. Completion of second layer.

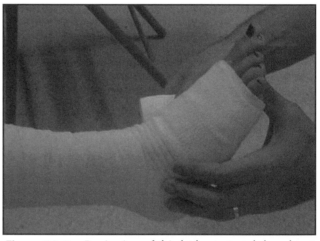

Figure 10-9e. Beginning of third (short-stretch bandage) layer in a figure-of-eight technique.

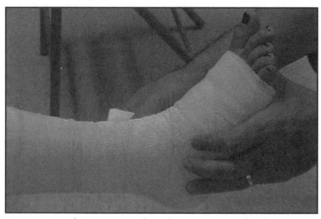

Figure 10-9f. Foot completed, starting up the leg.

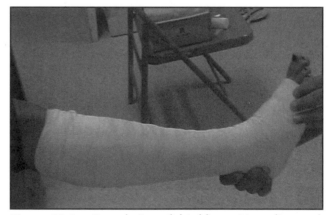

Figure 10-9g. Completion of third layer. Note diamond pattern generated by figure-of-eight technique.

tle increase in length, as opposed to ACE wraps, which elongate much more for the same increase in pressure. Many of the short-stretch bandages have calibrated markings to indicate the amount of pressure that will be exerted by the bandage at a given length. Typically, rectangles are elongated into squares when the appropriate length is achieved. An outside layer of cohesive bandage is frequently a component of the multilayer bandage system. Without the outer layer, what may be termed the "folding cup" phenomenon is likely to occur between clinic visits.

This phenomenon refers to the propensity for the upper turns of the elastic bandage(s) to become dislodged and slide down the leg in a manner ascribed to the collapsible camping cup. In a four-layer system, the second layer, which goes over the cotton batting, is a moderate-stretch

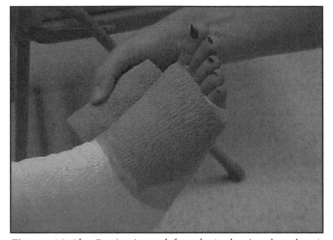

Figure 10-9h. Beginning of fourth (cohesive bandage) layer.

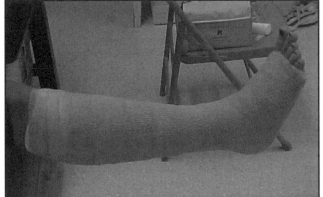

Figure 10-9i. Completion of fourth layer.

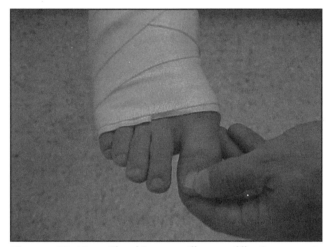

Figure 10-10a. Checking capillary refill. Pressure is applied to the great toe to cause blanching. Note close-up of diamond shape produced by figure-of-eight wrapping.

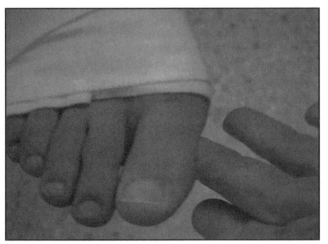

Figure 10-10b. Release and "pinking up" of nail bed due to normal capillary refill.

bandage; the third layer is a short-stretch bandage; and the fourth layer is a cohesive bandage. This type of bandage should be left in place as long as feasible, which typically is about 7 days.

Both half-overlapping spirals and figures of eight have been suggested for various layers of the bandaging systems. Half-overlapping spirals are simpler to apply but unravel more readily and may not control venous hypertension as well, whereas a figure-of-eight is difficult for the novice (can be performed almost as quickly as a spiral wrap by an experienced clinician) and appears to control venous hypertension more effectively. The cotton batting layer is generally applied with half-overlapping spirals with extra padding over irregular surfaces. Moderate stretch may be applied with half-overlapping spirals. Short-stretch bandages are expected to be wrapped in a figure-of-eight, and cohesive layers may be applied either way. An Unna's boot should be applied in a figure-of-eight to allow some movement between layers and to alleviate excessive pressure.

Wrapping should produce a greater pressure at the ankle and be progressively decreased as the bandage is wrapped more proximally. This pressure gradient can be automatically developed during the wrap by applying equal tension to the bandage as wrapping proceeds. Based on the law of LaPlace, tension equals pressure times radius ($\tau = P \times r$, where τ = tension in the bandage, P = pressure generated by the bandage on the limb, and r = radius of the bandage). Therefore, wrapping the bandage with a constant tension on the bandage as it is advanced from the foot toward the knee results in a greater pressure at the foot where the radius of the turns of the bandage is small and lower near the knee where the radius of the leg becomes largest.

Contraindications for Compression Therapy

The most important aspect of treating venous insufficiency is to first rule out arterial insufficiency. Although a

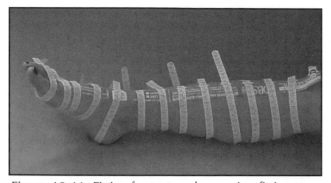

Figure 10-11. Fitting for custom hose using fitting tape provided by the manufacturer. Note the heel strap, which is used as a reference point in the manufacture of the stocking. Also note the irregular spacing on the foot. This is caused by the requirement to have the second-to-last strap around the metatarsal heads and the last strap at the base of the toe. On the leg, the straps should all be parallel to each other and perpendicular to the spine of the series of straps. Note the fourth strap from the knee is incorrectly applied for the purpose of this figure.

clear diagnosis of venous insufficiency may be made, arterial insufficiency must be ruled out thoroughly because some people may have both. Various experts suggest that an ABI of below 0.8 to 0.7 is a contraindication. Compression therapy will exacerbate arterial insufficiency and may threaten the limb. Other absolute contraindications include phlebitis and suspected deep venous thrombosis. Relative contraindications include those that may mobilize fluid from the lower extremities to a central circulation that cannot handle the extra fluid (congestive heart failure and pulmonary edema) and diminished sensation. In the case of diminished sensation, the concern is malfunction of the pump or foreign objects in the compression sleeve.

SUMMARY

Both arterial and venous insufficiency can create ulcers requiring skilled assessment and therapy. A thorough differential diagnosis is critically important. Arterial insufficiency can be an emergent surgical problem, and the treatment for venous insufficiency is contraindicated in the presence of arterial insufficiency. Arterial insufficiency may occur anywhere but is most common where vessels are the most distal—on the toes and heels. Venous insufficiency ulcers are located most commonly just proximal to the medial malleolus, sometimes proximal to the lateral

malleolus, and rarely elsewhere. Arterial insufficiency can be painful at rest, increasing with elevation, and the wounds tend to be pink rather than red. Venous insufficiency may cause an uncomfortable pressure in the leg, which is relieved by elevation; and the wounds tend to be red and very wet with hemosiderin staining of the skin surrounding the ulcer. Failure to treat the underlying venous hypertension is a frequent cause of failure to heal or recurrence of the leg ulcers. Compression therapy includes compression wrapping and sometimes pumping and fitting for custom stockings when edema is removed.

STUDY QUESTIONS

1. Which type of vascular ulcer tends to be dry? To be wet? What is the physiological basis of the moisture of these wounds?

2. Who is more likely to develop venous insufficiency—a tall person or a short person? A person who moves or one who stands all day?

3. Contrast arterial and venous ulcers in terms of how malnutrition of tissue occurs.

4. Why is compression contraindicated in the presence of arterial insufficiency? What simple test can be used to screen for arterial disease?

5. Why is compression therapy contraindicated in the presence of congestive heart failure?

REFERENCES

1. Lopez A, Phillips T. Venous ulcers. *Wounds.* 1998;10:149-157.

2. Rudolph DM. Pathophysiology and management of venous ulcers. *Journal of Wound, Ostomy, and Continence Nursing.* 1998;25:248-255.

3. Burnand KG, Browse NL. The cause of venous ulceration. *Lancet.* 1982;31:243.

4. Coleridge Smith PD, Thomas P, Scurr JH, Dormandy JA. Causes of venous ulceration: a new hypothesis. *British Medical Journal.* 1988;296:1726-1727.

5. Steins A, Junger M, Zuder D, Rassner G. Microcirculation in venous leg ulcers during healing: prognostic impact. *Wounds.* 1999;11:6-12.

6. Thomas Hess C. Management of the patient with a venous ulcer. *Advances in Wound and Skin Care.* 2000;13:79-83.

7. McGuckin M, Stineman MG, Goin JE, Williams SV. *Venous Leg Ulcer Guideline.* 1997; University of Pennsylvania; Philadelphia, Pa.

8. Blair SD, Wright DD, Backhouse CM, et al. Sustained compression and healing of venous ulcers. *British Medical Journal.* 1988;297:1159-1161.

Assessment of Wounds

OBJECTIVES

- List observations necessary for assessing wounds.
- Describe appropriate methods for documentation of the following and discuss the potential implications associated with: color of wounds, odor, drainage, extent, surrounding skin.
- Identify tissue types within a wound.
- Define and describe how to document tunneling, undermining, and sinus tracts.
- Describe and distinguish signs of infection and inflammation both locally and systemically.
- Perform differential diagnosis of wounds of different etiology.
- Provide a prognosis for different wounds; list factors that may alter the anticipated number of visits or time for reaching goals.

Previous chapters have been directed toward assessing a patient and describing characteristics of wounds of different etiology. The purpose of this chapter is to develop a systematic method of wound examination and testing to develop a differential diagnosis and a prognosis for reaching appropriate goals. Given two wounds with identical characteristics, patients with different cultural, work, and family backgrounds may have different goals or prognoses. In addition, comorbid conditions may have tremendous impact on prognosis. A systematic means of wound examination is described with the mnemonic "CODES." These five critical areas are color, odor, drainage, extent, and surrounding skin.

COLOR

This item refers to the color within the wound. The color of surrounding skin is discussed later. Three basic colors may be observed in a wound: black, yellow, and red. Black tissue within a wound represents desiccated necrotic tissue. With certain exceptions, black tissue should be debrided to allow migration of new cells to fill the defect and resurface it with epithelial cells. Mechanical, chemical, or sharp debridement should be used. An exception to debriding black tissue is the presence of dry gangrene, usually on the foot, caused by severe ischemia. Such advanced arterial insufficiency often requires amputation, and autoamputation of toes may occur. Debridement in the case of dry gangrene is unlikely to assist in healing due to the lack of delivery of nutrients necessary for healing. Rather, it exposes necrotic tissue to the risk of infection.

Yellow may represent one of three possibilities. *Pus* (purulent exudate) within a wound has a thick texture, usually an odor, and may have a color ranging from a greenish tint to a darker yellow. Purulence is a clear sign of infection with pyogenic (pus-producing) organisms, which may require the temporary use of topical antimicrobials or systemic antibiotic drugs, along with more aggressive debridement of the wound.

A second yellow substance is *fibrin*. Fibrinogen leaks from vessels during inflammation and is converted to fibrin. Fibrin is the end product of the blood coagulation cascade, forming an insoluble fiber that, along with platelets, creates thrombi. Fibrin forms a difficult to remove hardened sheet on wound beds, which may require debridement with specific chemicals or sharp instruments.

The third material is termed *slough* (pronounced sluff). This is partially solubilized necrotic tissue. It ranges from a grayish to brownish-yellow color depending on how well autolytic debridement (breakdown of necrotic tissue by enzymes produced by cells in the wound) is proceeding. Autolytic debridement is also associated with soupy brownish drainage and stringy tissue. It should not be confused with purulence. Although slough left under an occlu-

sive dressing (a dressing holding fluid under it) for a number of days may have an odor, this odor is milder than that associated with infection and will be lost when the wound is cleansed, whereas an infected wound will continue to have a foul odor after the wound is cleansed.

A beefy red color is observed in a clean, granulating wound. A wound with this color needs to be protected from both environmental factors and from harsh handling by the clinician or other caregiver. Appropriate dressings for clean, granulating wounds are discussed in Chapter 15. A lighter pink color indicates poor arterial circulation. A dusky red is an indication of impending necrosis suggesting infection of the granulation tissue.

ODOR

A foul-smelling wound is usually, but not always, infected. Infection, by definition, is the presence of greater than 100,000 organisms per gram of tissue. A wound with a strong foul odor from a distance or with the dressing still in place, however, is very likely to be infected. Large quantities of slough, may have an odor, and a clinician must be prepared to distinguish the odor of an occluded wound from infection. Certain organisms produce characteristic odors. Although words may fail to describe odors well, a fruity odor is characteristic of infection with *Pseudomonas aeruginosa*. Pseudomonas is also characterized by bluish-green color on the wound surface and greenish drainage. Treatment for Pseudomonas infection is frequently a topical application of acetic acid, the active ingredient of vinegar, which also has a characteristic odor. Proteus produces a characteristic ammonia odor.

DRAINAGE

Drainage should be described both in terms of quantity and quality. Terms used to describe the quantity are rather subjective. A continuum of terms such as desiccated, minimum, moderate, and maximum (or copious) is used. The terms *desiccated* and *maximum* are easy to distinguish. A wound bed that is dry needs intervention to increase its moisture to a level compatible with healing. Treatment of desiccation is described in Chapter 15. The term *maximum* or *copious* drainage may be used when the primary dressing (dressing directly in contact with the wound) and secondary dressings are soaked with drainage. A small area of moisture on the primary dressing may be described as *minimum*. Moderate drainage may be appropriate when the primary dressing is nearly full but not saturated with drainage. However, judgment of quantity may be difficult when the time that the dressing has been in place is not constant. For example, a dressing may be changed overnight or during early morning rounds with no indication of how long the dressing has been accumu-

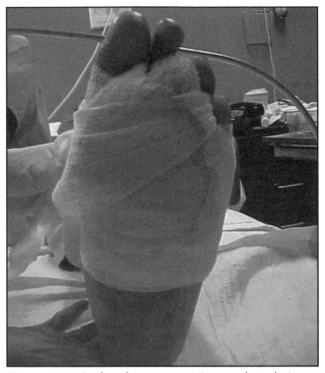

Figure 11-1. Red and green sanguinopurulent drainage of a diabetic foot infected with *Pseudomonas aeruginosa*. (Also shown in Color Atlas following page 274.)

lating drainage. Copious drainage needs to be managed by selecting an appropriate dressing or combination of dressings to absorb drainage and protect the surrounding skin from excessive moisture. Optimizing healing is often a balancing act of maintaining wound moisture without maceration of surrounding skin and requires good clinical judgment.

The color and consistency of drainage is also important. Clear drainage is caused by leakage of fluid from blood vessels during inflammation. By definition, a clear fluid consisting of water and small particles such as electrolytes is a *transudate*, whereas *exudate* contains larger elements such as cells and proteins. If the equivalent of serum (the fluid part of blood with removal of proteins) is present, the adjective *serous* is used. Because serum and transudate represent the same type of fluid, the term *serous exudate* should not be used. Moreover, distinction between exudate and transudate cannot always be made visually. On the other hand, purulent exudate is acceptable terminology. This fluid obviously has cells and proteins in it. The safest term to use is *drainage* if the clinician is unsure if the fluid is transudate or exudate.

Soupy brownish drainage is associated with autolytic debridement (breakdown of necrotic tissue using enzymes produced by macrophages and other cells). An example of copious bluish green sanguinopurulent drainage (bloody/purulent) due to *Pseudomonas aeruginosa* infec-

tion is depicted in Figure 11-1. Copious serous drainage indicates either venous insufficiency or inflammation and a need to reduce handling of the wound and to provide adequate absorption to prevent maceration. A desiccated wound indicates the need to use a dressing to retain fluid within the wound and to add moisture to a wound using dressings described in Chapter 15.

EXTENT

The extent of a wound may be assessed in many ways. The two basic methods are to measure representative distances or to measure volume. Measurement of only the surface area of a wound is suitable in the absence of subcutaneous tissue involvement. A means of establishing consistent directions for the measurement is the clock notation. Using the clock notation, we indicate the cephalic direction on the trunk or proximal direction on a limb as 12:00 and the caudal direction on the trunk or distal direction on a limb as 6:00. Three generally accepted means of measuring across a wound are in existence. One method is to measure the greatest width and greatest length regardless of the shape of the wound. In some facilities, the greatest length and width are multiplied to provide a crude approximation of surface area of the wound. A second method is to measure the greatest dimension across the wound and the distance perpendicular to this measurement, and multiply the numbers. The third means is to measure width and length regardless of size. In this third method, length is defined as the distance across the wound from 12:00 to 6:00 and width is defined from 3:00 to 9:00. Figures 11-2a and 11-2b show examples of each method. Other individuals have termed length as the greatest distance across a wound and width as the dimension perpendicular to length.

Tools for measuring the distance across the wound include sterile cotton-tipped applicators, transparent grids, and plastic materials such as sandwich bags. Sterile cotton-tipped applicators offer the advantage of low cost. The wooden end is held to one edge of the wound as the thumb of a gloved hand is slid to the opposite side of the wound. The cotton-tipped applicator is then held close to a ruler to measure distance in centimeters. If the wound is less than 1 cm across, the distance may be reported in millimeters instead. A number of companies supply clear plastic templates for wound measurements. Some of these are found in sterile dressing packages; these may be placed directly on the wound for measurement. Otherwise, clean plastic templates may be held over a wound, but not in direct contact, to measure it. These devices have a centimeter scale along one edge and a calibrated system in the middle. Many of these systems are a series of concentric circles or ellipses. Care must be taken to determine if the numbers written on the wound template refer to the radius

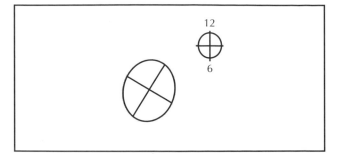

Figure 11-2a. Methods of measuring length and width with a cotton-tipped applicator. Measuring the greatest distance across the wound and perpendicular to the greatest distance, a clock is drawn to give a frame of reference with 12:00 as either superior or proximal and 6:00 as either inferior or distal.

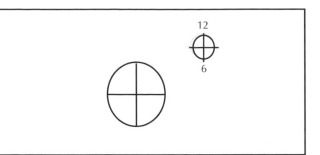

Figure 11-2b. Measuring the length of the wound as 12:00 to 6:00 and width of the wound as 3:00 to 9:00.

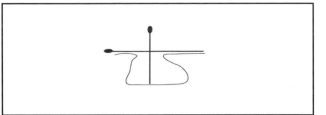

Figure 11-3. Measuring wound depth with a cotton-tipped applicator. A second cotton-tipped applicator is placed across the wound to indicate the zero point for depth, rather than estimating the top of the wound by eye.

or the diameter of the concentric circles or ellipses. Wound templates are placed over the wound and allow both length and width to be read rapidly.

A more exact system is to use a plastic sheet material such as plastic wrap or a sandwich bag to trace a wound for a permanent record. Simple measurement of length across a wound is not sufficient to determine cross-sectional area of a wound. Multiplying length times width usually over-estimates the surface area, unless the wound happens to be rectangular. A highly irregularly shaped wound may need to be measured at multiple locations. In such cases, a map of the wound should be drawn in the medical record with representative distances marked clearly on the map. A tracing of the wound can be retraced on a computer or by the use of a planimeter to compute surface area accurately. The problem with using a single sheet of plastic is the potential for contamination. A sandwich bag or a doubled-over piece of plastic wrap allows the top layer to be kept for the permanent record and allows disposal of the surface in contact with the wound.

Volume of a wound should be determined for wounds with significant subcutaneous involvement such as stage IV pressure ulcers. The volume of shallow wounds such as burns, stage II or III pressure ulcers, arterial ulcers, or venous insufficiency ulcers does not provide useful information. The simplest means of providing an index of volume is to measure wound depth with a cotton-tipped applicator (Figure 11-3). If a wound has substantial depth, a means of localizing the skin surface is to place a cotton-tipped applicator across the wound and place the wooden stick end into the wound next to the cotton-tipped applicator. Having a measurement of length, width, and depth provides a crude approximation of wound volume. If a wound has multiple depths, a map of the wound may need to be drawn with depths indicated on the map. A more precise means of volume determination is to fill the wound with either sterile saline or hydrogel from a premeasured

syringe. Volume of the syringe is recorded again after the wound is filled from the syringe. Volume is simply calculated by subtracting the final volume of the syringe from its initial volume. A related means is to use dental impression gel, such as Jeltrate (Dentsply International, Inc., Milford, Del). An equal volume of warm water is added to the powder from the canister and mixed. Before the material hardens, it can be placed into the wound to harden. Jeltrate is biocompatible and easily removed from a wound after it hardens. The impression of the wound can be placed in a graduated cylinder to determine wound volume.

Undermining, tunneling, and sinus tracts represent areas of tissue injury under intact skin. Undermining can be visualized as a cliff caused by necrosis of more metabolically active tissue that is more susceptible to hypoxia. In addition, shearing injuries are likely to produce undermining. The term *tunneling* describes a linear erosion between fascial planes. *Undermining* is demonstrated in Figure 11-3, which also depicts measuring depth with a cotton-tipped applicator. Undermining is often associated with pressure ulcers. To document undermining, a broken line is drawn to indicate the distance of undermining and to denote the radius involved. One may also use clock notation to indicate the area of undermining. For example, in Figure 11-4 undermining is present from 1:00 to 6:00.

A *sinus tract* is caused by erosion of subcutaneous tissue from one wound into another wound, often an abscess. A

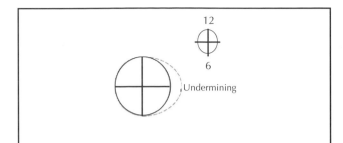

Figure 11-4. Documenting undermining. The typical arc of undermining below an edge of a pressure ulcer is denoted with a dotted line. Numbers representing the distance of the undermining may be written on the diagram or as text in a note.

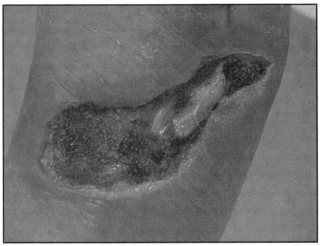

Figure 11-5a. Documenting tissue types. A dorsal foot wound with 100% granulation tissue. Note that much of the granulation tissue has a pink color, indicative of diminished arterial flow. Also note the presence of tendons within the wound bed. Tendons must not be confused with necrotic tissue. (Also shown in Color Atlas following page 274.)

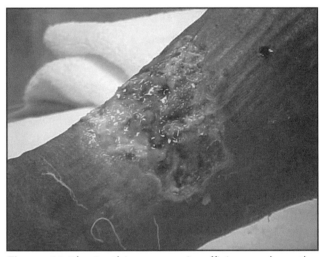

Figure 11-5b. In this venous insufficiency ulcer, the wound consists of approximately 10% black necrotic tissue, 40% yellow necrotic tissue, and 50% granulation tissue.

tunnel is a blind linear erosion of subcutaneous tissue. The locations of tunnels and sinus tracts may be documented using clock notation and the distance the tunnel or sinus tract extends under the skin. An example is a 5 cm tunnel at 11:00.

Within the wound, an estimated percentage of the wound bed of different tissue types or colors should be documented. One may use the terms: 1) granulation tissue versus necrotic tissue; 2) granulation tissue, slough, and eschar; or 3) red, yellow, and black and give percentages adding up to 100%. Examples of these ways of reporting include: 1) 40% granulation tissue and 60% necrotic tissue; 2) 40% granulation tissue, 30% slough, and 30% eschar; or 3) 40% red, 30% yellow, and 30% black (Figures 11-5a and 11-5b). The shape of the wound, if not drawn, should also be described. A round or elliptical wound is a reliable sign that the wound was caused by tissue loading such as pressure or shear. Vascular wounds

tend to have irregular shapes. Arterial insufficiency produces a dry depression due to the loss of moisture from the necrotic tissue.

SURROUNDING SKIN

Due to total focus on the wound itself, the surrounding skin is often neglected to the detriment of wound healing. Surrounding skin is the primary source of new epithelial cells to resurface wounds. Unhealthy surrounding skin will slow healing tremendously, even if the wound fills with granulation tissue. Moreover, potential problems with wound healing frequently show in surrounding skin first. The areas of concern are maceration, inflammation, hydration, nutrition, callus or hyperkeratosis, and induration. The color of skin may also provide important information.

Maceration is a result of excessive hydration of skin (see Figure 3-7). It can be seen in normal skin following long exposure to moisture, such as long baths or swimming. The macerated skin becomes swollen and lighter in color, in addition to an appearance of fissuring. Surrounding skin becomes macerated from using dressings that cannot keep drainage off the surrounding skin, not changing dressings frequently enough, or failure to use moisture barriers or skin sealants that protect the skin from moisture. An additional consideration is rough handling of the wound or placing cotton gauze in direct contact with the wound, leading to chronic inflammation of the wound bed.

Inflammation is readily detectible by its cardinal signs of heat, redness, swelling, and pain. Surrounding skin may be inflamed from either infection or rough handling of the wound. The clinician needs to be able to distinguish between these two possibilities. The presence of purulence and odor indicates infection. The lack of purulence and odor does not rule out infection. Culture or needle biopsy of a wound may be necessary to rule out infection.

Skin hydration and turgor are examined together. With normal aging, both hydration and turgor may be lost. Normally hydrated skin conforms to the surface below and resists compression. This is tested by pinching a fold of skin. Dehydrated skin without turgor folds into a tent shape and remains tented. In certain areas of the body, notably the neck, tenting is present in elderly individuals without pinching the skin. Elderly skin is at high risk for damage due to trauma, in particular the indiscriminate removal of the tape.

Skin nutrition is assessed by visual inspection for hair, nails, and thickness of skin. Hair loss, thickening of nails, and thinning of skin is common with aging, diabetes mellitus, and arterial insufficiency.

Hyperkeratosis or callus formation is the excessive thickening of skin frequently caused by chronic shearing of the skin. Formation of callus is normal on the hands of manual laborers. It is also a sign of abnormal shearing force when it is detected on feet. With loss of sweating, altered foot structure, and biomechanics of diabetes, callus formation is common. Callus must be trimmed from the foot to prevent excessive localized pressure. Callus frequently forms around neuropathic ulcers. Due to its hardness, it creates high pressure on the skin surrounding the wound and may enlarge the wound if it is not removed. Debridement of callus is discussed in Chapter 13.

Induration is the process of the skin "becoming hard." It is a red flag for the clinician to look for undermining, tunneling, sinus tracts, or infection. It is detected by palpation of the surrounding skin of a wound. If induration is palpated, the area under the skin should be examined for one of the processes listed above.

The color of the surrounding skin should also be documented. Redness indicates inflammation or infection. White indicates lack of blood flow or arterial insufficiency. Blue coloration or cyanosis is a sign of severe lack of oxygen in the tissue due to arterial insufficiency, heart failure, or respiratory disease. A blackened area surrounding a wound represents necrosis, probably due to severe arterial disease. A yellowish-brown, variegated coloration, especially when it is located on the lower part of the leg near the malleoli, is indicative of venous insufficiency as described in Chapter 10.

TESTS AND MEASURES

Appropriate tests and measures to assist in diagnosis and prognosis include temperature, ankle-brachial index (discussed in Chapter 10), culture (discussed in Chapter 19), and tests described in Chapter 5 for sensation, mobility, strength, range of motion, gait, need, and use of assistive devices.

Temperature may be assessed simply by palpation and comparison to other parts of the body. A more reliable indication of temperature, however, is use of either a thermistor or radiometer to measure temperature. These devices are very accurate, precise, and reliable. A thermistor measures temperature using a probe that varies in resistance to the current applied to it with temperature. Radiometers measure infrared radiation to determine temperature. Thermistor systems are relatively inexpensive if used on a large number of persons. The thermistors can be cleaned and disinfected between patients. The advantage of a radiometer is its ability to measure temperature without coming in direct contact with a wound. These devices, however, are very expensive.

DIAGNOSIS

Generally, acute wounds are not difficult to diagnose. Certain types of chronic wounds, however, need to be identified by etiology to determine the proper plan of care to address the underlying cause. Mechanical causes may include open fracture, degloving, laceration, incision, and abrasion (road rash). Thermal injuries include burn, scald, and frostbite. In addition, the cause of the burn, whether contact, flash, or ignition of clothing, should be noted. Chemical and radiation burns and dehiscence of a surgical wound can also be determined from history as well as toxic ulcerations (eg, those caused by brown recluse spider bites). Differential diagnosis is particularly important in determining whether the patient has a pressure ulcer, a neuropathic ulcer, or if the ulcer is caused by venous or arterial insufficiency. The history, physical examination, and special tests should be sufficiently rigorous to determine the cause. However, diabetes can predispose an individual to arterial, pressure, and neuropathic ulcers; and because venous insufficiency is so common, a person can have a combination of conditions.

Pressure ulcers should be classified according to NPUAP definitions as stage I, II, III, or IV based on the depth of structures involved, as described in Chapter 9. Before a stage is determined, however, the base of the wound should be visible. Several days of debridement may be required before an accurate staging can be performed.

The Wagner grading system is commonly used for neuropathic ulcers (see Chapter 8). However, the grading system does not grade the severity of the wound, but the severity of the injury to the foot. It combines aspects of neuropathy and arterial insufficiency. By definition, a Wagner grade 0 indicates intact skin, although the skin may be poised to break down. Grade 1 represents a superficial ulcer, grade 2 represents a deep ulcer, and grade 3 includes infection as indicated by abscess or osteomyelitis. Gangrene of the forefoot is documented as grade 4, and grade 5 represents gangrene of most of the foot.

Burns should be classified by the depth of tissue injury. Older terminology of first-, second-, and third-degree burn continues in common use today. Injury limited to damage of the epidermis with inflammation of the dermis is documented as a superficial or first-degree burn, which is equivalent to sunburn. Injury to the superficial dermis causes sufficient inflammation for fluid to accumulate between the dermis and epidermis, thereby producing the blisters characteristic of superficial partial-thickness or second-degree burns. The two other classes of burns are more difficult to distinguish from each other. Both may have a charred, pearly, or khaki, hardened appearance. The difference between a deep partial-thickness and a full-thickness burn is observable if preservation of hair follicles and blood vessels can be determined. In a deep partial thickness burn, hair follicles and blood vessels in the deep dermis are still viable. Tugging on a hair can be used to distinguish the two. However, in certain types of burn injuries, especially those involving flames, hairs may be singed and not available for testing. In a full-thickness burn, a tugged hair slides easily from the follicle. Resistance to tugging indicates a deep partial-thickness injury. Blanching with pressure indicates the presence of viable blood vessels and therefore a deep partial-thickness burn, whereas a wound with a full-thickness injury is not blanchable. Burns are explored further in Chapter 19.

Other types of wounds should be classified by the depth of injury into superficial, partial thickness, full thickness, or full thickness with subcutaneous involvement. Many individuals, however, incorrectly attempt to use the NPUAP definitions for wounds with causes other than pressure. A superficial wound exhibits damage to the epidermis only and may display some erythema. No treatment other than protection is usually needed. These wounds are usually caused by mild abrasion of the skin. Partial-thickness wounds have evidence of damage through the epidermis and into the dermis. These injuries include skin tears, deeper abrasions, blisters, partial-thickness graft donor sites, and others. Full-thickness wounds injure the skin through the entirety of the dermis. Causes include full-thickness skin graft donor sites, venous insufficiency ulcers, surgical wounds, neuropathic wounds, and degloving or avulsion injuries. Full-thickness wounds with

subcutaneous involvement injure tissues below the skin, including subcutaneous fat, muscle, tendon, ligament, and bone. Surgical wounds, arterial insufficiency, pressure, and open fractures are common causes of this type of wound.

Next, the clinician must determine the current phase of healing and whether a wound is failing to progress from one phase to the other or becomes chronic in a given stage of wound healing. A nonhealing wound may be chronically in the inflammatory, proliferative, epithelializing, or remodeling stage. The wound may also fail in one of these steps: inflammation, proliferation, epithelialization, or remodeling.

Critical decision-making points are whether the wound is infected; requires debridement; requires filling of depth, undermining, tunnels, or sinus tracts; and the degree of drainage. Many of these points are addressed together; however, in some cases the clinician may need to work with competing goals to optimize wound healing. For example, sharp debridement accomplishes the goals of treating infection and the presence of large quantities of necrotic tissue. On the other hand, use of autolytic debridement and preventing maceration of surrounding skin may be difficult.

The assessment for wound infection has been described frequently by the mnemonic "IFEE." An infected wound often has the characteristics of induration, fever, erythema, and edema. The odor and color of drainage from the wound can aid in this determination. The presence of dusky or brownish patches within the wound is also very suggestive of wound infection.

Debridement can be a difficult decision process and is discussed extensively in Chapters 12 and 13. Filling or packing a wound is discussed in Chapter 15 and is dependent on the presence of undermining, tunneling, sinus tracts, and the risk of abscess formation. Deciding on a dressing based on the drainage of a wound is also discussed in Chapter 15. In addition, a choice of using skin sealants and moisture barriers is described in Chapter 15.

A diagnosis and prognosis based on the *Guide to Physical Therapist Practice*[1] can be made. These patterns are straightforward, except when other systems are also affected (eg, with multiple trauma). Pattern A, primary prevention should be applied to individuals at risk for neuropathic ulcers, pressure ulcers, and venous insufficiency ulcers. Prevention of arterial insufficiency ulcers may be limited to detection of arterial insufficiency and referral to a vascular surgeon. Pattern B is applied to those with superficial skin involvement and may be limited to patient education. Pattern C describes partial-thickness wounds and may involve multiple interventions including a brief course of direct intervention and patient education. Full-thickness injuries are described by Pattern D, and Pattern E includes involvement of fascia, bone, or muscle. Both Patterns D and E require substantial direct intervention including debridement, dressing changes, possible adjunctive therapies, work or lifestyle modifications, and patient education.

Prognosis is the predicted optimal level of improvement in function and amount of time to reach that level based on the information available. Goals refer to remediation of impairments and may address characteristics of the wound and specific deficits in related areas (eg, limited mobility). The prognosis is based on multiple factors and is not limited to the wound itself. For example, a person who remains on his feet all day will have more difficulty in healing a venous insufficiency or neuropathic ulcer. Home resources and the ability to learn how to handle the wound at home are also important prognostic indicators. An example of a prognosis is that the wound will be clean and stable and ready for grafting in 10 visits and the patient will return to all previous roles in 6 weeks. The goal of the clinician's intervention also needs to be considered. In many cases, involvement may simply be limited to providing a clean, stable wound ready for grafting or delayed primary closure. Another common goal is to have the wound stable enough for the patient and any caregivers to manage at home with or without home health assistance. In longer-term health care settings, complete healing may be the goal of therapy. Goals may include prevention of pressure ulcers, protection of a wound, prevention of contamination or infection, management of drainage, management of edema, complete healing (more reasonable for long-term care rather than in an acute care facility), clean and stable wound (typical for acute care) with self-care, follow-up with home health or long-term facility, clean and stable wound ready for surgical closure or a clean and stable wound ready for grafting. Outcomes should be addressed relative to history, such as return to family, work, and social roles, or may include need for modified assistance using equipment, continued care in a different type of facility, or the need for assistance at home. These may include minimizing limitation of function, optimizing health status, preventing disability, and optimizing patient satisfaction.

Interventions are discussed in the plan of care (see Chapter 20). Within the assessment, the clinician may need to note that debridement of necrotic tissue may initially increase the size of the wound. An argument should also be developed for the plan of care in terms of frequency of treatment, particular type of dressing, method of cleansing wound, and type of debridement.

SUMMARY

Assessment of the wound requires clinical judgment based on objective tests, history provided by the patient or caregiver, and direct observation by the clinician. Whereas acute wounds usually present no problem with determining the cause, many chronic wounds may not present an obvious cause. In addition, the clinician needs to determine why the wound failed to heal and why any previous treatment failed. Observation of the wound can be based on the CODES system. Measurement of surface area is sufficient for superficial or full-thickness wounds. For wounds with substantial subcutaneous involvement, either wound volume or depth characteristic of the wound need to be documented. A discussion of the systems for characterizing wounds of different types is provided.

STUDY QUESTIONS

1. Why is the color of the wound important in the diagnosis and prognosis for a wound?
2. What is the importance of the condition of the surrounding skin of a wound?
3. What types of wounds require measurement of the volume or depth?
4. What influence does the history have on diagnosis of a chronic wound?
5. Why must social and work history need to be considered to develop a prognosis?

REFERENCE

1. American Physical Therapy Association. Guide to physical therapist practice. *Physical Therapy.* 1997;77:1177-1619.

Interventions

Having taken a history, performed a physical examination, and evaluated the wound, the clinician is prepared to make decisions appropriate for the given wound and patient. These decisions are elaborated in the plan of care. Although many combinations of interventions are possible and any number may be appropriate for a given wound, an understanding of the patient's situation will limit the possibilities. Moreover, the clinician should anticipate a progression of interventions, including contingency plans, foreseeing possible outcomes of the interventions, and determining appropriate referral to other health care providers and type of patient education. Different interventions and a description of appropriate indications for them are presented in the subsequent chapters of this unit. The issue of informed consent, as well as other ethical issues, needs to be addressed for all interventions. The four basic ethical principles are *beneficence*, *nonmaleficence*, *utility*, and *autonomy*. Beneficence is the cornerstone of the patient/clinician relationship. The patient trusts the clinician to provide services for the benefit of the patient. With this in mind, we are ethically bound to provide the optimum plan of care (see Chapter 20) for each patient as an individual. Nonmaleficence implies that the patient can trust the clinician to not intentionally injure him or her. Utility is based on the principle of risk/benefit ratio. Based on this principle, the clinician designs a plan of care that provides the greatest benefit relative to the risk. Although utility is a greater issue in prescribing medicine or performing surgery, the clinician involved in wound management needs to explore the risk and benefits of the plan of care and understand the patient's willingness to incur more or less risk to increase the chances of benefit. The fourth principle, autonomy, is the basis of informed consent. As described for utility, certain risks and benefits may be derived from interventions and education provided by the clinician. The patient has a reasonable expectation to be informed sufficiently to consent to any interventions. Included in informed consent are the risks associated with the procedure, benefits expected to be derived from the procedure, and the risk of choosing to forego the proposed intervention. The level of informed consent is likely to vary tremendously from facility to facility and for different procedures. A minimum of an oral informed consent should be obtained for each procedure, whereas some facilities may desire a written and signed informed consent form for each procedure. In particular, surgery or procedures that may be perceived as surgery, such as sharp debridement, should have a written, signed informed consent form.

Debridement

OBJECTIVES

- List indications and contraindications for debridement.
- Describe what tissues require debridement and risks of debridement.
- Describe indications for nonselective and selective debridement.
- Describe types of mechanical debridement including whirlpool and pulsatile lavage with concurrent suction, and list indications.
- List types of chemical debriding agents and their indications.
- Describe how to optimize an environment for autolytic debridement and give indications for autolytic debridement.

Debridement is a time-honored and frequently performed aspect of wound management. However, for each individual patient, the clinician should ask, why should I debride this particular wound and what is the optimal method?

Reasons for Debridement

Optimizing wound healing is a reasonable goal for any case. Because desiccated tissue acts as a barrier to cell migration, its removal via debridement is a clear benefit to patients. However, even moist necrotic tissue is problematic. Slough occupies space within a wound and thereby decreases the ability of cells to migrate. Devitalized tissue prolongs inflammation and delays the onset of proliferation of new cells to fill a wound. Inflammation, in turn, leads to leakage of blood vessels in the wound bed, leading to loss of protein and fluid through open wounds. Leakage of proteins causes additional problems. Fibrinogen leaking onto the surface of the wound is converted into the hard, insoluble protein coat of fibrin on the surface of a wound. Loss of protein from the vascular space leads to edema and malnutrition both locally in the dependent areas in which edema occurs and in general in the form of protein malnutrition.

Debridement is also important to decrease the potential for infection. Dead tissue acts as a medium for infection, and devitalized tissue may hide infection, abscesses, tunnels, and sinus tracts. Rapid debridement can bring a wound into bacterial balance. In one series of patients, pressure ulcers that had a bacterial burden of greater than 100,000 per gram were sharply debrided. Of these, 96% remained at less than 100 per gram. According to Robson,[1] the ideal environment is one in which the bacteria are in balance—not bacteria-free. Low levels of bacteria may accelerate certain aspects of wound healing, but a burden greater than 100,000 per gram severely retards healing. In particular, the production of proteases capable of breaking down growth factors and the attraction of neutrophils appear to be responsible. The presence of beta hemolytic streptococci is particularly problematic in even low numbers. Fibrinolysins, leukocidins, hemolysins and hyaluronidase allow the bacteria to protect themselves from the immune system and spread through tissue. In addition to the benefits of debridement, we must also consider the risks associated with not debriding. These include slow healing, osteomyelitis, the need for amputation of an infected limb, advancing cellulitis, sepsis, and in extreme cases, death. On these bases, debridement generally meets the definition of medical necessity.

Wound Cleansing

Wound cleansing during the initial visit and at each dressing change has been recommended by the AHCPR.[2] Prevention of injury during cleansing is emphasized.

Wound cleansing is discussed further in Chapter 18. Some authorities recommend against using any direct scrubbing action on the wound. Others have even challenged the notion that wound cleansing must be done with every dressing change. However, the clinician who must assess the wound during a dressing change must cleanse the wound sufficiently to make appropriate decisions for further management. The AHCPR recommendation is for use of normal saline or certain types of specialized detergents with a mild irrigation pressure that allows wound cleansing without traumatizing the wound bed or driving bacteria into the wound. The recommended safe and effective ulcer irrigation pressure range is between 4 and 15 psi. Whirlpool treatment is only recommended by the AHCPR for cleansing pressure ulcers with thick exudate, slough, or necrotic tissue, but never on clean ulcers; whirlpool therapy should be discontinued when the ulcer is clean. Irrigation or whirlpool can be useful, in particular, to clean residues of materials such as silver sulfadiazine from full- and partial-thickness burns and to encourage range of motion exercises in the moving water. Wound cleansing may also be done with a minimal amount of mechanical force with gauze, cloth, sponges, and either normal saline or special detergents. The AHCPR clearly recommends that clinicians not use antiseptic agents or disinfectants such as sodium hypochlorite, Dakin's solution, H_2O_2, iodine, acetic acid, or skin cleansers such as hexachlorophene and chlorhexidine, or povidone iodine scrub on pressure ulcers. Although these agents may be appropriate for initial cleansing of the acute wound, this recommendation against use of antiseptic agents on pressure ulcers should be extended to other chronic wounds. Lack of understanding the differences between gross contamination of acute wounds and colonization of chronic wounds is likely the source of referrals for cleansing wounds with these agents used for acute wounds.[2]

Debridement

AHCPR guidelines are vague on this issue. The guidelines call for removal of any necrotic tissue from the wound if consistent with goals, to select the method most appropriate to the patient's condition and goals and the need to assess and control pain. The guidelines also state that any one or a combination of sharp, mechanical, enzymatic, or autolytic debridement techniques may be used unless an urgent need for drainage or removal of devitalized tissue with sharp debridement arises. Indications for urgent sharp debridement include advancing cellulitis or sepsis.

Sharp debridement is the most rapid means of debridement and is the most appropriate for debriding thick, adherent eschar and extensive quantities of necrotic tissue from ulcers. Sharp debridement is discussed in more detail in the next chapter. Smaller wounds may be sharply debrided at bedside. However, extensive sharp debridement must be done in an operating room or special procedures room. Although not all wound care requires sterile technique, sharp debridement must be done with sterile instruments. A clean, dry dressing should be applied for 8 to 24 hours if bleeding occurs. After bleeding ceases, moist dressings, if appropriate, should be used again. In addition, sharp debridement is reserved for clinicians who meet licensing requirements and have demonstrated skill in this technique. Because of the availability of different methods for individuals with different treatment goals and in different settings (eg, inpatient versus home health) the recommendation for debridement of pressure ulcers cannot be more specific.

Heel ulcers have received special consideration in terms of debridement. AHCPR guidelines state that "heel ulcers with dry eschar need not be debrided if they do not have edema, erythema, fluctuance, drainage." However, the guidelines also state clearly that such wounds should be assessed daily for complications that may require debridement. One source of the controversy is the singling out of heel ulcers. Wounds with dry eschar on other body parts are not addressed specifically. Another important recommendation that is discussed further in Chapter 17 is pain management. AHCPR guidelines very specifically recommend the prevention or management of pain associated with debridement as needed.

TYPES OF DEBRIDEMENT

Four basic types of debridement are typically described: *sharp, mechanical* (nonspecific), *chemical,* and *autolytic.* The type of debridement suitable for a given wound—as with any intervention—depends on the complete clinical picture including characteristics of the wound, characteristics of the patient, social and work responsibilities, available resources, and the setting in which the patient is being seen. Important factors to consider in deciding which type of debridement to use include the type of wound (etiology); the amount of necrotic tissue, which may not be observable initially; the condition of the patient, including terminal illness; the care setting, which includes time constraints on discharge; and clinician or caregiver experience. The clinician must examine the depth of the wound for necrotic tissue using good lighting and should be familiar with different tissue types. The clinician should consider patient preferences. Issues related to patient preference include the time frame for the plan of care, pain and psychological issues, and who will be performing the dressing changes.

Mechanical Debridement

To remove necrotic tissue from a wound quickly, mechanical shearing or scrubbing forces can be applied. Most of these techniques cannot discriminate healthy and necrotic tissue and are often discussed as a means of non-

specific debridement. One simple technique is scrubbing the necrotic tissue with a gauze or other type of sponge. Rather than using direct scrubbing on the wound, some clinicians will utilize hydrotherapy and irrigation. Hydrotherapy and wound irrigation are useful for softening and mechanical removal of eschar and debris. A recommended method is irrigation through a 19-gauge angiocath or equivalent to produce an optimal irrigation pressure. Too little pressure is ineffective in removal of necrotic tissue, whereas excessive pressure may drive bacteria into the wound.

Wet-to-Dry Dressings

A very popular technique, but largely used inappropriately, is the wet-to-dry dressing. A moistened gauze sponge (frequently 4 x 4) is placed into the necrotic area and is allowed to dry completely. The adherent necrotic tissue is pulled out of the wound with the 4 x 4. This procedure can be very painful and is very nonspecific in that healthy tissue may be removed along with the necrotic tissue. Wet-to-dry dressings should be changed every 4 to 6 hours using adequate analgesia. Moreover, the clinician should avoid placing a dry dressing on granulation tissue. Removal of dry dressings from granulation tissue causes bleeding and damages the new tissue. Done properly, this technique can provide rapid debridement prior to operative repair. The patient can be discharged to home when the wound is clean and stable, although sharp debridement may produce a better outcome. Wet-to-dry dressings are not cost-effective for small wounds or wounds with little necrotic tissue, nor do they have any place in a setting that does not have severe time constraints. Ethical considerations contraindicate wet-to-dry dressings unless a clear benefit to the patient can be demonstrated. Pain and the loss of healthy tissue must be counterbalanced with an improved outcome such as earlier discharge from the hospital to meet ethical standards. The use of wet-to-dry dressings under circumstances in which a gentler method yields a similar outcome must be considered unethical. The purpose of the wet-to-dry dressing is also undermined when clinicians soak the dressing off the wound. If an order is received for a wet-to-dry dressing and the clinician determines that this approach is inappropriate, the clinician should arrange a discussion with the referring physician explaining the appropriate options.

Dextranomers

Filling wounds with dextranomers may also be considered a means of mechanical debridement. Dextranomers are beads placed in a wound to absorb exudate, bacteria, and wound debris. Dextranomers are rinsed out of the wound and changed daily. However, when very rapid debridement is required (eg, with advancing infection), sharp debridement is indicated and nonselective, mechanical debridement should be stopped.

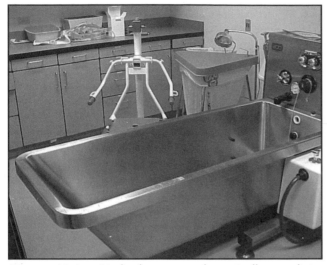

Figure 12-1a. Hydrotherapy tank typically used in wound care. The unit has a built-in water jet that allows the entire body to be submerged.

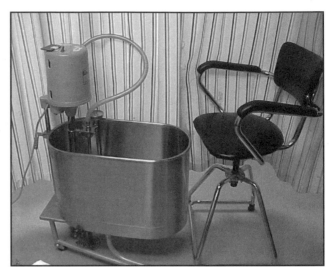

Figure 12-1b. Hand/foot tank may be used for wounds on the distal leg and foot, and the distal forearm and hand.

Hydrotherapy

A typical hydrotherapy session is carried out in a whirlpool tank (Figures 12-1a through 12-1c) for 20 minutes with water at a temperature generally in excess of body temperature with agitation directed toward the wound requiring debridement. A number of benefits, but also a number of detrimental effects, have been described for whirlpool treatments. In addition, several of the benefits commonly ascribed to whirlpool treatment have no sound physiological basis.

Benefits of whirlpool therapy include moisture to soften and agitation to loosen adherent necrotic tissue, increased temperature to increase blood flow and presumably increase metabolic rate, and proliferation of granulation tissue and epithelial cells. Clear detrimental effects include maceration of surrounding skin, dependent position of the lower extremities, potential occlusion of venous and arterial vessels in a limb hung over the edge of a whirlpool tank, increasing the demand for blood flow in a limb with arterial insufficiency, and increased damage to burned tissue by the elevated temperature of a whirlpool. Systemic effects include a drop in blood pressure in patients with compromised cardiovascular systems or those taking antihypertensive medications. In addition, the benefits listed above must be analyzed more critically in light of a particular patient. First, other methods of softening and loosening adherent necrotic tissue are available, and these methods may actually be faster or more cost effective. Wounds on certain areas of the body are not accessible to the agitated water. Elevated temperature does, in fact, increase circulation to a limb with normal, healthy blood vessels. Increased temperature raises metabolic rate, which, in turn, increases release of mediators of

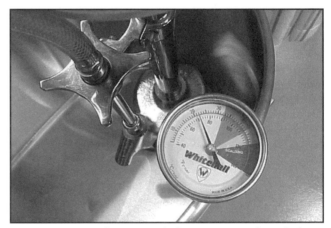

Figure 12-1c. Close-up of the air control and thermometer for the hand/foot unit.

increased blood flow to the area. This effect, however, only occurs in a person with the ability to dilate blood vessels appropriately. In a person with arterial insufficiency, demand for blood flow is increased with increasing tissue temperature, thereby aggravating the arterial insufficiency.

Moreover, as discussed in Chapter 2, growth of granulation tissue occurs most rapidly at normal body temperature. The elevated temperature of most whirlpools will not increase the growth of tissue but is more likely to retard growth. Failing to pay attention to the temperature of water in the whirlpool may also lead to burns in individuals insensitive to temperature. Additives for infection are frequently cytotoxic and may retard wound healing. This is discussed in Chapter 18.

Wound Irrigation

Irrigation is a mainstay of treatment of acute wounds by trauma surgeons and emergency physicians. It is also used

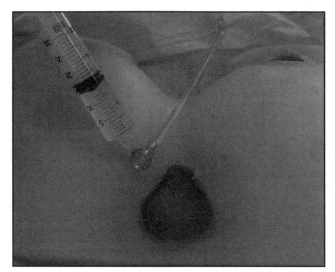

Figure 12-2. Irrigation syringe designed specifically for wound cleansing. A valve system allows the syringe to be filled from a source of sterile saline and the saline to be injected at the appropriate pressure for wound cleansing.

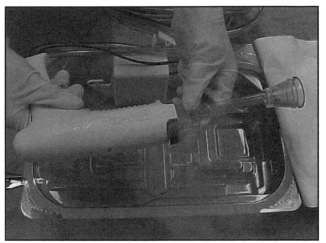

Figure 12-3. Inserting the tip on a pulsatile lavage system.

for treating infections such as osteomyelitis and abscesses. Irrigation and debridement (I & D) are used to clear infectious material and are usually accompanied by the placement of a drain, frequently a Penrose drain. A Penrose drain is simply a length of flexible tubing to allow fluid to drain from a surgical wound and represents a new wound to clean and drain an area of infection. The purpose is to allow infectious material to be carried from the wound with the fluid produced by inflammation. When fluid draining from the wound becomes clear and the quantity of fluid draining is small, the drain is removed and the wound is closed (third intention) or allowed to granulate (secondary intention).

Many devices are available for irrigation. Irrigation technique may range from simple pouring of normal saline over a wound, to a directed stream using an irrigation bulb, to pulsatile lavage with concurrent suction. Pulsatile lavage is discussed later. Irrigation bulbs produce very little pressure and have been deemed insufficient for debridement, although they may be used for gentle rinsing of wounds. As discussed, AHCPR guidelines have specifically endorsed irrigation through a 19-gauge angiocath or equivalent to produce an optimal irrigation pressure (Figure 12-2). Devices designed specifically for cleansing teeth, such as Waterpik (Waterpik Technologies, Fort Collins, Colo) have been used for debridement. These devices first gained popularity during the Vietnam conflict but are not designed to produce appropriate pressure. Irrigation devices should also have a splash shield to prevent spraying necrotic tissue and contaminated fluid over the treatment area. Several devices have recently been developed incorporating both the irrigation pressure

desired and a splash shield. Pulsatile lavage devices deliver appropriate pressure and include splash shields and suction to aid in the removal of loosened necrotic tissue and to minimize the spray of contaminated fluid in the treatment area.

Pulsatile Lavage with Concurrent Suction

These devices operate under the same concept as carpet cleaners. They simultaneously irrigate with controllable pressure and remove excess fluid from the wound. This technique has become very popular recently and in many facilities has nearly replaced whirlpool treatments. Three major product manufacturers produce battery-operated, compressed gas-driven, and external alternating current (AC) pump devices. Pulsavac (Zimmer, New York, NY) was the first to gain widespread recognition. The AC pump device is in its third version (Pulsavac III) and a battery-operated portable version is now available. Versions of these devices are shown in Figures 12-3, 12-4, and 12-5. The original Pulsavac device was somewhat cumbersome to set up, requiring threading of tubing through the machine, but has been redesigned to improve its usability. Davol (Cranston, RI) has both a handheld battery-operated unit and a unit driven by compressed gas. The Stryker device (Portage, Mich) comes only in a battery-operated unit.

Controversy exists as to the reuse of units. As originally developed, all pieces coming directly in contact with either the patient or body fluids were designed for disposal with infectious waste. In the case of hand-held battery-operated units, everything used was to be thrown away after treatment. One of the battery-operated units had been redesigned with the suction tubing built into the disposable tip, rather than running through the handpiece. With this arrangement, the handpiece could be conserved and reused on the same patient for multiple uses.

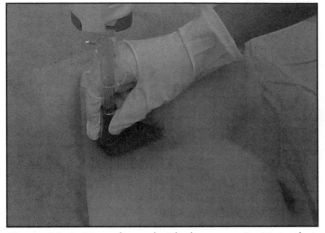

Figure 12-4. Use of a pulsatile lavage unit. Note that one hand is used to both guide and contour the tip to the wound.

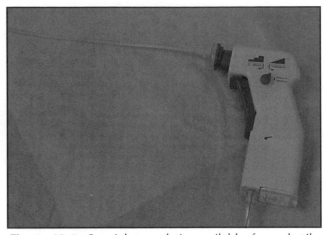

Figure 12-5. Special tunnel tip available for pulsatile lavage.

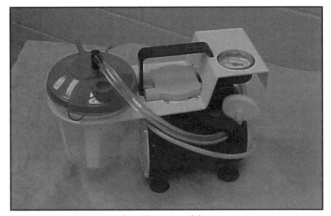

Figure 12-6. Example of a portable vacuum pump.

Four basic components exist in all types of pulsatile lavage units—*suction, adjustable pump, tip,* and *handpiece.* Suction is provided by either wall suction or a portable pump (Figure 12-6). In the case of wall suction, a pressure regulator must be placed on the wall outlet. Pulsatile lavage devices offer a distinct advantage in the hospital environment, in which patient care is performed within the patient's room. All hospital rooms have wall suction available and many have pressure regulators available in the rooms. In many outpatient locations, however, wall suction is not available. Portable pumps may be purchased for approximately $400. Often, these are mounted onto a cart ($200), which can also be used to store supplies. A suction canister is placed between the pulsatile lavage unit and either the wall suction pressure regulator or the portable pump. The canisters are designed to collect fluid and prevent the movement of fluid into the suction pump. Care should be taken to prevent overfilling suction canisters. This can be done by selecting a large enough canister to hold a fixed volume of fluid used to irrigate the wound. Care should also be taken to avoid spilling the contents of the canister. Individual facility policy should be followed for the disposal of suction canisters. Usually an extension hose is necessary to connect the suction line of the handpiece to the suction canister. Setting up the suction aspect of the device does not require sterile technique and should be done ahead of time before removing dressings from the patient.

The adjustable pressure source may be separate from the handpiece or built into it. The advantage of separate units is decreased cost of the handpiece and greater control of impact pressure. Companies provide these pumps to facilities that purchase a given number of supplies for them within a given time frame. Therefore, these can be cheaper for high-volume clinics to use. The pumps are mounted on poles and are fairly portable. The all-in-one handpiece

is much simpler to set up and is more portable, but the impact pressure cannot be adjusted as finely, and the operator cannot know with certainty how much pressure the device is delivering. In the case of a separate pump, the handpiece switch performs only an on/off function.

Handpieces with built-in pumps may have either fixed or variable settings. Placing the device into the variable mode allows the operator to vary the lavage pressure by altering the grip on the handle between high, medium, and low pressures or high and low settings. The fixed mode locks the lavage pressure into the high, medium, or low setting and requires the operator to depress a button to unlock the setting, similar to locking features on power tools such as drills.

A variety of tips, usually two sizes with splash shields, are available (see Figures 12-3 and 12-4). A long, flexible tip with a measuring guide is available for some models to allow lavage and suction of tunnels and tracts (see Figure 12-5). The markings allow measurement of the depth of the tract or tunnel for evaluation purposes and to ensure that the tip is placed the correct distance into the defect for appropriate cleaning. Splash shields are now usually very flexible and their contours can be manipulated to approximate the shape of the wound. One hand is generally left on it to guide the tip across the surface of the wound and to manipulate the shape of the splash shield to optimize cleansing. Manipulating the tip shape also minimizes the amount of fluid running out of the wound or being sprayed from the wound into the environment. While using pulsatile lavage, personal protective equipment should be worn to minimize risk of splashing (see Chapter 18).[3]

Several preparatory steps must be carried out before the actual process occurs. The bags of saline need to be warmed to skin temperature by approved methods. Some have proposed microwave ovens, and others have used hot packs. The patient needs to be draped appropriately, especially if the procedure is performed in the patient's bed. Sufficient clean towels are placed where fluid is likely to run off the patient, and sterile towels are placed around the wound. Also check the operation of the vacuum pump. You do not want to be surprised to find an inadequate vacuum source during the procedure. The procedure should be explained thoroughly to the patient. The carpet cleaner analogy is generally sufficient. Any necessary medications should have been given to the patient in advance so that desired plasma concentrations exist at the time of the procedure. Topical application of local anesthetic may be used as needed by individual patients.

The first step is to attach the suction canister to the vacuum source—either the wall suction or a portable suction pump—and set the regulator to the proper negative pressure. The bag(s) of normal saline should be prewarmed to skin temperature and hung on a pole to allow spiking. The handpiece, whether an external pump or battery-operated unit, is removed from the package and placed on a sterile field. The appropriate tip is then applied to the handpiece. The tip cannot be inserted incorrectly on the handpiece; it will only fit if the suction and spray are aligned properly. A different size or shape exists on the vacuum and spray openings. Identify the suction tubing coming from the handpiece and attach it to the vacuum canister either directly or using an extension tube. Next, the other tube is identified and inserted into either a single bag of sterile saline or a dual spike adapter. The dual spike adapter allows simultaneous use of two bags of sterile saline. Check for a lock pin on the handpiece before starting. At the time of this writing, the Davol Simpulse uses a black lock pin. The handpiece trigger is squeezed as the device is held over a waterproof container until the tubing fills with sterile saline and begins to exit the tip. Be certain that the vacuum pump is operating at the desired level before beginning lavage.

During the procedure, carefully follow the contours of the wound to avoid pulling the tip across the wound surface. Also take care to avoid occluding the hole built into the splash shield. This hole prevents the "latching on" of the tip to the wound, as well as damage and pain to the wound site. Contouring the flexible splash shield will minimize splashing and running over of fluid from the wound. If the wound begins to fill with saline, stop the lavage and troubleshoot the lack of suction.

Following the procedure, the lavage is turned off by releasing the trigger and then the suction is discontinued. Any tubing that has carried fluid from the wound must be discarded, as well as the tip inserted into the handpiece. Batteries may be retrieved from the Davol Simpulse unit, but not the Zimmer battery-operated unit. The fluid within the suction canister is disposed of in a manner consistent with facility procedure. Facility procedure may allow the dumping of the contents in a sink or commode and the disposable canister in a biohazard bag. A glass canister is placed in a container approved for return to central sterile supply (Table 12-1).

The Pulsavac devices with external pumps have additional steps to thread tubing through the pump. The process is simpler with the Pulsavac III, which uses a cassette arrangement for the tubing. Instructions are detailed on the machine and a representative will provide instruction in person as needed.

Chemical Debridement

The use of exogenous versions of naturally occurring enzymes is currently enjoying renewed popularity. At the time of this writing, proteolytic enzymes and collagenase are the only chemicals available. Collagenase is effective because collagen makes up such a large proportion (75%) of dry weight of skin. It is generally believed that breakdown of collagen enhances migration of cells. However, enzymes of any type are only effective within a certain range of pH. Moreover, enzymes can be inactivated by other chemicals and by poor environment. Therefore, thorough cleansing of wounds should be done before application of enzymes. The use of chemical debriders is limited by the need for a physician's order and prescription. Because these proteins are effective only on the surface available to them, the clinician needs to crosshatch eschar to increase surface area. Crosshatching with a scalpel increases the number of edges of eschar over which the chemical debriders can function. When done properly, the chemical converts one large mass of eschar into a large number of small areas of eschar, which will lift off the wound or be solubilized. With certain debriders, the manufacturers recommend concurrent use of topical antibiotic prophylactically to prevent bacteria from entering blood as tissue breaks down. Chemical debriders require the use of moist dressing to maintain a favorable environment for the chemical to work on the necrotic tissue. Because of the risk of sepsis with chemical debridement, the clinician needs to monitor for signs of sepsis. Chemical debridement is also indicated as an alternative for a patient who cannot tolerate sharp debridement. It is also indicated for

---

Table 12-1

PULSATILE LAVAGE PROCEDURE

- Warm bags of sterile saline
- Drape patient
- Attach suction canister to regulator or portable pump
- Set the suction to desired vacuum and check for normal operation
- Hang bag(s) of saline
- Place handpiece and tip on sterile field
- Attach appropriate tip on handpiece
- Attach vacuum tubing to vacuum source
- Spike the bag(s)
- Remove lock pin if applicable
- Squeeze trigger to fill the incoming line with saline
- Begin lavage
- At the end of the procedure, release the trigger
- Ensure wound is not full of fluid
- Turn off vacuum source and detach handpiece tubing from vacuum source
- Discard appropriate items in appropriate biohazard containers

---

the patient who has no time constraints or risk of infection. Chemical debridement may also be used in the acute care setting to complement mechanical debridement. Chemical debridement works well in long-term facilities, home care, and outpatient settings but only if the ulcer is not infected. The breakdown of tissue within the wound increases the risk of bacteria entering the circulation and causing sepsis. A more absorbent dressing must be used with chemical debridement, such as a clean, moist dressing applied over the wound, because of the increased drainage associated with chemical debridement as the chemical solubilizes the necrotic tissue.

At the time of this writing, three agents are available. All three are indicated for a wide variety of wounds with necrotic tissue. Adverse reactions seem to be limited for all of these. Sensitivity to any of the ingredients and stinging or irritation of periwound skin in the presence of heavily draining wounds are listed by the manufacturers. Santyl (Smith & Nephew, Inc., Largo, Fla) is a specific collagenase and the other two—Accuzyme (Healthpoint, Ltd., Fort Worth, Tex) and Panafil (Healthpoint, Ltd., Fort Worth, Tex) are combinations of papain and urea. Panafil comes in two varieties—white and green. Panafil white and green are both a combination of papain and urea, but Panafil green also contains chlorophyllin-copper complex to reduce wound odor. All of these agents are indicated on necrotic wounds and are safe for non-necrotic tissue. These debriders are packaged in tubes and are placed directly on the necrotic tissue in a thin layer. Moist dressings are to be placed over the chemical debriders.

However, if left in place too long, moist dressings can desiccate and adhere to the wound. If the dressing becomes adherent, gentle irrigation to remove the adherent dressing is reasonable. Some clinicians use petrolatum-gauze products such as Adaptic (Johnson & Johnson, New Brunswick, NJ) or Xeroform (Sherwood Medical Company, Mansfield, Mass) over the chemical debrider to minimize desiccation and adherence. These agents should be discontinued when the necrotic tissue is cleared from the wound, if signs of sensitivity are present, or the product fails to remove necrotic tissue within a 2-week trial period. These should also be discontinued in the presence of bacterial supergrowth or tunneling to other body cavities.[4]

Autolytic Debridement

This type of debridement relies on the ability of the clinician to trap endogenous enzymes in an optimized environment by using occlusive dressings. The wound environment is also optimized by filling cavities loosely to prevent abscess formation, but not tightly to prevent granulation. If the wound is dry, the clinician should hydrate the wound to allow enzymes access throughout the wound bed. For a dry wound, a combination of hydrogel and film may be used as long as the surrounding skin does not become macerated. Foam or hydrocolloid dressings may be used to promote autolytic debridement in cases of greater drainage. However, occluding a wound for several days in an effort to promote autolytic debridement creates a risk that others may mistake exudate for pus. Autolytic debridement is another alternative for the patient who cannot tolerate sharp debridement or other methods but who also has no time constraints or risk of infection. Because the wound must be occluded with a synthetic dressing and occlusion promotes the growth of bacteria, autolytic debridement is contraindicated in infected ulcers.

WHEN NOT TO DEBRIDE

Not all necrotic tissue needs to be debrided. Specific examples include stable heel wounds and severe arterial insufficiency. In addition, technical issues need to be considered. Some authorities recommend not debriding stable heel wounds. General guidelines for not debriding heel wounds include eschar that is firmly adherent, lack of inflammation of surrounding tissue, lack of drainage from below the eschar, and eschar that does not feel soft or boggy. Small wounds a few millimeters to centimeters with eschar may heal just as rapidly without debridement. Necrotic tissue caused by arterial insufficiency should not be debrided. In these wounds, a lack of blood flow not only retards healing but prevents the immune system's handling of bacteria that may enter the wound. Moreover, exposure of necrotic tissue to surface bacteria presents the risk of potentially serious infection.

As a general rule, the clinician should never debride what cannot be seen. As tempting as it may be to rapidly remove what is believed to be necrotic tissue, the clinician risks not only damage to healthy tissue but also introducing bacteria into the blood. Reasons to stop debridement include exposure of tendons, bones, and blood vessels; penetration of a fascial plane; excessive bleeding; the patient can no longer tolerate debridement; and the clinician's desire to stop based on past experience. Only physicians are licensed to cut healthy tissues; therefore, if a sinus tract or tunnel needs to be deroofed, the patient should be referred to a surgeon.

Sharp debridement requires greater skill and in some states may require certain credentials and documented training. This topic is covered in the next chapter.

SUMMARY

The process of debridement is preceded by the development of a plan of care addressing why debridement is necessary and which method is most suited to reach the outcomes outlined. Three types of debridement are described; sharp debridement is discussed in the next chapter. Sharp, mechanical, chemical, and autolytic debridement are options determined based on the characteristics of the wound, characteristics of the patient and facility, and time constraints placed on wound debridement. In many cases, sharp debridement is preferred to

manage risk of infection. Sharp debridement requires the use of sharp instruments to cut along the border between viable and necrotic tissue; it also requires a high skill level. Mechanical means of debridement include use of hydrotherapy, scrubbing, and irrigation. Serial instrumental debridement refers to the use of sharp instruments to cut loosened necrotic tissue and requires a much lower level of skill than sharp debridement. Serial instrumental debridement is often preceded by hydrotherapy to soften and loosen necrotic tissue. Autolytic debridement is a means of allowing the wound to clean itself with endogenous enzymes under an occlusive dressing. Chemical debridement involves the use of enzymes requiring a physician's prescription to degrade necrotic tissue. Autolytic and chemical debridement is useful when time constraints and infection are not issues. Debridement is not performed on dry gangrene caused by arterial insufficiency and may not be necessary for stable heel ulcers.

STUDY QUESTIONS

1. What considerations are made before deciding to debride?
2. What are the major reasons for performing sharp debridement?
3. Why might autolytic debridement be preferred by some patients?
4. What is the rationale for not debriding dry gangrene?
5. Under what circumstances might hydrotherapy be a preferred method of debridement?
6. Discuss problems in using hydrotherapy for wounds caused by arterial insufficiency, venous insufficiency, and burns.
7. What are some of the major advantages of using pulsatile lavage? Disadvantages?

REFERENCES

1. Robson MC, Mannari RJ, Smith PD, Payne WG. Maintenance of wound bacterial balance. *Am J Surg.* 1999 Nov;178(5):399-402.
2. Bergstrom N, Bennett MA, Carlson CE, et al. Treatment of Pressure Ulcers. Clinical Practice Guideline, No. 15. Rockville, MD: US Department of Health and Human Services. Public Health Service, Agency for Health Care Policy and Research. AHCPR Publication No. 95-0652; December 1994.
3. Irion GL. Sharp debridement and consequences of coding and the APTA position statement. *Acute Care Perspectives.* 2000;8(2)1-6.
4. Arnall DA. Enzymatic debriders in wound care management. *Acute Care Perspectives.* 2000;8(2):12-18.

Sharp Debridement

13

OBJECTIVES

- List indications and contraindications for sharp debridement.
- Describe regulations and training necessary for sharp debridement.
- List materials and instruments used for sharp debridement.
- Discuss anatomical considerations for typical areas requiring sharp debridement.

The method of choice when a wound has a risk of infection or progression of infection is sharp debridement. It may also be the method of choice for removing large quantities of necrotic tissue rapidly. This method may not be suitable for some individuals. In particular, this method needs to be used with caution in patients with bleeding disorders or anticoagulation.

Sharp debridement is the most efficient means of removing necrotic tissues. However, it is also very demanding of resources including training of the clinician, tools, cost, and possibly the need for an operating or special procedures room. The clinician performing this procedure must have special credentials, training, and licensure. Those typically allowed to perform sharp debridement include physicians, physician's assistants, physical therapists, and advanced practice nurses. These individuals are required to have licenses issued by individual states. In addition, payers may require evidence of advanced training to receive reimbursement for sharp debridement. State practice acts may limit which health care providers are allowed to perform sharp debridement and may list additional requirements.

SHARP DEBRIDEMENT IN THE OPERATING ROOM

In certain cases, sharp debridement needs to be performed by a surgeon. These cases include those in which the procedure may cause severe pain, if extensive debridement is required, if the degree of undermining/sinus tract/tunneling is undetermined, if bone must be removed, if debridement must be done near vital organs, or the patient is septic. Surgical debridement should also be considered if the patient is immunosuppressed.

BEDSIDE DEBRIDEMENT

In cases other than those described above, clinicians other than surgeons may perform the procedure. Tools typically used include curved scissors, Adson or other type of forceps with teeth, scalpels with #11, #15, or #10 blades (Figure 13-1), silver nitrate sticks, and local anesthetic. The clinician may choose to use either lidocaine or benzocaine spray, lidocaine gel or eutectic mixture of local anesthetic (EMLA), which consists of 2.5% lidocaine and 2.5% prilocaine. The clinician should attempt to provide an optimal environment for the procedure. Most important is provision of good lighting. A comfortable position for both the patient and clinician should be assumed to prevent fatigue or other problems in both the patient and the clinician.

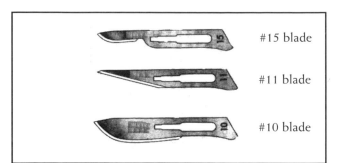

Figure 13-1. Types of scalpel blades.

BASIC TECHNIQUES

In all cases, sharp debridement should be considered a highly selective form of debridement. As such, the clinician should endeavor to minimize damage to healthy tissue. Because of the risk of bleeding from adjacent healthy tissue, the clinician should start debridement at the bottom of the wound and work toward the top. Bleeding may obscure the clinician's vision. Other considerations include working from the center of the wound where the wound is less sensitive to pain, to its periphery, which is more likely to be sensitive. A general rule to follow is to debride the areas likely to bleed or to be painful last. Using local anesthesia and silver nitrate sticks, however, should minimize these problems. Another consideration is to stay within a given plane to avoid spreading bacteria into lower layers. Following sharp debridement with a high risk of bleeding, a dry dressing should be placed on the wound for 8 to 24 hours if significant bleeding occurs during the procedure. The dressing may then be changed to an appropriate occlusive dressing (see Chapter 15).

In many cases sharp debridement can be done once for a wound. However, it may become necessary to stop sharp debridement and continue later, particularly with a large wound, a wound with painful areas, and wounds that bleed. Moreover, a brief period of other forms of debridement may need to follow sharp debridement to prepare a wound for surgical closure. Care must be taken to avoid cutting in undermined or tunneled areas and in areas of purulent drainage. The clinician should take care to never cut what cannot be seen. Reasons to stop debridement include exposure of tendons, bones, and blood vessels; penetration of a fascial plane; excessive bleeding; the patient can no longer tolerate debridement; and based on the clinician's experience to stop.

INSTRUMENTS

Sharp debridement requires the use of personal protective equipment both to protect the clinician from body fluids and to protect the wound from contaminants on the

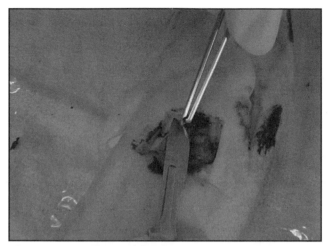

Figure 13-2. Sharp debridement practice on a pig's foot.

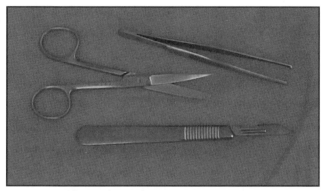

Figure 13-3b. High-quality permanent instruments.

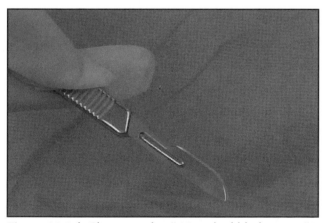

Figure 13-3d. Close-up of a #10 scalpel blade on a #3 handle, showing proper handling.

clinician. The face should be protected with either a visor or goggles and a mask. A cap, gown, and gloves are also needed. For the procedure itself, instruments used include scissors, forceps, scalpel, and hemostats. Scalpels should be used sparingly; they can cause too much inadvertent cutting and are difficult for the novice to control.

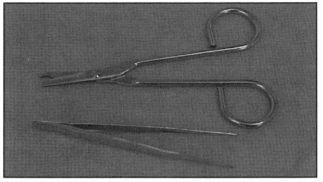

Figure 13-3a. Instruments used for sharp debridement: suture removal kit.

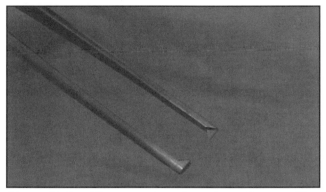

Figure 13-3c. Close-up of toothed tissue forceps. The teeth improve the handling of necrotic tissue.

However, they are useful for trimming callus and scoring eschar. An individual should have substantial experience in using a scalpel in a safe setting, such as practice on a pig's foot (Figure 13-2), scoring eschar, and trimming callus before using a scalpel on the edges of necrotic tissue.

Forceps and scissors are available in either disposable or permanent (resterilizable) forms (Figures 13-3a through 13-3d). Generally speaking, disposable forceps and scissors packaged in suture removal kits are poor-quality instruments and not suitable for sharp debridement near viable tissue. Quality forceps that will hold tissue securely cost $40 or more plus the cost of sterilization for each time they are used. Forceps should minimally have serrated tips; however, many individuals who use these instruments on a regular basis express a preference for Adson forceps with teeth on the tips. Scissors with good quality cutting edges are even more expensive and can cost from $30 for small scissors up to $80 or more. For the person who will use these instruments frequently, the cost becomes small because of the durability of the instruments. Several types of scissors are used by different clinicians. Scissors may have blunt or sharp tips, or one sharp and one blunt tip (blunt/blunt, sharp/sharp, or blunt/sharp, respectively). The advantage of blunt tips is the reduced risk of inadvertent injury caused by a sharp tip. The novice may wish to start with a pair of blunt/blunt curved Mayo scissors because of the safety issue. Some clinicians, however, prefer curved sharp/sharp iris scissors. Iris scissors are smaller; therefore, the clinician is able to reach into tighter areas of the wound but at greater risk of accidental injury to healthy tissue. An alternative to using iris scissors in such a location is to use a scalpel blade. However, the beginner may wish to stay away from such tight areas until he or she is comfortable with less challenging debridement. Curved scissors are preferred to flat scissors for two reasons: when cutting with the tips up, less risk of accidental injury by the tips occurs; secondly, the clinician may cut closer to the wound surface with either the tips pointing up or down.

Scalpel blades, like scissors, are available in several different types, and operator preference plays a large role in the type used. The type of blade is identified by number. The blades may be curved or straight, large or small. Certain types of blades are more useful for particular tasks, whereas others are versatile. In addition, different types of blades fit onto different types of handles. Both the #3 and #7 handles fit a series of useful blades for working in tight areas—the smaller #10, #11, and #15 blades. The #3 handle is familiar to most people. It is shaped to fit in the palm of the hand as well as being held with a pencil-like grip and has a serrated portion to aid grip with the thumb and index finger. The #7 handle also fits these blades, but it is a thinner handle and may not be as easy to grasp for the novice. The #4 handle is appropriate for the larger #20, #21, #22, and #23 blades.

The #10 (#3 handle) and #20 (number 4 handle) blades are versatile with a rounded edge and nearly straight tip. The #11 blade is a straight blade with a narrow tip. A small but versatile blade is the #15. It is a small blade with a curved point and somewhat rounded edge. Any of the blades can be used for the basic sharp debridement techniques of scoring, shaving, and cutting. The #11 blade with its straight edge can be more difficult to handle for scoring or other cuts perpendicular to the surface, whereas the #10, #20, or #15 blades allow a more natural wrist and finger flexion motion for scoring. For shaving, a #11 blade can be equally effective in a cutting motion that is parallel to the surface. For fine work, a #15 blade works nicely, but because of its size it is not suitable for removal of a large amount of easily accessible necrotic tissue and will dull rapidly. Eventually, most operators will likely develop a personal preference for either a #10 or #11 blade. The advantage of using a #10 blade over a #20 blade is the ability to use the same handle for a #15 or #11 blade.

Just like scissors and forceps, scalpels may be either disposable or permanent. In either case, the blades themselves are always disposable. Disposable scalpels come with blades already attached. The handles are usually plastic and tend to have an awkward feel. Disposable scalpels have the advantages of lower cost and avoiding the inconvenience of sterilizing instruments. The personal preference of many is the heavier permanent handle with ridges on the handles to improve the grip. The downside of permanent handles, in addition to the cost, is the risk associated with changing blades. Some bold individuals will change these by hand. The prudent person changes the blade with either hemostats or a scalpel blade remover available from surgical instrument suppliers. Another advantage is the flexibility of changing blades during a procedure. Changing blades during a procedure requires foresight to have blades that fit the same handle and having them available during the procedure. Because sterile technique is followed during sharp debridement, the scalpel blade package will need to be opened by another individual not involved in the sterile technique.

BLEEDING

Bleeding is largely unavoidable if sharp debridement is to be accomplished efficiently. Although necrotic tissue does not bleed, a clear margin between necrotic tissue and tissue that may still bleed is often not observable, especially with increasing depth of the ulcer. When bleeding occurs, hemostasis is desired. With careful debridement, bleeding is usually stopped easily. Hemostasis is only problematic when clearly healthy tissue is cut. Even individuals with bleeding disorders will eventually stop bleeding, and the amount of bleeding is usually insignificant from a hemodynamic standpoint. On the other hand, we do not wish to have a wound act as a hematoma and promote inflammation.

Several means are available to promote hemostasis. Silver nitrate sticks are available from many sources. They are similar to cotton-tipped applicators, with a small amount of silver nitrate on their tip, rather than cotton. They need to be touched briefly to small bleeds and may need to be moistened slightly with saline. Flooding the rest of the wound with saline minimizes the damage done to other areas of the wound. Pressure may be applied with a small piece of alginate dressing. For larger bleeds, pressure may need to be applied with 4 x 4 cotton gauze sponges.

ANATOMIC CONSIDERATIONS

Although debridement may be required on any body part, it tends to be needed more commonly in a few locations. These locations include common areas for pressure ulcers, such as the sacrum, ischial tuberosity, greater trochanter, and sites common for neuropathic ulcers such as the metatarsal heads. A particular concern is avoiding damage to flexor tendons of the foot. As discussed in the previous chapter, debridement should be considered carefully for arterial insufficiency ulcers, and venous insufficiency ulcers may require a short course of debridement.

SERIAL INSTRUMENTAL DEBRIDEMENT

This type of debridement needs to be distinguished from sharp debridement. Although sharp instruments are used for both of these techniques, a higher level of skill is needed for sharp debridement. Serial instrumental debridement is generally preceded with some form of hydrotherapy to moisten and loosen necrotic tissue. Only clearly necrotic tissue is cut with the sharp instruments. Traction is first placed on the necrotic tissue with forceps. Frequently, traction alone is sufficient to remove much of the tissue. If a piece of necrotic tissue remains adherent, it can be cut with scissors and may, on occasion, be cut with a scalpel. As with sharp debridement, painful areas or areas that tend to bleed should be debrided last. A session of serial instrumental debridement should be concluded similar to that of sharp debridement—patient tolerance, bleeding, pain, clinician fatigue, reaching a tissue plane, and exposure of blood vessels. This type of debridement will require more sessions than sharp debridement, more preparation of the wound, and will generally cost more to perform than sharp debridement. The only clear advantage of serial instrumental debridement is the skill level. Whereas sharp debridement is not considered appropriate to be performed by a physical therapist assistant, serial instrumental debridement may be.

SUMMARY

Sharp debridement is the preferred method for rapid removal of necrotic tissue, especially in cases of high risk of infection or neuropathic ulcers. Cutting is performed along the margins between necrotic and viable tissue, and bleeding is likely to occur. Bleeding may need to be controlled by silver nitrate sticks, alginate, or gauze. Dry dressings are placed on bleeding wounds for several hours to prevent hematoma formation.

STUDY QUESTIONS

1. Under what circumstances is sharp debridement mandatory?

2. What restrictions are placed on the performance of sharp debridement?

3. Name contraindications for bedside sharp debridement.

4. Name criteria for terminating a session of sharp debridement.

5. Under what circumstances is sharp debridement likely to require multiple sessions? Single sessions?

6. List advantages of #10, #11, and #15 scalpel blades.

7. List advantages and disadvantages of using iris scissors.

8. What are the advantages of curved scissors with blunt tips?

9. Contrast sharp debridement and serial instrumental debridement.

Physical Agents

14

- Discuss indications, contraindications, and parameters for use of electrical stimulation with high-voltage pulsed current (HVPC).
- Describe the use of diathermy in wound healing.
- Discuss the use of ultraviolet C in wound management.
- Discuss the indications for negative pressure therapy.
- Discuss the theory of and uses of hyperbaric oxygen therapy.
- Describe the role of infrared radiation in assisting wound healing.
- Discuss the theory behind and mechanism of using arterial assist.
- Discuss the theory of using therapeutic ultrasound and parameters for wound healing.

ELECTRIC STIMULATION

High-voltage pulsed current (HVPC), formerly known as high-voltage pulsed galvanic (HVPG), is the only type of stimulation presently available that has been consistently shown to improve wound healing. A number of early studies are supportive of low-intensity direct current; however, devices of this type are not generally available. On the other hand, microcurrent types of devices, which use currents with intensities in the microamperage range and various waveforms, have not been shown to be effective in promoting wound healing.

In electrotherapy, several parameters must be used to describe a treatment protocol. Intensity may be quantified either in units of current (milliamps) or the electromotive force causing charge to flow (volts). For most devices intensity refers to current in milliamps. HVPC devices, on the other hand, are set in volts. Some devices will only have a knob or other adjustment marked *current* or *intensity* with a relative scale. If these devices are used, the intensity is adjusted to give a response that is determined by what the clinician observes, such as a minimally observable contraction or to the patient's subjective response.

Intensity determines the type of neuron recruited by current. Although transcutaneous current recruits neurons based on size, the distance of the neuron from the source of current is also important. Based on size alone, the first neurons recruited by transcutaneous current would be the motor neurons signaling muscles to contract and neurons from muscle spindles and Golgi tendon organs that indicate muscle length and tension. The next group of neurons recruited would be sensory neurons indicating mechanical stimulation of the skin. Small sensory neurons carrying information about pain, temperature, and crude touch would be recruited last. However, based on distance between surface electrodes and different types of neurons, sensory information would be perceived at a lower intensity than a motor response. Because of these two factors, the typical recruitment pattern produced by transcutaneous current is:

1. the larger sensory neurons located within the skin
2. the large motor neurons beneath the skin
3. pain-receptive neurons in the skin.

These three levels of intensity are termed *sensory*, *motor*, and *noxious*, respectively. Although the patient's perception tends to be dominated by the type of neuron newly recruited at each level of intensity, these levels are cumulative and overlap. For example, to develop a strong muscle contraction, a current is usually uncomfortable.

The second parameter is the frequency of pulsed current. In the case of direct current, frequency is meaningless. The frequency of pulsed current is usually given in Hertz (Hz) (cycles per second). The frequency of pulsed current determines the quality of muscle contraction. Low frequencies create single twitches. Intermediate frequencies create undulating contractions called *unfused tetanic contractions* in which a slight relaxation occurs between stimuli. High frequencies produce tetanic contractions. The need to use the relative terms *low, intermediate,* and *high* is due to the properties of different muscles. For example, hand and forearm muscles may tetanize at 15 Hz, whereas quadriceps may require 50 Hz for a tetanic contraction. For the purposes of wound healing, the frequency is generally much in excess of that needed for a tetanic contraction. A continual tetanic contraction would be very uncomfortable for the patient; therefore, electrodes are placed away from muscles, if possible, and intensity is adjusted to a value that barely produces a muscle contraction.

The third parameter is the pulse duration or width. In general, increasing pulse width produces the same effect as increasing pulse intensity. Compared with devices used for neuromuscular electrical stimulation and transcutaneous electrical nerve stimulation, the pulses used for wound repair are very short, but the intensity is very high.

Waveform describes the combined effects of intensity, duration, and rise and fall times of pulses. The waveform of HVPC is generally described as triangular, although this term imprecisely describes the waveform. The pulses have a rapid rise and a slower decay and are paired. This waveform is often termed *twin peaks*. The rapid presentation of the second peak causes the two spikes to behave as a single electrical event. Therefore, in HVPC terminology, each set of two spikes is considered as a pulse with two phases. The timing between the two phases is adjustable on some devices as either the interphase or intrapulse interval. A shorter intrapulse interval increases the effectiveness of the pulses but can be more uncomfortable for the patient.

Polarity describes the direction that ions or electrons travel relative to electrodes. A cathode attracts positive ions and repels electrons. Anodes attract electrons and negative ions and repel positive ions. As a twist in terminology, the anode is termed the *positive electrode* because of its effect of driving positively charged particles away from it, and the cathode is termed the *negative electrode*. A number of studies have been performed with either positive or negative polarities for the electrodes attached to the wound. In addition, some clinicians have started with a positive electrode over the wound and, based on a number of criteria, switched to a negative polarity. Other parameters include the duration of individual treatment sessions, the frequency of treatments, and the number of treatments given.

General Technique for HVPC

A typical HVPC device is depicted in Figures 14-1a through 14-1c. Twin-peak HVPC is used at an amplitude

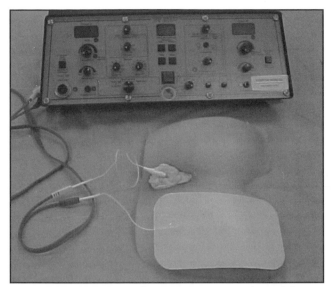

Figure 14-1a. Set-up of HVPC on a wound model.

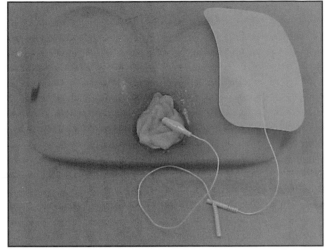

Figure 14-1b. Set-up of HVPC on a wound model. Close-up of electrode placement.

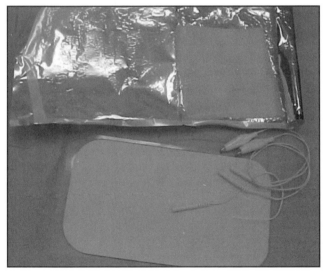

Figure 14-1c. Set-up of HVPC on a wound model. Close-up of electrodes.

and frequency of approximately 100 V and 100 Hz, with pulse duration of approximately 50 µ/seconds. However, pulse duration and the interphase (intrapulse) interval is fixed on many devices. A variety of means of setting up the patient have been described. In a typical set-up, the positive electrode is placed over the wound with the negative electrode attached to the patient distally. Usually, the electrode that is not over the wound is larger in surface area to minimize current density and, therefore, any electrical effects in the area used to complete the electrical circuit.

Electrodes

Several types of electrodes have been described. One approach to a wound with subcutaneous tissue loss is to

place saline-moistened gauze into the wound and attach the lead wire with an alligator clip. A number of manufacturers distribute hydrogel-impregnated gauze for this purpose (see Figures 14-1a through 14-1c). The other lead wire is attached to a larger electrode to minimize any effects. If this second electrode is large enough, one may consider the second electrode to be the "indifferent" electrode. Note the large indifferent electrode in use in Figure 14-1a. A typical protocol is to use a positive electrode in the wound for 1 hour either daily or three times per week, depending on the circumstances of the patient. When the wound does not continue to close at the accelerated rate, the polarity of the electrodes is switched to negative. The reversal of electrode polarity is to continue until the wound is either healed or progressing and stable enough to allow care to be completed at home. The size and distance between electrodes is adjusted based on the depth of the desired current. Superficial wounds should be treated with smaller electrodes placed closer to each other than deep wounds. In the case of a deep wound, larger electrodes placed farther apart are used to drive current more deeply through the tissue of interest.

Electrode arrangements can be monopolar, bipolar, or multipolar. Due to the nature of electricity, any current will be bipolar (ie, electricity will flow from one area to another). The simple bipolar arrangement consists of two equally sized electrodes that will produce an equal flow of charge per surface area (current density) at both electrodes, although the polarity will be different. With alternating current or biphasic pulses, the polarity of the electrodes alternates on a regular basis. A monopolar arrangement is not truly monopolar but behaves as if only one electrode is active. The monopolar effect is generated by creating a greater current density of the electrode of interest. Current density of the indifferent electrode is reduced

---

Table 14-1

TYPICAL HVPC PROTOCOL

Polarity
- Initially negative
- Switch to positive when necrosis is gone
- Switch to negative if healing reaches plateau

Pulse Rate
- 100 Hz, some as low as 30 Hz

Amplitude
- Several volts below contraction
- Expected in range of 100 to 200 Volts
- Depends on nature of tissue beneath electrode
- May be less than 100 Volts depending on patient tolerance

Waveform
- Twin-peak HVPC

Location
- Bipolar: One electrode on either side of wound
- Monopolar: Active (negative) in wound, large dispersive distant on intact skin

---

by using a much larger electrode. The current is dispersed over a greater surface area; therefore, the indifferent electrode is commonly called a *dispersive electrode*. A multipolar arrangement is produced by arranging multiple electrodes for each polarity; this may be done using a bifurcated lead or a multichannel device. If the tissues below each electrode of a multipolar arrangement are equivalent, this arrangement will allow the patient to tolerate a larger current than a monopolar or bipolar arrangement. The impedance of tissue beneath each electrode may vary tremendously from one place on the body to another. Certain areas will cause discomfort or will diminish current. In general, the clinician should avoid dry skin, callused areas, bony prominences, and motor points. Placement of electrodes over these areas will either cause patient discomfort and cause the clinician to reduce current to suboptimal levels or will force the clinician to increase current to the point of patient discomfort. No conclusive data exist on optimal locations of electrodes. Several researchers have suggested that the dispersive electrode should be placed proximal to the wound (Table 14-1).

Diathermy

Application of very high-frequency (~1000 Hz) pulsed radio wave creates heat in tissue. Heat may be used to bring tissue temperature, especially on the extremities, to core temperature, which is the temperature at which cells replicate the most rapidly. A similar type of response occurs with exposure to pulsed electromagnetic fields (PEMF). PEMF is also applied at a very high frequency to increase tissue temperature. Two types of diathermy exist, but microwave diathermy is no longer widely practiced. The benefit of diathermy as a heating agent is the ability to generate heat deep within the tissue, whereas other modalities, such as hot packs and whirlpool therapy, limit application of heat mainly to superficial tissues. Protocols suggested for applying diathermy to wounds call for a lower intensity—below that required to heat tissues. The mechanism by which diathermy is alleged to facilitate wound healing has not been elucidated. The literature at this time does not contain sufficient randomized clinical trials to support the use of diathermy to augment wound healing.

A major advantage of diathermy is the ability to deliver the energy to the tissues surrounding the wound without actually touching the wound. Lack of patient contact with the device both protects the wound and the equipment from contamination. The diathermy drums (Figures 14-2a and 14-2b) are placed near but not touching the wound. Care must be taken to avoid metal in the area being exposed to the radio waves. Metal can become very

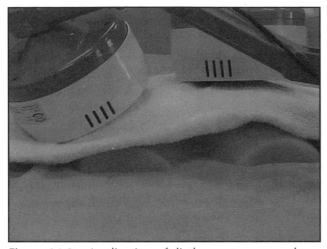

Figure 14-2a. Application of diathermy to a wound.

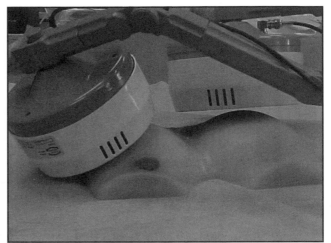

Figure 14-2b. Application of diathermy to a wound.

hot and burn the patient or may cause metal components of prostheses or orthoses to fail. As with electrical stimulation, diathermy is provided for approximately 1 hour either daily or three times per week, depending on the patient.

Although a number of manufacturers produce diathermy devices, at the time of this writing, the Magnatherm (International Medical Electronics, Kansas City, Mo) device has been promoted specifically for enhancing wound healing. The protocol described by the manufacturer is described below. A number of precautions must be observed when using diathermy. One critical precaution is to remove any metal from the patient and ensure that no metal comes within the electromagnetic field. Check the patient for jewelry, ask specifically about any metal implants including pacemakers and prosthetic joints, have the patient remove any clothing with zippers or other metal fasteners. Also check for zippers on pillows or any metal on the surface of the treatment table. The patient will need to be kept relatively still for more than 30 minutes and must, therefore, be positioned comfortably. Usually, positioning should not be a problem, because the arms on most diathermy devices are easily adjusted to accommodate most positions.

Moisture in wounds, especially under dressings, may be heated sufficiently to burn the patient. Dressings need to be removed and drainage absorbed as much as possible before treatment begins. Wounds need to be cleansed thoroughly before treatment begins to remove any substances that might absorb heat. If a wound needs to be covered, dry gauze may be used. In addition, the diathermy drum will need to be separated by either a folded towel or multiple towels to a thickness of about 1 to 1.5 cm. Some individuals have recommended that surgical caps be used to cover the drums. If this alternative is used, ensure that the drum does not make contact with the open wound, especially if the wound is wet. The drum typically needs to be kept an additional centimeter above the wound.

According to the Magnatherm protocol, the patient is to receive 5 minutes of treatment at a frequency of 5000 Hz at power level 12. This high frequency will produce heating of the tissue. The protocol finishes with 25 minutes of exposure at the nonthermal frequency of 700 Hz and power level 12, depending on the size of the wound and complicating factors. Treatment is scheduled for twice daily for 15 to 30 minutes for 1 to 4 weeks. Following treatment, the wound needs to be dressed as quickly as possible to retain the thermal effect of the treatment. The clinician should choose a dressing that is suitable for frequent dressing changes, yet optimizes the wound environment. A dressing such as a hydrocolloid sheet or semipermeable film would be inappropriate. A reasonable choice for this type of wound would be a foam dressing. However, changes twice daily (BID) of this type of dressing are greatly in excess of the DMERC Surgical Dressing Utilization Schedule, which allows three per week. Daily hydrogel sheets (without border) are allowed, but the potential for maceration of surrounding skin needs to be managed, possibly requiring the use of a skin sealant. Petrolatum-impregnated gauze may be suitable for daily or BID changes, but this type of dressing will require more vigorous cleansing between dressing changes. Another choice is to coat the wound with hydrogel filler and cover with dry gauze.

ULTRAVIOLET C

Ultraviolet C (UVC) had once been used topically from cold quartz lamps for its fungicidal effect. Current recommendations for generating a bacteriocidal effect for cold quartz lamps is exposure for 72 to 180 seconds with the lamp 1 inch from the wound surface. Recently, a form has been approved by the FDA for bacteriocidal use on

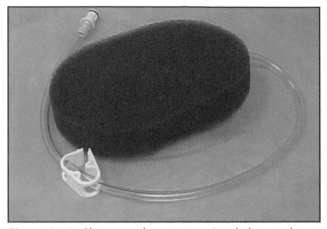

Figure 14-3. Close-up of vacuum-assisted closure dressing.

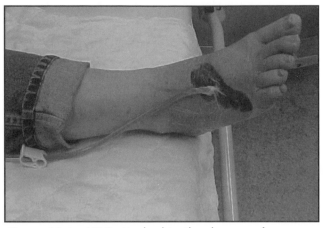

Figure 14-4a. VAC attached to the dorsum of a neuropathic foot.

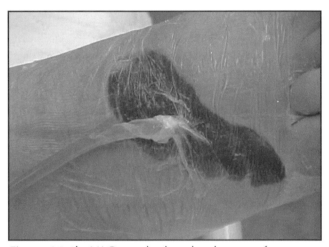

Figure 14-4b. VAC attached to the dorsum of a neuropathic foot.

open wounds. UVC has a wavelength between 200 to 290 nm. In contrast to Ultraviolet A (UVA), which is used to activate chemicals in the skin such as psoralens for treating conditions such as psoriasis and Ultraviolet B (UVB) used to activate melanocytes, UVC is directly toxic to certain susceptible bacteria. Wavelengths between 250 to 270 nm have the greatest bacteriocidal effect with a peak wavelength of 266 nm. The new UVC device has guide bars so the wand can rest over the wound, rather than requiring the operator to hold the lamp a given distance from the wound. UVC is particularly effective against multiply-resistant *Staphylococcus aureus* (MRSA) and vancomycin-resistant *Enterococcus faecalis* (VRE). It has a 99.9% kill rate with an 8-second exposure of UVC (Med Faxx V-254, Wake Forest, NC) at a wavelength of 254 nm and an output of 15.54 mW/cm^2 at a distance of 1 inch. The VRE were reduced 99.9% with only 5 seconds of exposure. Exposure for 90 seconds and 45 seconds were required for 100% kill of MRSA and VRE, respectively.

NEGATIVE PRESSURE THERAPY

In many deep wounds, accumulation of drainage within the wound slows the delivery of nutrients necessary for healing. A constant, negative pressure device applied to the wound with a drainage system can be used to enhance the wound environment by removing excessive drainage. One such device is available at the time of this writing. The vacuum-assisted closure (VAC) (Kinetic Concepts, Inc., San Antonio, Tex) consists of a pump, tubing, reservoir, and special foam type of dressing (Figure 14-3). The dressing is cut to fit the wound and is placed into a cavity with a film cover to seal the vacuum created by the pump (Figures 14-4a and 14-4b). Constant suction is applied to the wound until the wound decreases in size sufficiently so that the foam dressing can no longer fit in the wound. The

original device was too bulky to allow mobility, and therefore was limited to application while the patient was in bed. A newer system called the Mini-VAC is more portable. It can be carried in a pouch around the patient's waist and allows nearly full mobility.

Indications for the VAC include chronic open wounds such as venous ulcers, neuropathic ulcers, arterial ulcers, acute and traumatic ulcers, meshed grafts, dehiscent wounds, and flaps. Contraindications include fistulas (abnormal openings between body compartments) to organs or body cavities, necrotic tissue with eschar, untreated osteomyelitis, and malignancy in the wound. In addition, several precautions exist. These include active bleeding, use of anticoagulants, and abnormal hemostasis.[1]

Four additional considerations have been described in the Burdette Tomlin Memorial Hospital VAC Policy.[2] These considerations are support surface selection, nutritional status, special nutritional needs of diabetic patients, and terminal illness. In general, pressure ulcer risk assessment should be performed for all hospitalized patients using validated tools such as the Braden or Norton scale. Patients identified at risk should be placed on appropriate support surfaces and a turning schedule and monitored. Nutritional risk also needs to be addressed. In particular, loss of fluid and protein through application of the VAC is likely to occur. In hospitals, a dietician should be consulted and the diet adjusted in accordance with the total clinical picture. A number of factors may need to be considered in addition to the loss of fluid and protein in the fluid evacuated from the wound. The diabetic patient will need more careful monitoring, including the management of insulin, diet, and physical activity. VAC therapy may be used on wounds of terminally ill patients if overwhelming drainage or odor of a wound cannot be managed by more conservative means such as dressing changes.

Application of the VAC

The system consists of a pump, which is durable equipment, and the foam dressing and canister, which are considered consumable supplies. Application should be done following standard infection control procedures. The wound should be cleansed or debrided as needed prior to application; necrotic wounds with eschar are contraindications for VAC. The surrounding skin is also cleaned thoroughly so the semipermeable dressing used in the VAC application will adhere to the skin surrounding the wound.

The procedure should be explained thoroughly to the patient and the patient positioned so the dressing can be placed in the wound without risk of it falling out during application. The patient should also be made as comfortable as possible and lighting should be adequate. Once the patient is in position, a new canister is placed in the VAC pump and the open-cell foam dressing is cut with aseptic technique to a size slightly smaller than the wound. The foam dressing is then placed in the wound and the evacuation tube is connected to the dressing. At this point, the semipermeable film dressing that comes with the foam dressing material is placed over the foam and the tubing, and is smoothed to ensure a seal around the wound and dressing. When a good seal appears to be in place, the evacuation tube is connected to the canister in the VAC pump.

The green on/off button is located on the top left corner of the control panel of the pump. The VAC therapy button below the green on/off button is then depressed and the display should read "Therapy On" and "-125 mmHg". VAC therapy is delivered for 48 hours continuously, then the dressing is removed and the wound is cleansed and reevaluated. As needed, VAC therapy is continued. The canister may be used for up to 1 week or until full.

VAC therapy is discontinued when goals set for VAC therapy are reached. Goals may include wound closure, sufficient cleanliness of the wound, or reduction in wound size to allow delayed closure. VAC therapy is generally stopped if no positive results are demonstrated in 1 to 2 weeks despite optimal care. Stopping VAC therapy may require a physician's order.

HYPERBARIC OXYGEN

As discussed in Chapter 2, oxygen is a required nutrient for survival of most tissues over an extended time. Specific to wound healing, oxygen is necessary for collagen production, neutrophil function to reduce risk of infection, and for macrophage function in autolytic debridement. Moreover, high oxygen levels destroy anaerobic bacteria. Especially important is *Pseudomonas aeruginosa.* On the other hand, high oxygen levels slow formation of new capillaries, cause arteriolar constriction, present a risk of oxygen toxicity, and damage to tissue. The basic concept of hyperbaric oxygen (HBO) is to increase the oxygen available for wound healing. Claims made for HBO include increased antibiotic efficacy, fibroblast proliferation, collagen production and strength, increased production of growth factors and growth factor receptor sites, and elevated tissue partial pressure of oxygen.[3]

Two types of HBO have been described. Systemic administration requires placing the patient in a chamber to accommodate the entire body. The gas composition inside the chamber is changed to 100% oxygen and is pressured to further increase the amount of oxygen within the chamber. A second type of HBO is topically administered by use of a plastic bag or other device attached to the skin over a wound.

Increases in PO_2 of inspired air at normal atmospheric pressure have a negligible effect on the amount of oxygen carried by the blood due to saturation of hemoglobin. Under normal circumstances, nearly 100% of oxygen carried by the blood is bound to hemoglobin. Once hemoglobin is saturated with oxygen, very little additional oxygen can be added to the blood. However, administration of 100% oxygen under 2 to 3 atmospheres of pressure can produce such a tremendous increase in arterial PO_2 that the amount carried by the blood improves. HBO has been demonstrated as an effective treatment for a large number of conditions, including decompression sickness, gas embolism, carbon monoxide poisoning, and gas gangrene (clostridial myonecrosis).

Specific types of wounds appear to respond well to HBO. Crush injuries incurred within a few hours may benefit from the combination of pressure to reduce edema in the enriched oxygen environment and decreased leukocyte adherence. A similar problem may occur with skin flaps and grafts. These grafts may be compromised by neutrophil accumulation during ischemia. HBO has also been suggested for treatment of radiation necrosis and refractory ischemic ulcers. Unfortunately, the failure of wounds to heal is generally more complex than insufficient delivery of oxygen to tissues, which makes indiscriminate application of HBO to ischemic ulcers suspect. Moreover, the amount of time spent in a hyperbaric chamber is limited. Poor delivery of oxygen to tissues is generally caused by arterial disease, which may be improved by surgery, rather than intermittent exposure to a source of enriched oxygen.

Different types of systemic HBO chambers are available in different facilities. The type generally used for wound management consists of a clear tube accommodating one individual. Large chambers that accommodate multiple individuals are used for underwater physiology or treatment of decompression sickness (the "bends" or caisson disease) from too rapid ascent during deep sea diving or excessive exposure to hyperbaric environments. Typical systemic HBO treatments consist of 100% oxygen pressured to 2.0 to 2.5 atmospheres for 2 hours daily or twice a day. One hundred percent oxygen is pressurized up to two to three times atmospheric pressure. Normal partial pressure of oxygen in the environment is approximately 760 x 0.21, or 160 mmHg. Partial pressure of oxygen in a whole body chamber may be as high as 1500 to 2000 mmHg. However, exposure to such high partial pressure of oxygen can cause oxygen toxicity, which needs to be monitored. Different facilities, however, may have different protocols. Protocols may be different for various types of wounds as well.

HBO appears to produce dramatic effects in individuals with long-standing, chronic wounds but is also often ineffective. Whole body HBO is still recommended by those in this field, as opposed to extremity chambers or spot-chambers for areas such as the sacrum.

A large number of case studies have been published, but randomized clinical trials showing efficacy of HBO are lacking. Perhaps, factors determining which patients will be successfully treated with HBO will be uncovered in the near future. At this time, a number of recommendations have been made against using HBO because of the cost and inability to demonstrate a consistent, positive result.[4]

Topical Hyperbaric Oxygen

Topical HBO (THBO) has not been generally accepted for the treatment of any specific types of wounds at this time. Medicare reimbursement is not allowed for THBO. The key difference between systemic and THBO is the means of supplying oxygen to the wound. With systemic HBO, the goal is to enrich the content of oxygen dissolved in plasma to increase the supply of oxygen to the tissue and produce effects such as decreased leukocyte adherence to microvessels. With topical administration, the goal is to increase oxygen diffusion from the localized chamber through the wound. One benefit of THBO is reduced likelihood of adverse effects.[5]

This modality may be used on a number of wound types but is limited to open wounds due to the exchange of gases at the surface of the wound only. In addition, the wound must be well-debrided for the treatment to be effective. The presence of eschar or necrotic tissue diminishes the effectiveness of the treatment because oxygen must diffuse from the topical chamber into the viable tissue below. Types of wounds receiving THBO include neuropathic ulcers, venous insufficiency, post-surgical infection, arterial insufficiency, pressure ulcers, amputation wounds, burns, frost bite, skin grafts, and flaps. The purpose of THBO is to augment immune function and increase granulation. The increased pressure and proper positioning can also reduce the edema associated with venous hypertension. THBO is not to be used in the presence of deep venous thrombosis, phlebitis, or severe ischemic ulcers. Precaution is to be used for patients with congestive heart failure.[6]

INFRARED RADIATION

Infrared was once commonly used on open wounds via heat lamps in an effort to dehydrate wounds as a means of preventing infection. Many research articles have been written about using infrared radiation on burn wounds and comparing infection rates to older antibiotics. With the advent of silver sulfadiazine, desiccation of wounds was no longer a suitable option for treating burns and other open wounds. Some had continued to promote infrared radiation as a means of stimulating tissue growth by heating the wound. Current research, however, indicates that tissue growth occurs most rapidly at normal body temperature, and for that reason the practice of heating a wound became questionable.

Hypothermia also slows growth due to vasoconstriction and decreased phagocytic activity. Recently, a new device has been developed to allow controlled warming of a wound to the body's internal temperature. The device, called Warm-Up (Augustine Medical Inc., Eden Prairie, Minn) was approved by the FDA to regulate the temperature of wounds to optimize healing. The device consists of a foam ring with a film covering to allow visualization (Figure 14-5). A card with a radiant heater and temperature sensor is placed into a pocket in the film covering above the wound. The manufacturer recommends using the device three times a day for 1 hour; the unit automatically shuts off after 2 hours. The recommended procedure consists of placing the warming card into the pocket on the wound cover and turning on the device for 1 hour, removal of the card for 1 hour, and repeating the warming for another hour. This cycle is to be repeated three times each day. To control the temperature of the wound, the card is plugged into the controller unit. The controlling unit is portable and can be either battery-operated or run with wall current. The AC adapter is also a battery charger.

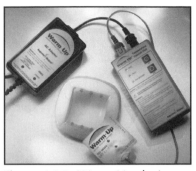

Figure 14-5. Warm-Up device.

The sensor maintains the temperature of the wound, and the film and foam dressing material maintains humidity at an optimal level to promote growth of granulation tissue and re-epithelialization of the wound. The dressing, consisting of the foam ring and semipermeable film cover, should be left in place for as many days as possible based on the amount of drainage. Although the foam ring is capable of absorbing drainage, fluid accumulation can occur within the dressing if left in place too long, leading to maceration of the surrounding skin and slow wound healing. The recommendation is to leave the dressing in place up to 5 days but to change the dressing if the foam becomes overwhelmed with drainage. Daily changes may be necessary for a few days on some wounds; however, avoidance of wound handling may lead to decreased drainage and fewer dressing changes after the first few days.[7]

At this time, the Warm-Up is indicated for pressure ulcers of all stages and neuropathic and venous insufficiency ulcers.[8,9] Wounds are expected to be thoroughly debrided before use of the device, but the presence of necrotic tissue is not a contraindication for use of the Warm-Up. Because heating increases the demand for oxygen, the device should not be used in the cases of severe arterial insufficiency. The manufacturer states that arterial wounds with dry gangrene or any ischemic ulcer without adequate circulation should be carefully evaluated before using this device. Also, because the device promotes growth with an optimum temperature and humidity, infected wounds and osteomyelitis should be treated prior to beginning Warm-Up therapy. In addition, full-thickness burn injuries are a contraindication for this therapy. A greater reduction of wound size was demonstrated for pressure ulcers compared with "standard" treatment using "moisture-retentive" dressings. This study[10] did not, however, compare healing using the same dressing across heating and nonheating groups. Therefore, the contribution of the foam ring with a semiocclusive covering could not be separated from the effect of heating alone. The results of two other studies using venous insufficiency ulcers, however, are indicative of improved healing with this system.

ARTERIAL INSUFFICIENCY

Few devices have been developed to address arterial insufficiency. Generally, this condition is treated either medically or surgically. Arterial insufficiency develops when arterial pressure is no longer capable of driving blood flow through excessively narrowed blood vessels, usually due to atherosclerosis. Two devices have been developed to assist arterial pressure in providing blood flow to affected lower extremities. The vasotrain is a negative pressure chamber that rhythmically develops negative pressure around the affected extremity, rendering arterial pressure more effective at driving blood flow though the lower extremity.

The ArtAssist (ACI-Medical, San Marcos, Calif) is a counterpulsation device similar to what is used for severe heart failure. The device is timed by the EKG to inflate during diastole to drive the blood present in the lower extremity vessels further distally and to deflate during systole to minimize the resistance of the lower extremity vessels and assist arterial pressure in driving flow through the vessels of the affected lower extremity.

THERAPEUTIC ULTRASOUND

Ultrasound refers to sound waves with a frequency greater than what can be perceived by the human ear (20 to 20,000 Hz). Ultrasound is generated by the application of a high-frequency current to a crystal. The crystal vibrates due to what is called the *reverse piezoelectric effect*. The piezoelectric effect is produced when pressure is placed on a crystal to produce an electrical current. This effect is the basis of the phonograph. Ultrasound used to create an image, such as echocardiography to examine the heart, or to view fetal development is called *diagnostic ultrasound. Therapeutic ultrasound* is the use of ultrasound to treat a patient. Ultrasound can be used to heat tissue or can be used at a lower intensity in an effort to assist healing of soft tissue injuries such as strains, sprains, and tendinitis. Ultrasound has been proposed as a means of assisting healing open wounds. However, this modality has not been recommended by AHCPR due to lack of randomized clinical trials to demonstrate its effectiveness.

A number of studies supporting the use of ultrasound have been published, however.[11] Several studies investigating the effects of ultrasound at the cellular level have been published as well. Some of these demonstrate severe cellular damage created by ultrasound. For ultrasound to be transmitted to the wound bed, a coupling medium is required. Ultrasound does not conduct well through air but does well through water or water-based gel. Two approaches may be used to conduct ultrasound. These approaches are to place the patient and the ultrasound head underwater and to fill a wound with sterile ultrasound gel, covering the wound with a hydrogel dressing (Second Skin, Spenco Medical Corporation, Waco, Tex, or Vigilon, C. R. Bard, Inc., Covington, Ga) with sterile saline below and ultrasound gel on the outer surface.

Application of Ultrasound to a Wound

Ultrasound can be provided at different frequencies, notably either 1 or 3 MHz. Higher frequency of ultrasound does not penetrate tissues as deeply as lower frequency ultrasound. Clinicians have suggested using 3 MHz ultrasound on superficial wounds and 1 MHz on deeper wounds. The method of determining duration of treatment is based on the size of the ultrasound application. The recommendation is to move the ultrasound head over a site 1.5 times the size of the applicator for 1 to 2 minutes, then proceed to another site. For a small wound, the treatment can be done in a reasonable time. However, for a large wound, the duration of treatment may become excessive. For example, using a typical 10 cm^2 applicator on a 300 cm^2 wound, twenty areas would be created, requiring 20 to 40 minutes. The suggestion has also been to gradually increase time to 3 minutes per treatment area.

For intensity, both pulsed and continuous modes have been described. Continuous ultrasound is more likely to create a heating effect, which may be desired or undesired. Acute injuries are typically treated with a low intensity (~0.5 W/cm^2), whereas chronic wounds may be treated with a somewhat higher intensity, approaching 1 W/cm^2. Intensity will depend on whether pulsed or continuous ultrasound is used and the duty cycle. One suggestion is to use pulsed ultrasound at an intensity of 1 W/cm^2 with a duty cycle of 25%. The suggestions given in the literature for the onset and frequency of treatment sessions is for BID treatments until the inflammatory phase is over, then reducing treatments to three per week. For chronic wounds, the same sources suggest three treatments per week.[11]

LEECHES

Application of leeches for medicinal purposes originated more than 500 years ago. Although the original goal was to restore health by bringing the body's four humors back into balance, current use is generally directed at overcoming venous congestion following reattachment surgery. For the same reasons, repair of injuries that approximate reattachment, such as gun shot wounds of the foot and crush injuries, may also be indications for leech therapy. The leech used in current practice is Hirudo medicinalis. These leeches can be ordered from a small number of suppliers for overnight delivery and kept for several weeks in a refrigerator until needed. The saliva of leeches also has anticoagulant properties, which may diminish the

risk of thrombosis of reattached digits, ears, and skin flaps. Although some patients may not relish the idea of leeches being attached to them, the leech bites are usually painless, but may leave a characteristic "Y" shaped scar. The leeches may also attempt to migrate to other areas so a protective barrier must be applied around the area of interest to prevent migration. A small risk of infection or allergy also exists.

As needed, leeches are removed from the refrigerator and the skin is cleaned thoroughly with normal saline. A barrier is made from a 4 x 4 gauze sponge with a hole cut in the center and is reinforced with a towel. The leech should be transferred to the area of interest with forceps and guided as needed to the correct area. If the leech does not show interest, the skin may need to be pricked to draw a drop of blood to the area. The leech will feed for about 20 minutes and perhaps longer. The leech should be allowed to release the skin and should not be forcefully removed. When full, the leech will detach, but if pulled, mouth parts of the leech may be left in the wound and cause infection. The detached leech is then placed in a cup, covered in alcohol, and discarded in an appropriate biohazard container.[12]

Application of leeches may be difficult for the clinician. Because patients may be reluctant to agree to leech therapy, an unsteady or squeamish clinician may cause the patient to refuse an important therapy. Hematocrit and appearance of the site should be monitored regularly to ensure that excessive blood is not lost and the reattached body part is maintaining good circulation.

LARVA THERAPY

The use of maggots (fly larvae) for tissue debridement has been traced to the Civil War. At that time, wound infection was a major cause of mortality. Wounds infested with maggots appeared to have a lower rate of infection and mortality than those that did not. The use of maggots declined with the introduction of antibiotics but has survived and enjoyed a recent resurgence.

Maggots used for wound debridement are the larvae of blowfly. Like leeches, they can be obtained from specialized laboratories at a cost of approximately $75 per bottle of 200 maggots. Appropriate wounds include any chronic wound that does not require surgical intervention for debridement. Any wound for which autolytic or enzymatic debridement is suitable may be treated with maggots. Maggots perform highly selective debridement of necrotic tissue as well as maintaining a suitable level of bacteria in the wound.

A number of protocols for using maggots have been developed. The maggots need to be contained over the wound and not allowed to migrate. They are typically left in place for 48 to 72 hours, so they need to be held in place more securely than leeches. One approach is to use two hydrocolloid sheets. A hole approximating the size of the wound is cut in the first hydrocolloid sheet and applied around the wound. The bottle of maggots is applied to the wound and covered with a mesh material. A second hydrocolloid sheet, also with a hole in it, is placed over the first to secure the mesh in place. The top hydrocolloid sheet is removed and discarded with the maggots and mesh between applications and the bottom sheet is left. The procedure is repeated up to twice per week until the wound bed is completely debrided. Two to six applications may be necessary.[12]

SUMMARY

Several adjunctive therapies have been promoted to aid wound healing. The AHCPR guidelines at the time they were written only supported a trial of electrical stimulation for stage III and IV ulcers that failed to respond to conservative care. Since that time, however, new technologies have been developed. The use of radiant heat to maintain a wound at body temperature and application of negative pressure to manage wound edema may prove to be useful. Ultraviolet radiation may be a useful alternative to the use of antiseptics for controlling the growth of bacteria on the surface of wounds. Ultrasound and hyperbaric oxygen lack compelling evidence to support their use for treating chronic wounds.

STUDY QUESTIONS

1. Which adjunctive therapies have received support from AHCPR?
2. Explain the differences between heating by ultrasound, diathermy, and regulated radiant heat.
3. List advantages of using maggots for wound debridement.
4. For what types of wounds would leeches be appropriate?

5. Contrast the purposes of systemic and topical hyperbaric oxygen therapy.
6. What potential benefits may be derived from HBO? What are some of the possible drawbacks?

REFERENCES

1. Crow L. New wound therapy offers treatment advantages for PTs. *Acute Care Perspectives.* 1999;7(2):10-11.
2. Horn J. Vacuum assisted closure (V.A.C.) policy. *Acute Care Perspectives.* 2000; in press.
3. Sheffield PJ. Tissue oxygen measurements with respect to soft tissue wound healing with normobaric and hyperbaric oxygen. *HBO Review.* 1985;6:18-43.
4. Health Care Financing Administration. *Coverage Issues Manual 35-10, Hyperbaric Oxygen Therapy.* Washington, DC: Health Care Financing Administration; 1999.
5. Rossi F, Elsinger E. Topical hyperbaric oxygen therapy for lower extremity wound care: an overview. *Podiatry Management.* 1997;November:110-111.
6. Burdette-Tomlin Memorial Hospital. *Policy and Procedure: Topical Hyperbaric Oxygen.* Cape May Court House, NJ. 2000.
7. Myer AH. Review of warm-up therapy. *Acute Care Perspectives.* 2000;8(2):22-25.
8. Santilli Sm, Valusek PA, Robison C. Use of a non-contact radiant heat bandage for the treatment of chronic venous stasis ulcers. *Advances in Wound Care.* 1999;12:89-93.
9. Cherry GW, Wilson J. The treatment of ambulatory venous ulcer patients with warming therapy. *Ostomy and Wound Management.* 1999;45.65-70.
10. Kloth LC, Berman JE, Dumit-Minkel S, Sutton CH, Papanek PE, Wurzel J. Effects of a normothermic dressing on pressure ulcer healing. *Adv Skin Wound Care.* 2000;13(2):69-74.
11. Young SR, Dyson M. Effective therapeutic ultrasound on the healing of full-thickness excised skin lesions. *Ultrasonics.* 1999;28:175-180.
12. Hudson M. What's old is new again. Leech and maggot therapy: wound care in the 90's. *Acute Care Perspectives.* 1999;7(2):15-17.

15 Dressings

OBJECTIVES

- List basic purposes of dressings.
- Distinguish desired characteristics for dressing acute and chronic wounds.
- Discuss appropriate conditions for occluding wounds.
- List types of nonocclusive dressings; discuss appropriate conditions for nonocclusive dressings.
- Discuss properties of different types of occlusive dressings including hydrogels, semipermeable film, hydrocolloids, foam, alginate and hydrofibers, and composites.
- Discuss appropriate conditions for using each type of occlusive dressing.
- Describe alternatives for individuals who cannot tolerate adhesives.
- Discuss the types of secondary dressings and list purposes for using them.
- Discuss different types of tape relative to their appropriate use, including use on fragile skin.

Table 15-1

PURPOSES OF DRESSINGS

- Physical protection of wound
- Prevention of contamination
- Promote autolytic debridement
- Fill dead space to prevent formation of hematomas, abscesses, tunnels, sinus tracts
- Management of drainage by absorption, evaporation, or occlusion
- Retain moisture in wound bed including cells, enzymes, and growth factors

---

Throughout history, man has placed a wide variety of substances in, over, and on wounds in an effort to improve healing. Today, we enjoy a wide variety of very good materials for use as wound dressings. However, many of those responsible for choosing wound dressings base decisions on the physiology of the wound and properties of the dressing. The purpose of this chapter is to develop a decision-making process by which a wound dressing may be chosen. More important, the process must extend to making decisions about whether a previous choice may no longer be appropriate. Four categories of products must be considered for their appropriateness on any given wound: dressings, wound fillers, products to protect the surrounding skin, and secondary dressings to hold dressings in place.

PURPOSES OF WOUND DRESSINGS

Armed with an understanding of the cause of the wound and possible complicating factors, we can begin the process of selecting a wound dressing. The next step is to understand the purposes of dressings in general, as well as the properties and purposes of specific classes of dressings. As we will see, even within a class of dressings, substantial differences in properties may make one brand of dressing more appropriate than another dressing.

Starting with the simplest purpose, dressings serve to physically protect the wound from the external environment and prevent contamination. As discussed previously, tremendous differences exist between acute and chronic wounds. With acute wounds, the greatest concerns are infection and hematoma formation. In contrast, chronic wounds are usually colonized, but contamination with microbes new to the wound increases the risk of infection. The major concern with chronic wounds is optimizing the wound's microenvironment without compromising the integrity of the surrounding skin. Because of these differences in goals, dressings are usually different for acute and chronic wounds. A second purpose for dressings is to promote breakdown and removal of necrotic tissue. A third purpose is to fill dead space in a wound to prevent the formation of hematomas, abscesses, tunnels, and sinus

tracts. Managing drainage, whether purulent exudate or serous transudate, is a fifth purpose. Dressings that hold fluid within wounds (occlusive dressings) promote healing by maintaining moisture, retaining growth factors and enzymes, and allowing autolytic debridement (Table 15-1).

Dressings may be classified by the way they are used to manage drainage. A dry-to-dry dressing is placed in a wound dry and removed when it is dry. These are used to absorb drainage and promote hemostasis in acute wounds. These dressings may be used to cover acute wounds closed by primary intention or small acute wounds. This type of dressing is usually not employed for large or chronic wounds.

A wet-to-wet dressing is moistened, usually with either normal saline or an antiseptic solution such as triple antibiotic, to soften eschar or treat an infected wound.

A third type is the wet-to-dry dressing (Figure 15-1), which is used for nonselective debridement of wounds with either large amounts of necrotic tissue or wounds that must be debrided rapidly.

Microenvironmental or occlusive dressings are designed to optimize the wound environment to promote healing. Several subtypes of occlusive dressings are discussed in Tables 15-2 and 15-3. In addition to differences in the ability to retain moisture (occlusiveness), they have several other important characteristics such as their ability to absorb drainage, to allow drainage to evaporate, and to maintain temperature of the wound bed.

USING DRESSINGS

A few general points about using dressings need to be addressed. The first important point is organization. Organizing the dressing change in advance is key to minimizing contamination of the wound. The clinician should gather all dressing materials and anything else that might be needed to evaluate the wound, especially if cleansing and debridement will precede the dressing change. Although a sterile field is not an absolute requirement (more discussion follows in Chapter 18), following the basic principles of maintaining a sterile field in a reason-

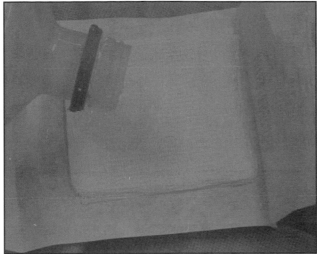

Figure 15-1. Wet-to-dry dressing.

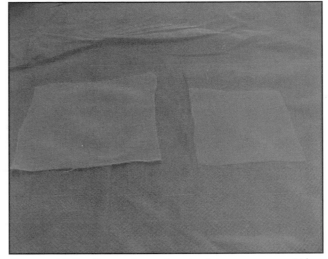

Figure 15-2. Examples of petrolatum gauze. (Also shown in Color Atlas following page 274.)

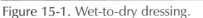

Table 15-2

TYPES OF DRESSINGS

Nonocclusive	*Occlusive*
Dry-to-dry gauze	Semipermeable film
Wet-to-wet gauze	Hydrocolloid
Wet-to-dry gauze	Hydrogel
Petrolatum gauze	Semipermeable foam
Contact layer	Alginate, hydrofiber
Composite	Composite

Table 15-3

CATEGORIES OF DRESSINGS BY THE CENTERS FOR MEDICARE AND MEDICAID SERVICES[1]

Alginates	Hydrogels: sheets
Biologicals and synthetic membranes	Impregnated
Collagens	Silicone gel sheets
Contact layers	Silver technology
Elastic gauzes	Transparent films
Foam	Wound fillers
Gauzes and nonwoven dressings	Liquid skin protectors
Hydrocolloids	Moisture barriers
Hydrogels: amorphous	Therapeutic moisturizers
Hydrogels: impregnated dressings	Skin substitutes

able manner is good practice to prevent contamination of the wound. Packages should be opened just before being used if possible. This can be achieved by having an assistant available, allowing the patient to be the assistant, or organizing the dressing change as carefully as possible.

BASIC TYPES OF DRESSINGS

Gauze products include telfa pads, gauze sponges, and bandage rolls. These dressings offer simple protection of the wound. Cotton gauze is reasonably absorbent and can

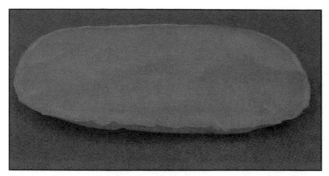

Figure 15-3a. Composite dressing: intact Exudry dressing.

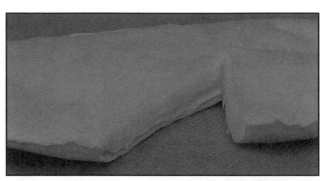

Figure 15-3b. Exudry dressing cut in cross-section to reveal layers.

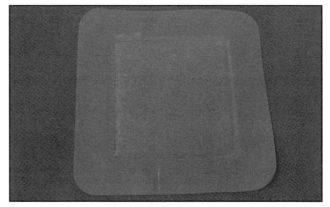

Figure 15-3c. "Island dressing" consisting of foam outer and surrounding surfaces with an absorptive center.

be layered to provide sufficient absorption of copious exudate. Dry gauze performs well as a bacterial barrier, but wet gauze may transmit bacteria into a wound. When gauze becomes soaked with drainage, it needs to be changed to prevent transmission of bacteria. Telfa and related products have nonstick layers between the wound surface and the absorbent material. However, one drawback is the potential for desiccation and adherence of drainage between the absorbent material and the wound bed. Gauze is also used for wet-to-dry dressings to promote nonselective debridement. Contamination with small pieces of cotton that shed from the dressing into the wound can promote chronic inflammation and stimulate copious drainage from the wound. Gauze products are permeable to bacteria, gas, and fluid and are, therefore, considered nonocclusive. They are indicated for protecting acute wounds closed by primary intent, infected wounds, when rapid debridement is necessary, or when absorption of copious drainage or absorption of bleeding to prevent a hematoma is important.

Petrolatum-impregnated gauze products (Figure 15-2) are sometimes used in an effort to protect the wound from adherence of the dressing. Although petrolatum decreases the risk of adhesion, drainage can also dry across the perforations as described for telfa pads; granulation tissue may grow through the perforations, causing adherence and bleeding during dressing removal. Petrolatum gauze may be useful for protecting a wound and retaining moisture in a wound that is not at risk for adherence to the petroleum and with planned frequent dressing changes. In particular, it can be useful as a dressing when ointments are used directly on the wound that require frequent dressing changes (eg, over silver sulfadiazine or chemical debriding agents to minimize desiccation).

Contact layer dressings and composites with contact layers are made of nonstick material similar to telfa but with much smaller perforations that allow some evaporation of excessive moisture, not larger molecules that cause adherence. Some products (eg, Exudry, Smith & Nephew, Largo, Fla) combine a contact layer with a layer of highly absorbent material. This type of dressing has characteristics that are suitable for acute or infected wounds without the drawbacks associated with gauze, telfa, and impregnated gauze (Figures 15-3a through 15-3c).

MICROENVIRONMENTAL (OCCLUSIVE) DRESSINGS

The basis of these dressings is that healing is most effective if the wound microenvironment is optimized. Optimization includes maintaining an appropriate moisture level and temperature, availability of macromolecules of healing (glycosaminoglycans, proteoglycans, collagen), availability of growth factors (macrophage- and platelet-derived), acceptable levels of nonpathogenic microflora, and protection of environment from pathogens.[2,3] Wound moisture is critical for migration of epithelial cells, movement of enzymes, growth factors, and structural molecules, but excessive moisture damages surrounding skin (maceration). An appropriate microenvironmental dressing also prevents scab formation. As discussed previously, desiccated fibrin and blood act as a dressing to retain moisture below and to keep out pathogens, but they slow epithelial cell migration as cells are forced below to resurface a wound. Promotion of autolytic debridement is

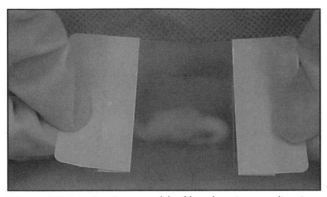

Figure 15-4a. Semipermeable film dressing application over alginate wound filler. Tension is maintained on the edges to prevent self-adherence.

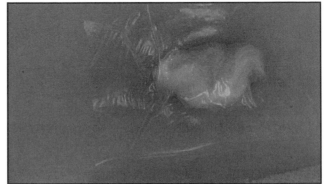

Figure 15-4b. Dressing in place. Placing a hand on the dressing to warm it for several seconds improves the adherence. The alginate filler is clearly visible beneath the dressing.

SEMIPERMEABLE FILM DRESSINGS

Many brands of semipermeable films are now available. An example is shown in Figures 15-4a and 15-4b. Opsite (Smith & Nephew, Largo, Fla) is probably the best known of these, and it has been redesigned to improve its handling.

These dressings are occlusive and will allow drainage to accumulate under them, but they cannot handle moderate or maximum levels of drainage. They allow some evaporation of fluid, but cannot absorb any drainage. If drainage becomes too great, the dressing can loosen and leak. Film dressings are particularly useful for superficial wounds or partial-thickness wounds with minimal drainage, or as a secondary dressing to hold a more absorbent material in the wound.[4] Most of these dressings are quite adherent and can damage the patient's skin if used inappropriately. A skin protectant such as Skin-Prep (Smith & Nephew, Largo, Fla) should be applied to the surrounding skin (see Skin Sealants on page 174). Proper technique must also be used to remove semipermeable films. If pulled directly from the wound, the skin may adhere more strongly to the film dressing than to itself, causing the skin to tear. Proper technique to remove a film is to lift a corner and stretch the semipermeable film tangentially to the wound, causing the dressing to stretch and loosen. Semipermeable films, in particular, and any dressing should be applied with care to avoid restricting adjacent parts of the body, particularly with sacral and coccygeal wounds. Care must be taken not to bridge the gluteal cleft with these dressings. If a semipermeable film is to be used in this area, a number of alternatives may be used. First, the dressing may be turned such that a corner of the dressing is placed in the cleft, between fingers, or toes, or other areas. A second option is to cut a dressing into a "valentine" shape and apply the dressing with the point in the cleft. Placing two dressings with one on either side and overlapping in the middle to cover the

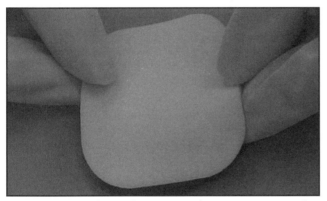

Figure 15-5. A foam dressing used to cover a wound.

also important because necrotic as well as desiccated tissue obstructs cell migration. Therefore, these dressings are useful for chronic wounds in an effort to enhance healing but not for infected wounds. Some of these dressings are useful for acute wounds with little necrotic tissue or drainage.

Occlusive dressings offer some very important advantages for the wound, the patient, and the clinician. Many of these dressings may be left in place for several days at a time, ranging from 3 to 10 days. Decreased handling of the wound minimizes inflammation, which in turn decreases drainage from the wound. Some of these dressings are nonadherent, whereas others are very adherent to the surrounding skin. The more adherent a dressing, the longer it should be left on the wound to minimize trauma to surrounding skin. Certain types of occlusive dressings, especially hydrogels, are soothing to irritated wounds, especially burns, chemical burns, and radiation burns. Occlusive dressings also retain fluid and macromolecules important for wound healing. However, among the occlusive dressings, only alginates and the related hydrofibers are indicated for infected wounds.

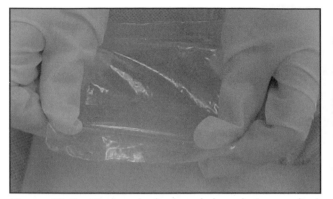

Figure 15-6a. Hydrogels: hydrogel sheet being applied over a wound.

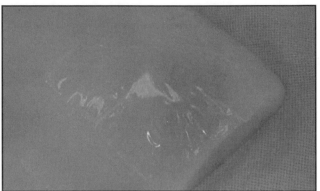

Figure 15-6b. Hydrogel sheet dressing in place.

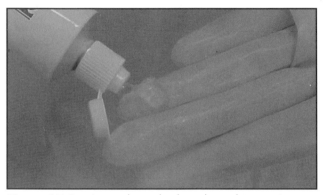

Figure 15-6c. Amorphous hydrogel used to moisten a dry wound bed.

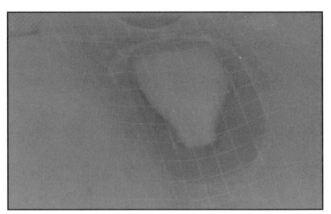

Figure 15-7a. Hydrocolloid dressings. Thin hydrocolloid sheet placed over an alginate filler.

entirety of the wound is another option. If placing a single piece of dressing material across an area such as the gluteal cleft cannot be avoided, start with the dressing folded and begin placing it in the center and delicately smooth outwardly so that full mobility is unimpeded.

SEMIPERMEABLE FOAMS

These dressings manage drainage by absorption, evaporation, and occlusion. An example is shown in Figure 15-5. They are the most absorbent of the occlusive dressings. However, a variety of foam thickness results in a wide variation of the amount of drainage that can be absorbed. They will retain large quantities of fluid in the wound, absorbing excessive drainage. Some brands allow substantial evaporation to occur as well. They are not as permeable to gas and water vapor as films but are less occlusive than hydrogels or hydrocolloids. Major advantages of foams, in addition to their absorbency, are the physical cushioning of wounds and thermal insulation to maintain temperature of the wound closer to the optimal temperature for the growth of fibroblasts and epithelial cells.

HYDROGELS

This material is available in two basic forms: sheets and amorphous. Examples of hydrogels are shown in Figures 15-6a through 15-6c. Hydrogels are not generally used to manage drainage, but they provide some occlusion, absorption, and evaporation. Rather than absorb drainage, however, hydrogels are used primarily to hydrate dry wounds. In addition, hydrogel can be very soothing on wounds, especially burns and radiation burns. Hydrogel sheets may also be used on partial-thickness or full-thickness wounds. Sheets are also available over-the-counter in nonsterile form, which are very popular for cyclists and other athletes prone to abrasions. Hydrogel sheets are nonadherent and can slide off the wound, requiring taping to keep them in place. They can also transmit bacteria. The sheets come with polyethylene film on both sides. The inner film is always removed and the outer film may be removed to increase evaporative loss of fluid from the wound. Amorphous gel is available in tubes and other squeezable containers for use in wounds with subcutaneous involvement. Amorphous gel is particularly suited to hydrate dry wounds, especially tendons and

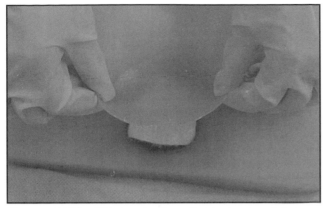

Figure 15-7b. Thicker hydrocolloid sheet cut into a valentine shape to place over a sacral wound.

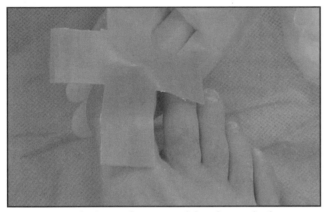

Figure 15-7d. Cross shape used for the end of a toe or finger.

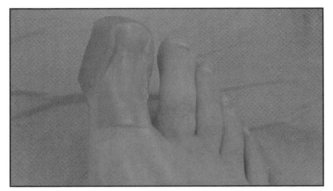

Figure 15-7f. Completed application. Holding a hand over the hydrocolloid sheet to warm it increases the conformability and adherence of the dressing to provide a good fit over the irregular shape of the great toe.

other specific structures. A thin layer of amorphous gel may also be used to line cavities; Medicare specifically states that hydrogel should not be used to fill a wound. Metronidazole gel is available for treating wounds infected with gram-negative bacteria. Amorphous hydrogel and hydrogel sheets can also be used as an interface for therapeutic ultrasound (see Chapter 14).

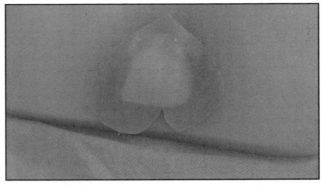

Figure 15-7c. Valentine-shaped hydrocolloid sheet in place.

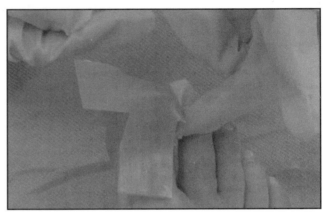

Figure 15-7e. Folding the tabs in place.

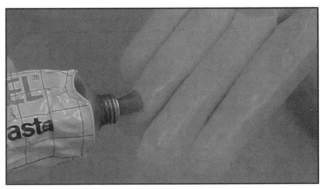

Figure 15-7g. Hydrocolloid wound filler.

HYDROCOLLOIDS

A material easily distinguished by its appearance, hydrocolloids are the most occlusive of the microenvironmental dressings. Many brands and types are available (Figures 15-7a through 15-7g). They have a characteristic appearance of dried-up cheese with a distinctive tan color. This material comes in a variety of thicknesses. The thicker varieties are opaque and a deeper tan. Thin hydrocolloid sheets are a lighter tan color and allow limited visualization of the wound. The material is also capable of absorbing moderate drainage in addition to occluding the wound. As hydrocolloid absorbs water, it becomes lighter

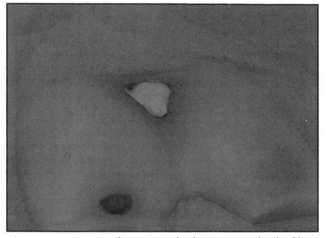

Figure 15-8a. Application of alginate or hydrofiber dressings. Alginate sheet was cut to fit a sacral wound.

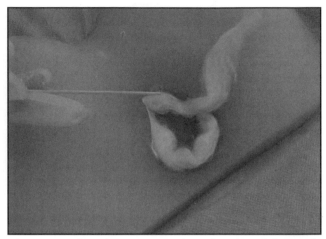

Figure 15-8b. Alginate rope loosely placed beneath undermined areas of a wound.

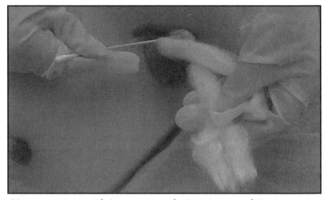

Figure 15-8c. Alginate rope being inserted into a tunnel.

in color and softer. These dressings are designed to be used for several days at a time, which leads to several precautions. First, these dressings should never be used on infected wounds. Occlusion promotes the environment for growth, whether fibroblasts, epidermal cells, or bacteria. The outer surface is impermeable to water, therefore hydrocolloid dressings can be worn in the shower with some prudence to avoid soaking the dressing constantly. The backing of hydrocolloid sheets is very adherent to allow the dressing to stay in place for several days between dressing changes. For this reason, hydrocolloids should only be used if the clinician is comfortable with allowing the wound to stay covered for 5 days or longer. When the dressing is removed, the product of several days' worth of autolytic debridement will have a mild odor and superficially resemble purulence. However, when the drainage is cleansed from the wound, the odor and soupy drainage will be gone, indicating that the wound is not infected. The edges of hydrocolloid sheets will frequently roll up, especially when placed in locations where shearing forces are present with bed mobility. In these cases, clinicians frequently tape the edges of hydrocolloid sheets.

Hydrocolloids are also available for filling cavities and managing drainage. Hydrocolloids can be formulated in pastes, granules, and spiral-cut sheets to fill a wound. These absorption products require a secondary dressing to hold them in the wound. The secondary dressing could be a hydrocolloid sheet or something simpler such as film or gauze. These fillers will allow the absorption of maximum drainage and decrease the need for dressing changes, which increases patient comfort, patient adherence to the plan of care, and decreases the opportunity for contamination and chronic inflammation caused by rough handling. Like semipermeable films, hydrocolloid sheets must also be removed carefully to prevent injury to the surrounding skin, and a skin sealant may need to be used to protect the skin from injury.

ALGINATES AND HYDROFIBERS

The most versatile of the microenvironmental dressings, alginates, are derived from long-chain sugars obtained from seaweed and have the property of changing from a fiber to a gel as they absorb fluid. Hydrofibers are improvements on the older-generation products. Examples are shown in Figures 15-8a through 15-8c (see also Figures 15-4a, 15-4b and Figures 15-7a through 15-7g). With an appropriate secondary dressing, alginates and hydrofibers can be used with maximum drainage. The gel that is formed when water is absorbed is removed easily from the wound bed as a single piece of gel. Some clinicians like to premoisten alginates to fill desiccated wounds. However, a simpler and more cost-effective approach is to line the wound with amorphous hydrogel instead. The secondary dressing used over the alginate or hydrofiber can be selected based on the drainage. A semipermeable film can be used with minimum exudate (see Figures 15-4a and 15-4b), whereas foam or absorbent secondary dressings may be used for copious drainage. If a hydrocolloid is used as the secondary dressing (see Figures 15-7a through 15-7f), the

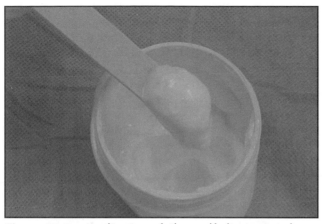

Figure 15-9a. Application of silver sulfadiazine to a burn injury of the hand. This figure shows scooping with a tongue depressor.

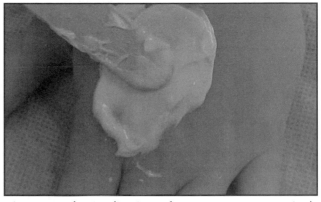

Figure 15-9b. Application of a 0.0625 to 0.125 inch layer.

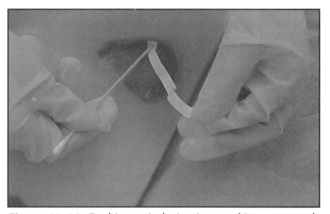

Figure 15-10. Packing strip being inserted into a tunnel.

clinician must be willing to leave the dressing in place for several days. Alginates come in the form of sheets and ribbons, have remarkable tensile strength, and can be placed in tunnels and sinus tracts (see Figures 15-8a through 15-8c). Some clinicians have a habit of fluffing the alginate sheets before filling a cavity, but this practice is unnecessary. One new product of particular note is alginate combined with collagen. The alginate absorbs drainage as the collagen is absorbed into the wound to promote healing.

SILVER SULFADIAZINE

This antibiotic, in the form of a thick, soothing ointment, may be considered a dressing. It is used primarily on burns with or without gauze to protect wounds, but may be applied to some types of acute wounds. Silver sulfadiazine should be applied under clean conditions, with a thickness of 0.0625 inch after hydrotherapy and debridement (Figures 15-9a and 15-9b). It also needs to be reapplied to areas from which it has been removed by patient activity. The ointment is to be left in place for 24 hours. It is contraindicated for pregnant women, infants younger than 2 months of age, or premature infants because of the risk of kernicterus, brain damage caused by bilirubinemia. Although frequently used for many days, it should be discontinued when the risk of infection has passed, usually with complete debridement.

MANAGEMENT OF CAVITIES

Wounds with substantial subcutaneous involvement may require either packing or filling to optimize healing. The term *packing* is frequently used incorrectly to describe a process of placing dressing materials into a wound. Packing refers to a specific type of wound filling that is used to keep a wound open as it is prepared for delayed primary closure (tertiary closure). Packing prevents the wound from filling with granulation tissue and reepithelializing, so tertiary closure can be performed once the wound is clean and stable. Wounds created for irrigation and drainage of abscesses and osteomyelitis are the usual type requiring packing. Filling, in contrast, is used strictly to allow dead spaces to heal from the wound bed to prevent the wound from covering an open area and forming an abscess. Filling is done loosely to promote healing from inside out and to manage drainage in wounds with undermined or tunnels, or those with sinus tracts. Alginate sheets or ropes (see Figures 15-8a through c) are removed easily and have greater biocompatibility than gauze packing strips or sponges. Collagen sheets and ropes have the added advantage of the collagen being absorbed into the wound and possibly enhancing healing rate.

The procedure used is also determined by the drainage of the wound and whether the wound is infected. Packing strips of various sizes, commonly 0.25 or 0.50 inch width may be packed in an infected tunnel or sinus tract (Figure 15-10). Frequently, the packing strip is soaked in antibiotic solution; packing strips containing iodine are also available for this purpose. Either packing strip or gauze sponges (2 x 2 or 4 x 4) may be loosely placed into an infected undermined or open area, or packed into a diabetic foot undergoing irrigation and drainage for osteomyelitis. Gauze sponges and packing strips will need to be changed at least daily and possibly twice each day to remove infectious material.

Cavities with dry wound beds can be lined with hydrogel to provide moisture to assist healing as well as fill the void. Wet wounds can be filled loosely with alginate or hydrofiber ribbon or sheet, hydrocolloid fillers, or dextranomers. Dextranomers are beads placed in wounds to absorb exudate, bacteria, and debris. Tunnels and sinus tracts may be filled with alginate or hydrofiber ribbons if they are clean. An appropriate secondary dressing is based on the desired frequency of dressing change and whether the wound is infected. An infected wound that needs to be changed daily or more often needs a nonocclusive secondary dressing such as an abdominal (Abd) pad, bandage rolls, or simply gauze sponge taped over the primary dressing. If a more occlusive dressing is needed to prevent desiccation, petrolatum gauze may be used. Secondary dressings for wounds that will be covered longer can either be films for low drainage or hydrocolloid for heavier drainage.

SKIN SEALANTS

Although several companies now manufacture these products, Skin-Prep is probably the best known. The liquid material is applied with either a gauze sponge or cotton-tipped applicator from a sealed package. Consisting of a plastic polymer and solvent, the material polymerizes as the solvent evaporates, leaving a film of plastic on the skin. Instead of the dressing adhering directly to the surrounding skin of the wound, the adhesive of the dressing sticks to the protective material placed on the skin. These products also have the advantage of protecting surrounding skin from moisture. Other types of moisture barriers are discussed in Chapter 16. Although skin sealants can be used under any self-adherent dressing, they are particularly important when semipermeable films are used. This type of dressing is not only very adherent, but usually needs to be changed more frequently than other types such as hydrocolloids.

SECONDARY DRESSINGS AND BANDAGING TECHNIQUES

Two basic types of bandage rolls are in general use. Bulky bandage rolls such as Kerlix (Kendall, Mansfield, Mass) are absorbent, cushion, retain warmth, and can be used to immobilize a body part. Lightweight bandage rolls are designed to have a more elastic weave and neater finish, and may be used if movement of a body part is encouraged. Examples of bulky and lightweight bandage rolls are

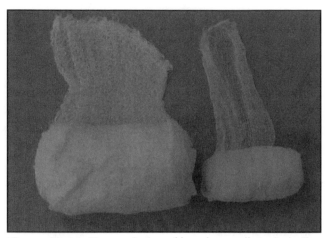

Figure 15-11. Two varieties of bandage roll. Left: bulky bandage used for absorbency. Right: lightweight bandage to promote movement and give a neater appearance.

shown in Figure 15-11. Bandage rolls should always be rolled on the patient's body from the bottom (Figure 15-12a). Rolling from the top causes bandage rolls to catch on themselves, causing uneven coverage and possibly dropping of the bandage roll. The primary dressing is the dressing placed in direct contact with the wound. A secondary bandage is used to hold the primary dressing in place, increase absorption, provide compression when needed, provide warmth and comfort to the area, and to physically protect or pad the area of the wound. Secondary dressings may consist of adhesive bandages, bandage rolls, gauze sponges (commonly 4 x 4) taped over the primary dressing, or one of a number of elasticized materials such as Stretch Net (DeRoyal Industries, Powell, Tenn), Tubigrip (Convatec, Skillman, NJ), ACE bandages, or certain compression bandages. A tertiary dressing is placed over a secondary dressing on occasion.

Bandaging has several purposes. In addition to the roles of secondary dressings to secure and protect primary dressings, increase absorption of drainage, and provide warmth, bandage rolls can also be used to apply pressure. Three basic techniques are commonly used. A simple spiral is used for holding dressings in place and coverage of the wound (Figure 15-12b). A figure of eight is commonly used for controlling the amount of pressure under the bandage. Bandages can also be fan-folded (Figure 15-12c) by folding it back over itself. Fan-folding is used to increase absorption and provide padding. Typically, bandage rolls are convenient to meet the needs of bandaging. They come in various widths, although 4-inch bandages appear to be most commonly used. In applications with smaller or larger areas, a 2- or 6-inch bandage may also be used. The weave of the bandage roll also determines its properties. A thinly layered interlocking weave provides elasticity to the bandage roll, whereas a loose, bulky band-

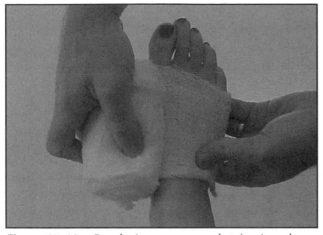

Figure 15-12a. Bandaging as a secondary/tertiary dressing. Proper technique is to roll the gauze bandage from the bottom.

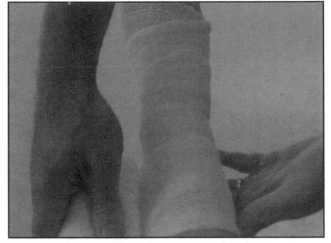

Figure 15-12b. Half-overlapping spiral technique.

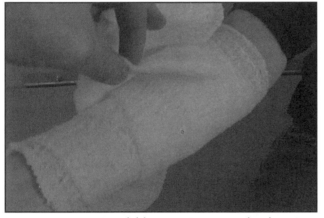

Figure 15-12c. Fan-folding to increase the layering, cushioning, and absorbency in the cubital fossa.

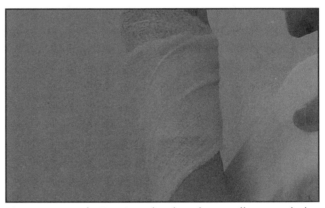

Figure 15-12d. Turning the bandage roll around the ankle to anchor it.

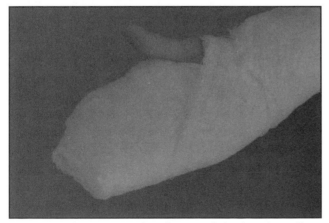

Figure 15-12e. Proper bandaging of the hand to allow free movement of an uninvolved thumb.

age provides more absorption and insulation. Elasticized cotton bandages such as Kling (Kendall, Mansfield, Mass) or Conform (Johnson & Johnson, New Brunswick, NJ) allow mobility, but they are less absorbent than soft bulky

bandage rolls such as Kerlix, which are more absorbent and provide better padding but less mobility. Soft, bulky bandage rolls may be used for the specific purpose of limiting mobility on occasion. When using a bandage roll on the hand or foot, create a lock by making at least one turn (Figure 15-12d) around the wrist or ankle. In general, keep the thumb separate from the other fingers to allow grasp (Figure 15-12e). Humidity can increase to a damaging level under bandage rolls. If toes or fingers are covered by a bandage roll, place 2 x 2s between toes or 4 x 4s between fingers to prevent maceration (Figure 15-12f).

Bandage rolls and other secondary dressings may be easily dislodged between dressing changes. A means of securing the secondary dressing should be in place. In particular, a piece of tape above the heel or on the wrist just proximal to the hand needs to be used to prevent loosening and migration of the bandage off the hand or foot (Figure 15-12g). However, any taping over either a primary or secondary dressing, including bandage rolls, should be done to avoid circumferential closure. That means that one end of a piece of tape should never be arranged so it adheres to the other end. If swelling occurs,

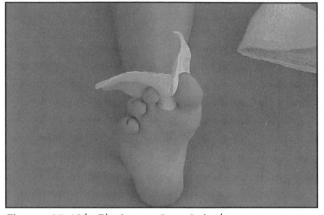

Figure 15-12f. Placing a 2 x 2 inch gauze sponge between the toes to prevent maceration.

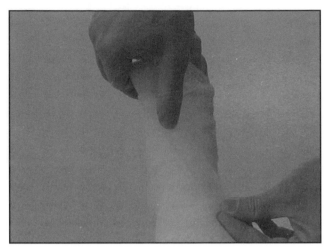

Figure 15-12g. Application of "racing stripes" across turns of the bandage roll to prevent unraveling.

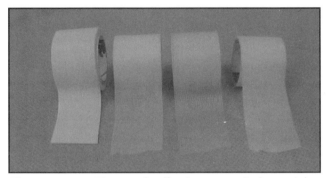

Figure 15-13. Types of adhesive tape. Left to right: Foam, paper, plastic, and silk.

circumferential taping may lead to limb-threatening ischemia. If needed, tape can be placed in a spiral such that the ends are still free to move relative to each other. Better yet is to prudently use short pieces of tape that serve the purpose of preventing the material of interest from being dislodged. Strips of tape perpendicular to the bandage roll also prevent turns of a bandage roll to unravel.

TAPE

Four basic types of tape are used in wound care (Figure 15-13). They will be discussed in order of harshness to the skin. *Silk* tape such as Durapore (3M, St. Paul, Minn), is the most adhesive of the four types. It may cause minimal damage when used carefully and occasionally on young, healthy skin; but it will tear weak, elderly skin and damage healthy skin with repeated use. It should be avoided for wound dressings because of cost and adhesiveness.

Plastic tape such as Transpore (3M, St. Paul, Minn), is still too adhesive and harsh for skin at risk for damage. It is convenient for use because it tears easily in both directions. Appropriate uses include taping secondary dressings to surfaces other than skin and anchoring a secondary dressing to itself, especially by means of "racing stripes" (see Figure 15-12g) on a bandage roll to prevent unraveling.

Paper tape including Micropore (3M, St. Paul, Minn), has low adhesion and is hypoallergenic. As such, it is usually gentle enough for repeated applications to healthy skin or occasional application to at-risk skin. It is a lower-cost tape, but comes off skin easily. Appropriate uses include taping a primary or secondary dressing directly to the skin.

The best type of tape to place directly on skin is an elastic *foam* tape such as Microfoam (3M, St. Paul, Minn). This type of tape has low but adequate adhesion. It is gentle enough for daily or BID changes on at-risk skin and is comfortable and water resistant. Due to its elasticity, it conforms to irregular surfaces and stretches with swelling. However, it should not be stretched as it is placed on the skin. The recoil of the elastic tape causes shearing and potential damage to the skin. This type of tape is expensive and loses adhesion when repositioned. Its uses include taping a primary or secondary dressing directly to skin, especially at-risk skin or for those receiving frequent dressing changes.

MONTGOMERY STRAPS

One may consider these as a special type of tertiary dressing used for approximating dehiscent wounds. Montgomery straps protect the healing wound from trauma caused by patient movement in bed, coughing, sneezing, and similar movement. They can be made with 2-inch silk tape laced with umbilical tape (Figures 15-14a and 15-14b). The skin can be protected by placing the tape onto hydrocolloid sheets placed on either side of the wound rather than placing silk tape directly on the skin. Montgomery straps are also available premade but are rather expensive. Usually an ABD pad is the secondary

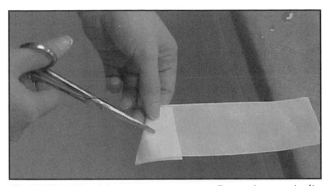

Figure 15-14a. Montgomery straps. Preparing an individual strap from 2-inch silk tape doubled over at one end and an opening cut for lacing in the doubled end.

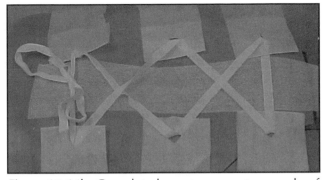

Figure 15-14b. Completed montgomery strap made of 2-inch silk and a 0.5-inch umbilical tape.

dressing with either a wet-to-dry or alginate primary dressing, depending on the state of the dehiscent wound.

TOLERANCE FOR ADHESIVES

Many individuals cannot tolerate the adhesives used on wound care products. One problem is the strength of the adhesive relative to the cohesiveness of the person's skin, especially in elderly individuals. Many individuals also have immune reactions to adhesives. Wound dressings that are particularly problematic are semipermeable films and hydrocolloids, although other types of dressings may include adhesives. Semipermeable films are particularly problematic because they tend to be changed more frequently than other dressings. Even dressings that do not contain adhesives can cause problems because of the need for taping to keep them in place or the use of secondary dressings containing adhesives.

A number of solutions are available. To protect skin from the mechanical aspects of aggressive adhesives, skin protectants such as Skin-Prep can be used. Skin protectants are described further in Chapter 16. Careful removal of semipermeable film by stretching and leaving hydrocolloids in place as long as possible then carefully removing them from the surrounding skin will minimize trauma. Alternatively, nonadherent dressings may need to be substituted for films and hydrocolloids. Films perform by occlusion and evaporation, whereas hydrocolloids retain moisture by occlusion and absorb some drainage. Foam dressings can occlude wounds and absorb even greater amounts of fluid than hydrocolloids but may dry out wounds more suited to film dressings; therefore, represent an alternative for hydrocolloids for a wound with moderate drainage and intolerance for the adhesive on a hydrocolloid dressing.

Nonocclusive gauze dressings will allow desiccation of wounds with moderate or minimal drainage and may adhere to the wound or cause inflammation of the wound.

Nonadherent types of nonocclusive dressings, such as telfa pads or petrolatum-impregnated gauze, may be adequate with minimal serous drainage but will adhere to the wound if exudate is allowed to dry through the pores in the dressing. Dressings with special contact layers are much less likely to adhere to wounds but may also desiccate a wound with minimal drainage. One solution is to use amorphous hydrogel under nonocclusive dressings for the person who cannot tolerate a semipermeable film dressing for a minimally draining wound.

For dressings that require taping to hold them in place, a foam tape is the most appropriate as long as the tape is not stretched as it is applied. Stretching foam tape causes shearing of the skin. Because foam tape is not as adherent as other types, a 2-inch width is usually necessary. Other options include the use of either bulky or elasticized bandage rolls, tubular bandages, or net bandages (Figures 15-15a through 15-15c). These may work well on areas of the body not subject to weight shifting and moving, but on highly mobile areas, the nonadherent dressing below is likely to shift.

ECONOMICS OF DRESSING CHANGES

One drawback of occlusive dressings is their cost. However, if we account for the faster healing under occlusive dressings and the greater frequency of nonocclusive dressings ($5.00 to $8.00 for a 4 to 7 day application) compared to the cost of gauze, the economic picture becomes quite different. Moreover, the greatest charges come not from the dressing itself, but the time for the dressing change to be performed. A wound being treated with nonocclusive dressings may cost $3.00 or more depending on the number of gauze layers and the size of them. Moreover, the dressing change may be done twice each day at a cost of up to $6.00 a day in materials compared to $5.00 to $8.00 for the entire 5 ± 2 days. These numbers are based on a cost of 4¢ for nonsterile 4 x 4s, 48¢ for sterile 4 x 4s, and $1.50 for a 4-inch bandage roll appli-

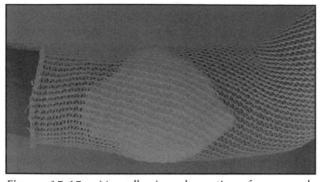

Figure 15-15a. Nonadhesive alternatives for secondary/tertiary dressings: stretch netting.

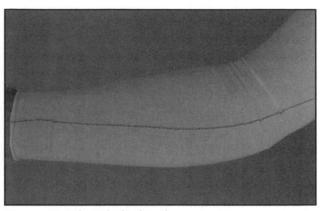

Figure 15-15b. Tubular bandage.

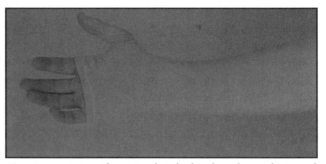

Figure 15-15c. Elasticized tubular bandage designed specifically for the hand and forearm.

cation. Clearly, an occlusive dressing left in place for a number of days decreases time charges and may actually cost less in materials.

For patients covered by Medicare Part B, additional reimbursement issues may need to be considered. Medicare Part B will reimburse only primary and secondary dressings for wounds that are caused by a surgical procedure, treated by a surgical procedure, or require debridement. Debridement must be performed by a licensed physician or health care professional as permitted by state law. Debridement may include any of those described in Chapter 12. Medicare will not reimburse for dressings used on skin conditions treated with topical medications; draining cutaneous fistulas; dressings used to protect a healed wound by reducing friction, shear, moisture; dressings over catheter insertion points; first-degree burns; skin tears, abrasions, venipuncture; or arterial puncture sites.

For reimbursement, dressings must be ordered by a physician, nurse practitioner, clinical nurse specialist, certified nurse midwife, or physician's assistant within state regulations. In addition, dressings will be covered only as long as medically necessary. For a number of procedures billed to Medicare, the cost of applying the dressing is considered incident to the charge and cannot be billed separately. Dressings sent home with the patient for home dressing changes can be billed through the Durable Medical Equipment Regional Carrier (DMERC) based on a fee schedule established for each state by the use of a Health Care Financing Administration Common Procedure Coding System (HCPCS). Each clinician should determine who the DMERC is for that state. No more than 1 month's supply may be ordered at a time. For these dressings, Medicare pays 80% of the fee schedule amount or the actual charge, if lower.

For dressings with adhesive borders, no payment for other dressings or tape is allowed. Use of more than one type of wound filler or more than one type of wound cover is not allowed. A combination of hydrating dressing with an absorptive dressing on the same wound at the same time is not allowed. Dressing size should be based on and

appropriate to the size of the wound. Medicare suggests that the size of wound cover be about 2 inches greater than the actual dimensions of the wound. In addition, Medicare does not cover skin sealants or barriers, wound cleansers or irrigating solutions, solutions used to moisten gauze, topical antiseptics, topical antibiotics, enzymatic debriding agents, gauze and dressings used to cleanse or debride a wound but not left on a wound, elastic stockings, support hose, foot coverings, leotards, knee supports, and pressure garments under surgical dressings. Note, however, that a number of the unallowable items are either incident to other charges such as debridement or treatment of venous insufficiency. For the most part, these regulations represent good clinical practice. However, note that at this time, dressings cannot be ordered by a physical therapist or occupational therapist (Table 15-4).

For optimal reimbursement, documentation of wound characteristics must be congruent with the treatment plan. The DMERC will review documentation accompanying claims to determine medical necessity. Of importance to documentation is any specific or unique condition of the patient requiring an unusual product or combination of products, why no other product can be used, or why this product was ordered. A letter of medical necessity from the ordering physician or other eligible clinician and the expected outcome of using the product are also necessary for reimbursement.

Table 15-4

DRESSING DECISION CHART BASED ON CHARACTERISTICS OF WOUND

Type	Characteristics	Potential Problems	Goals	Dressing
Venous insufficiency	Shallow, granulating, moderate to heavy drainage	Maceration, lack of re-epithelialization, edema of wound	Absorb drainage, reduce edema	Alginate/hydrofiber, foam or hydrocolloid, contact layer under multilayer compression bandaging
Neuropathic	Varied drainage depending on coexisting arterial disease, deep	Continued mechanical damage, possible concomitant arterial insufficiency, potential for infection	Prevent or manage infection, manage drainage, protect from trauma, debridement	Sharp debridement until necrotic tissue and infection cleared; determine dressing based on characteristics
Dry, shallow	Formation of scab	Lack of proliferation and autolytic debridement	Moisten	Hydrogel with transparent film
Moist, shallow	Signs of chronic inflammation	Maceration of surrounding skin	Absorb drainage	Hydrocolloid, foam
Dry, deep	Induration, erythema of surrounding skin	Lack of proliferation and autolytic debridement, dead space	Fill dead space	Hydrogel with transparent film
Moist, deep	Copious exudate, maceration of surrounding skin	Maceration, lack of healing due to edema	Absorb drainage, fill dead space	Hydrofiber/alginate filler covered with hydrocolloid or foam
Deep, infected	Odor, drainage, necrotic tissue	Spread of infection, lack of healing	Remove necrotic tissue, fill dead space	Sharp debridement, moist gauze; brief trial of topical antibiotic
Covered with eschar	Black or yellow covering, base of wound not seen	Potential for infection, slow healing	Remove eschar	Sharp debridement or cross-hatch with chemical debrider; determined by depth and drainage
Deep, filled with necrotic tissue	Mild odor, yellow	Potential for infection, slow healing	Remove necrotic tissue, fill dead space	Sharp debridement with dry dressing, chemical debrider with moistened gauze

---

Table 15-5

DMERC SURGICAL DRESSING UTILIZATION SCHEDULE

Type of Dressing	Drainage/Stage	Allowable Utilization
Alginate wound cover	Moderate to high, full thickness, stage III or IV, not allowed for dry wounds or wounds covered with eschar	One per day
Alginate wound filler	Same as above	12 inches per day
Composite dressing	No specific listed	Three per day
Contact layer	Used to line the entire wound	One per week
Foam	As primary on full thickness wounds and stage III or IV pressure ulcers; as secondary for wounds with heavy drainage	Three per week
Gauze (nonimpregnated)	None listed	Six pads per day without border or one per day with border
Gauze (impregnated with something other than water or saline)	None listed	One per day
Gauze (impregnated with normal saline or water)	None listed	Not covered; reimbursed at gauze rate
Hydrocolloid sheet	Full-thickness wound with minimum or no drainage; stage III or IV; not medically necessary for stage II	One per day without border; three per week for adhesive border
Hydrogel wound filler	Full thickness wounds with minimum or no drainage; stage III or IV; not medically necessary for stage II	Three 3-oz per wound per month

---

Characteristics, problems, and dressing decisions are expected to change through the course of healing. When wound characteristics change, the goals and dressing decisions should change. Dressing choice and frequency of dressing changes should be guided by Table 15-5. Dressing decisions also need to be based on preferences of the patient, financial considerations, and the ability of the caregiver to apply the dressing appropriately. The DMERC regulates payment for supplies and equipment as opposed to services provided under Medicare Part B (Table 15-5).

SUMMARY

A number of decisions must be made regarding what dressing is appropriate for a given wound on a given per-

son. A thorough history and physical examination, including issues that may dictate the need for more or less frequent dressing changes, and the ability to perform dressing changes must be done. With each dressing change, the appropriateness needs to be reassessed. The clinician must decide on the need for four products: wound dressings, wound fillers, skin moisturizers/protectants/sealants (see Chapter 16), and secondary dressings. Nonocclusive dressings are appropriate for acute wounds, infected wounds, and wounds requiring rapid debridement or frequent inspection. Clean, stable wounds or wounds requiring autolytic debridement are suitable for occlusive dressings. Occlusive dressings range in properties from semipermeable films that retain fluid and allow some evaporation, foams that absorb large quantities of fluid, hydrogels that hydrate dry wounds, and hydrocolloids that absorb some drainage but mainly hold drainage in place. Wound fillers are needed to occupy dead space in the wound. Alginates and hydrofibers are very absorbent, biocompatible, and suitable for wounds with heavy drainage. Hydrogels are useful for filling dry wounds. Various other products include dextranomers and hydrocolloid pastes, powders, granules, and spiral-cut sheets. The use of moisture barriers and skin sealants helps protect surrounding skin from excessive moisture and the adhesion of wound dressings. Most types of tape are too harsh for frequent use on skin, especially that of the elderly. Foam tape is preferred for direct skin contact. Silk tape is too harsh even for single use on healthy, young skin. Harsh tape can cause tears in elderly skin. Secondary dressings are used in combination with primary dressings to meet the goals of the dressing. They range from simple bandage rolls to occlusive dressings. The proper combination of wound dressing materials cannot be dictated from a chart or company representative but comes from consideration of all of the pertinent factors gleaned from a thorough history and physical examination.

CASE STUDIES

Based on the information given, choose an appropriate dressing, an interval for changing the dressing, and any progression in the dressing chosen:

1. An 80-year-old woman with a 40-year history of diabetes mellitus presents with shallow red wounds on the medial border of the left foot over the first metatarsal and below the medial malleolus. The wounds have minimal drainage and the surrounding skin is dry. What long-term interventions need to be made to prevent such wounds from recurring?

2. A 90-year-old debilitated man is seen at bedside and observed to have a deep wound filled completely with gray necrotic tissue. He is also dependent in mobility. In addition to wound care, what other interventions are needed to promote healing and prevent other ulcers from forming?

3. A 35-year-old, 5-feet-tall, 425-pound woman has a dehiscent abdominal wound with 25% granulation tissue, but 75% of dry necrotic tissue in the wound. What would you use initially? Once your initial goals are reached what would you do differently? What needs to be done with this person's nutrition at this time? At a later date?

4. A 25-year-old female cashier has had a wound superior to the medial malleolus for 2 years. The surrounding skin is indurated and stained a brownish-yellow color. The ulcer is irregularly shaped and shallow with nearly 100% granulation tissue within

the wound. In addition to dressing changes, what other interventions are needed? What long-term intervention is necessary?

5. A 20-year-old man received a gunshot wound to the thigh. The wound is filled completely with a grayish yellow tissue and is foul-smelling. The surrounding skin is hot, red, swollen, painful, and indurated with red streaks moving proximally. What type of dressing is needed? What other intervention is needed immediately given the signs evident on the surrounding skin?

6. A 25-year-old man decided to relieve the pressure in his overheated radiator by removing the radiator cap, and water sprayed over the entire anterior surface of the right upper extremity, chest, and axilla. The upper extremity displays redness from the elbow to the shoulder, and blistering from the elbow to the wrist. The radiator cap and rag protected his hand from burning. What dressing would you use initially? At what point would you discontinue this? What is likely to occur to the surrounding red areas on the arm, axilla and chest over the next few days? Why would you extend the medication onto these areas?

7. A 55-year-old man with a spinal cord injury has an ulcer on the ischial tuberosity with bone showing and surrounding areas of grayish yellow tissue. In addition to your dressing, what other interventions are necessary to prevent recurrence or occurrence on the other side?

8. An 85-year-old nursing home resident with poor mobility is left reclining in a chair almost all day long every day. He has a rounded triangular ulcer over the sacrum covered in hard black material. What needs to be done initially to remove the blackened material if signs of infection are present? What would you do if the wound appeared stable instead and you did not have any time constraints? What long-term interventions are needed to prevent recurrence?

REFERENCES

1. American Medical Association. *Current Procedural Terminology: CPT 2002.* 4th ed. American Medical Association; 2001.
2. Kerstein MD. The scientific basis of healing. *Advances in Wound Care.* 1997;10:30-34.
3. Kerstein MD. The scientific basis of healing: Erratum (missing table 2). *Advances in Wound Care.* 1997;10:8.
4. Hess, T C. When to use transparent films. *Advances in Skin and Wound Care.* 2000;13:202.

Topical Agents

16

- Discuss the use of endogenous and exogenous growth factors to accelerate wound healing.
- Discuss indications for skin care products including therapeutic moisturizers, liquid skin protectors, and moisture barriers.

Table 16-1

Categories and Ingredients of Skin Care Products

Category	Ingredients
Emollient	Aloe vera, glyceryl stearate, lanolin, mineral oil
Humectant*	Propylene glycol, glycerine
Preservative	Methylparaben, quanterium-15, propylparaben
Skin Protectant	Allantoin, calamine, cocoa butter, dimethicone, glycerine, kaoline, white petrolatum, zinc oxide

* May be considered a subcategory of skin protectant

Growth Factors

As of this writing, two forms of growth factor are available. Regranex is a recombinant form of human platelet derived growth factor (PDGF), whereas Procuren is obtained from amplifying the production of the patient's own growth factor under optimal laboratory conditions.

Regranex has been approved for neuropathic ulcers with good circulation. This indication is based on research performed years ago showing that PDGF is deficient in poorly controlled diabetes mellitus. Replacement of endogenous PDGF has been clearly shown to promote wound healing in individuals with diabetes mellitus unless they also have arterial insufficiency. Regranex is provided in a gel that is to be applied in a thin film. A thicker coating provides no increased benefit, and given its high cost, it should be applied carefully.

Procuren is an even more expensive means of providing growth factor. Blood is taken from the patients to extract and produce their own growth factor.

A number of researchers are investigating the use of several cytokines and growth factors to facilitate healing. In particular, granulocyte-macrophage colony-stimulating factor, platelet growth factor BB, and transforming growth factor β2 are being investigated for accelerating closure of acute wounds.

Skin Care Products

A number of skin care products are designed to promote proper moisture levels in skin by adding moisture to skin, retaining moisture in the wound, or by protecting the skin from exposure to excessive moisture or aggressive adhesives used on some dressings. Three categories of skin products are classified by the Centers for Medicare and Medicaid Services (CMS). These skin products are not used directly on wounds but to protect skin at risk for wounds or to protect surrounding skin from damage by excessive fluid or adhesives used for dressings. The categories are *therapeutic moisturizers, moisture barriers,* and *liquid skin protectors.* Other ingredients present in skin care products include antimicrobials, detergents, humectants, preservatives, and surfactants.

Several terms are used for these products. An *emollient,* by definition, is used to soften skin. Emollient is a lay term that typically refers to lotions used to moisturize dry skin but could be used to refer to skin protectants. *Humectants,* such as glycerin, are designed to protect skin integrity by absorbing moisture and retaining it in the skin. These agents could also be considered a type of skin protectant. Types of products are also classified among lotions, creams, and ointments. The type is determined chiefly by the concentration of solids and the fraction of water within the product.

A lotion has a high water content and low concentration of solids. Lotions are useful primarily for moisturizing skin that has lost moisture due to dry air or frequent hand washing. Lotion is important for both health care workers and for at-risk patients to prevent cracking of skin. Typical ingredients in lotions are water combined with mineral oil, stearic acid, glycerine, petrolatum, triethanolamine, magnesium aluminum silicate, glyceryl stearate, demethicone, carbomer, methylparaben, Dimethylol Dimethyl (DMDM) hydantoin, aloe vera, and tetrasodium ethylenediaminetetraacetic acid (EDTA). Several of these components are described in Table 16-1. In particular, aloe vera has been suggested to promote wound healing. Aloe vera gel is available commercially, but is not currently recommended by any wound guidelines. Aloe vera gel has also been shown to reverse the retardation of healing caused by the antiseptic, mafenide acetate.[1]

Using the CMS terms, a product used to prevent drying and cracking of skin on patients is termed a therapeutic moisturizer, which could include lotions or creams. Creams are thicker in consistency with less water than lotions and are frequently combined with solids such as

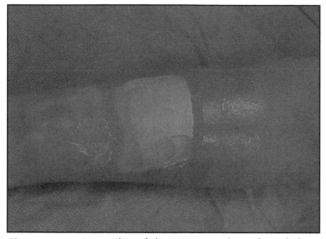

Figure 16-1. Examples of skin care products from left to right: moisturizing cream, protective cream, and protective ointment.

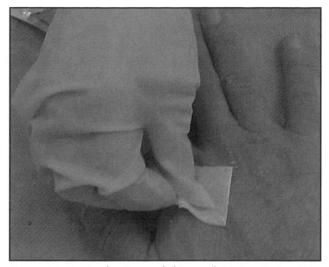

Figure 16-2. Application of skin sealant (protectant) to the hand.

zinc oxide. Ointments typically consist of substances that repel water and adhere to the skin. Ointments typically consist of petrolatum, mineral oil, lanolin, dimethicone, and glycerine. Ointments are used as moisture barriers for either protecting the skin around a draining wound or for protecting the perineum of individuals with urinary or fecal incontinence. Creams may on occasion be used as moisture barriers but are unlikely to work as effectively as ointments. Different types of lotions, creams, and ointments are shown in Figure 16-1. Common ingredients and their classifications are listed in Table 16-1.

The characteristics of various lotions, creams, and ointments can be tested easily by rubbing a small quantity on your own hand and dropping water on it. An ointment that will function well as a moisture barrier causes beading and run-off of water, whereas lotions designed as therapeutic moisturizers will allow water to remain on their surface. Depending on the purpose of the substance, characteristics of the patient, and cost, different brands of ointments, creams, or lotion may be better suited for a particular patient. Various products may have ingredients better suited for therapeutic moisturizer or for moisture barrier, and some have a combination of both properties—these substances have a wide price range.

Optimizing healing of wounds includes maintenance of an optimal level of wound moisture. Wound moisture is necessary for migration of epithelial cells, movement of enzymes, growth factors, and structural molecules. However, excessive moisture damages surrounding skin, producing what is termed *maceration*. Maceration may be prevented by less frequent and gentler dressing changes and treatment of the wound to decrease inflammation. However, less frequent dressing changes allow more drainage to accumulate beneath the dressing. A dressing and wound filler must be selected to allow the most gentle handling of the wound, yet keep moisture off the sur-

rounding skin. In many cases, the clinician is faced with the choice of more frequent dressing change and promoting inflammation or leaving a dressing in place and causing maceration. Moreover, when autolytic or chemical debridement is used, drainage will be very heavy, leading to moisture accumulation in the wound and spilling over onto the surrounding skin. In these cases, the clinician should use a moisture barrier to protect the skin and a very absorbent dressing. A number of products are available for this purpose. An ointment with a large petrolatum component and dimethicone is useful as a barrier to water and causes beading and run-off necessary to keep fluid off the skin. Therapeutic moisturizers and moisture barriers are frequently supplemented with substances such as lanolin, vitamins A and E, aloe, collagen, elastin and other ingredients claimed to be beneficial to skin.

Liquid skin protectors, also known as skin protectants and skin sealants, may be used for one of two purposes. Specifically, they are designed to protect skin from adhesives used for wound dressings. They consist of molecules (butyl ester of polyvinylmethyl ether/maleic anhydride acid copolymer) in a liquid vehicle that polymerize when exposed to the air. Application of skin protectant is shown in Figure 16-2. Isopropyl alcohol is commonly used in skin protectants, which can cause some discomfort. Nonsting formulations that do not use alcohol are also available. With a skin protectant in place, the adhesive of dressings does not contact the skin directly. When the adherent dressing is removed, the skin is less likely to be damaged. In addition, the polymer retains moisture in the skin and keeps moisture off the skin. Because of the stronger adhesive used on transparent films and hydrocolloid dressings, they are the most likely to cause damage during removal and prudent practice includes use of skin protectants. Therefore, the problem of protecting the skin from moisture leaking from the wound onto the surrounding skin and protecting the skin from aggressive adhesives can be accomplished with these products.

Common skin protectors include Skin-Prep, Allkare (Convatec, Skillman, NJ), Sween Prep (Coloplast Corporation, North Mankato, Minn), and 3M No Sting Barrier Film (3M, St. Paul, Minn). Skin protectors come in swabs, wipes, and squeeze containers. Regardless of the type of applicator, the material must be allowed to dry. Although adhesive removers are available, removal of skin protectors is not necessary with each dressing change. They should simply be reapplied as necessary. Adhesive removers are made of SD alcohol, propylene gylcol monomethyl ether, decahydronaphthalene, ethyl acetate, and stearic acid. Frequent use of these can dry and damage skin. The use of a skin protectant can actually reduce the need for adhesive removers. Adhesive removers are typically used for removing dressings with aggressive adhesives. Use of a skin protectant under the adhesive allows the dressing to be removed without adhesive remover by gently lifting a corner and stretching the dressing material parallel to the skin surface.

Therapeutic moisturizers and moisture barriers prevent adhesion of dressings. Several means are available for securing dressings in these cases.

A simple approach is to extend the dressing beyond the skin protected by these moisture barriers. This approach requires that the moisture barrier be extended exactly to the adhesive border of the dressing or to skin that can tolerate the increased moisture that may reach beyond the moisture barrier. A sufficiently absorbent dressing or a dressing supplemented with another absorbent material (eg, alginate beneath a hydrocolloid dressing) may be sufficient to prevent moisture from reaching the unprotected surrounding skin. Another approach is to secure a nonadherent dressing with elasticized netting or tubing. The clinician needs to exercise judgment as to the appropriate body part and person. For example, using this approach on the heel or elbow of a person who frequently shifts position in bed is likely to allow the dressing to shift off the wound, whereas this approach would work well on a nonweightbearing surface, away from joints in a person with limited mobility. Another approach is to use either an elasticized bandage, an elasticized bandage roll, or a bulky bandage roll to secure a nonadherent dressing. Elasticized bandages or bandage rolls have the advantage of also managing edema, but on the other hand, may cause excessive pressure and limit the ability to monitor the wound. Bulky bandage rolls have the advantage of absorbing drainage that may leak from under the dressing to protect surrounding skin. Elasticized netting, tubing, and bandages come in a variety of sizes to allow wounds on any body part to be managed this way. A fourth approach is to use a liquid skin protectant to protect the skin from both moisture and aggressive adhesives.

WOUND CLEANSERS

AHCPR guidelines include cleansing of wounds with each dressing change. From a philosophical standpoint that the clinician should be performing a limited evaluation with each dressing change, a clear argument for cleansing with each dressing change can be made. On the other hand, some argue that cleansing with each dressing change is unnecessary in attempting to minimize tissue trauma and prevent chronic inflammation. Because each patient presents a different set of priorities and priorities are likely to change through the healing process, the clinician should make a careful judgment of which approach to follow. A reasonable philosophy to follow is that a dressing should be chosen to minimize the frequency of dressing change, but with each dressing change the wound bed should be clearly visualized to aid in the decision of when and how the wound should be dressed next. If possible, the dressing should be chosen to fit the number of days before the next evaluation, and evaluation requires cleansing the wound depending on the ability of other caregivers to perform adequate dressing changes.

A number of products are available for cleansing wounds. Many forms of nonspecific mechanical debridement also cleanse wounds (eg, whirlpool, irrigation, pulsatile lavage). This discussion is limited to products designed for cleansing, not debridement. Cleansers are designed to remove materials other than adherent necrotic tissue, which includes drainage, desiccated tissue, blood, adherent macromolecules, and foreign materials. Cleansers range from normal saline to complex mixtures of detergents, chelators, surfactants, and preservatives including poloxymer, hydroxypropyl methylcellulose, potassium sorbate, DMDM hydantoin, methylparaben, D-panthenol, zinc gluconate, magnesium gluconate, and malic acid. Normal saline is least likely to cause tissue trauma and inflammation. Application of saline as a cleanser may be done by simply pouring normal saline over the wound or by using low pressure means such as an irrigation bulb. Cleansing may also be accomplished by the use of angiocaths and similar devices (discussed in Chapter 12). Cleansing under pressure could also be considered a form of debridement depending on the goal of the use of pressurized saline wash. Some individuals have suggested using hydrogen peroxide as a cleansing agent, citing the effervescence as a means of lifting materials from the surface of the wound. This approach is generally not recommended because of the cytotoxicity of hydrogen peroxide. Ingredients commonly found in wound and skin cleansers are listed in Table 16-2.

Commercially available cleansers have a range of tissue toxicity; a number of these agents are listed in the AHCPR guidelines for treatment of pressure ulcers. Soaps and detergents dissolve in both water and lipid-containing substances such as cell membranes. Therefore, no soap or detergent is completely safe on wounds. In Chapter 18,

Table 16-2

INGREDIENTS IN WOUND AND SKIN CLEANSERS

Category	Ingredients
Antimicrobial	Benzalkonium chloride, benzethonium chloride, benzoic acid, hexylresorcinol, malic acid, methylbenzethonium chloride
Chelators	Disodium EDTA
Detergents	Ammonium lauryl sulfate, sodium lauryl sulfate
Surfactants	Poloxymer, polysorbate 20

infection control, soaps, and detergents are discussed as antimicrobial methods. Surfactants allow soaps and detergents to bind to molecules in the wound. Surfactants are able to reach between water molecules to bind organic materials. Chelators such as EDTA bind metal ions to remove them from the fluid. Metal ions reduce the effectiveness of soaps and detergents; therefore, chelators soften hard water and improve the effectiveness of soaps and detergents. The combination of detergents, chelators, and surfactants make specialized wound cleansers more effective than normal saline. Some dressings actually have these ingredients built into them in an attempt to accelerate the healing process by removing foreign and degraded materials from the wound fluid.

SKIN CLEANSERS

Skin cleansers are designed for use on at-risk skin and are often designed, promoted, and used as complementary products with skin protectors or therapeutic moisturizers. They are designed to be more gentle and effective than typical skin soaps and detergents. In particular, they are used for individuals with fecal and urinary incontinence. Both urine and feces are acidic, and fecal material is often very adherent. Frequent episodes of fecal incontinence throughout the day can lead to rapid breakdown of the perineal skin. Unfortunately, frequent cleansing itself with bath soap and scrubbing to loosen fecal material can add to skin damage. Skin cleansers, as described for wound cleansers, contain detergents, surfactants, and chelators. In addition, they are designed to neutralize the acid pH of urine and feces to reduce damage to the perineum.

SUMMARY

Topical agents other than debridement and antiseptics are discussed in this chapter. Currently, two forms of

growth factors are available. Regranex is indicated for slow healing neuropathic ulcers in the presence of adequate blood flow. It contains PDGF, which is deficient in diabetes mellitus. Procuren is currently only available through a limited number of specialized facilities. It is an amplification of the patient's own PDGF. Skin products include therapeutic moisturizers to prevent damage to skin by drying, moisture barriers that protect the surrounding skin from wound moisture, skin protectants that prevent damage from adhesives and fluid, and skin and wound cleansers. Skin and wound cleansers contain special ingredients to facilitate cleaning of wounds.

STUDY QUESTIONS

1. What is the purpose of using PDGF for neuropathic wounds? Why is it not indicated for other types of wounds?

2. Why do skin protectors need to be used under dressings such as semipermeable films and hydrocolloids?

3. What is the purpose of a therapeutic moisturizer? What might occur if they are not used when indicated?

4. How can one maintain an optimal fluid level in a wound without damaging the surrounding skin? What are common ingredients in this type of product?

5. What purposes do surfactants and chelators play in wound and skin cleansers?

REFERENCE

1. Heggers JP, Elzaim H, Gardield R, et al. Beneficial effect of aloe on wound healing in an excisional wound model. *The Journal of Alternative and Complementary Medicine.* 1996;2:271-277.

Pain Management

- Discuss options available for medical management of pain and how individual characteristics must be evaluated based on the characteristics of the patient and the medications.
- Describe the electrical modalities available for management of wound-related pain including contraindications.
- Discuss the use of topical agents used by providers other than physicians for management of pain associated with wound management.

In the management of wounds, the focus on healing can easily obscure the need for management of pain associated with the wound. Although pain management is very specifically addressed in the AHCPR guidelines, it has not yet seemed to reach the consciousness of health care providers. Too often, pain is considered an inevitable consequence of dressing changes and debridement. Moreover, the responsibility for pain management is delegated to the physician and nurse, leaving everyone else to ask, "Has the patient received his or her pain meds yet?" Three types of pain management are addressed specifically in this chapter—*medical management, electrotherapy,* and *topical medications*. In addition, we have the responsibility to assess the causes of pain and take reasonable steps to eliminate or minimize pain through means such as positioning, selection of dressings, as well as the types of interventions described below.

MEDICAL MANAGEMENT

General Anesthesia

Although this text is directed toward a broad audience, the majority of individuals reading this text will not be in a position to prescribe drugs to manage pain. However, everyone involved in wound management is in a position to recommend the use of analgesic medications and is responsible for understanding how the prescribed drugs interact with the patient, the wound, and the ability of the patient and the patient's caregivers to manage the wound.

Complex debridement may be performed in an operating room with the patient under general anesthesia. However, several issues need to be considered for general anesthesia. General anesthesia is not appropriate if the patient needs to be conscious (eg, to have verbal interaction with the surgeon during the procedure). Another form of anesthesia should be used if post-recovery residual effects, cardiopulmonary consequences, maternal/fetal transfer of general anesthesia is problematic, or the patient clearly expresses a preference to be conscious.

Two methods of general anesthesia are used: inhaled and intravenous. In many cases, both are used. Inhaled general anesthesia is performed through an endotracheal tube attached to the source of anesthetic gas (GETA). Either a gas or volatile liquid is placed into the device. An anesthesiologist or nurse anesthetist is responsible for monitoring the patient's response to anesthesia. Inhaled anesthesia is often preferred because of the ease of adjustment. Volatile liquids such as halothane, enflurane, isoflurane, and methoxyflurane are aerosolized for GETA.

Intravenous (IV) anesthesia is useful due to its rapid onset of inducing general anesthesia. Intravenous anesthesia alone may be sufficient for short procedures; for longer procedures, general anesthesia is maintained with gas. Drugs used for IV general anesthesia include barbiturates

such as thiopental. Adjuvants to general anesthesia include preoperative sedatives such as barbiturates, opioids (Demerol), and benzodiazepines, especially Valium (Roche Laboratories, Nutley, NJ); and for certain procedures, neuromuscular blockers are indicated. Valium is also sometimes used as an adjuvant during local anesthesia to relax a patient. These adjuvants also improve the ease of administering general anesthesia through an endotracheal tube.

Inhalation anesthetics dissolve in membranes, altering the membrane fluidity and interfering with the opening of sodium and other ion channels. Because inhaled general anesthetics are highly fat soluble, they are stored throughout the body and wash out slowly in obese individuals. If the general anesthetic effects linger, leading to longer periods of immobility, an increase in the risk of pressure ulcers, accumulation of secretions in the lungs, and other problems associated with lack of mobility may occur. General anesthetics can cause confusion and sleepiness, and some patients develop temporary psychosis. Patients may also have temporary muscle weakness if a neuromuscular blocker is used; however, these are unlikely to be used for surgical debridement.[1]

Intravenous general anesthetics such as thiopental bind to receptors on chloride ion channels. Binding to these receptors decreases the probability of neurons depolarizing. At the proper dose, these drugs produce sedation or anesthesia. At greater doses, medullary paralysis and death may result.

Local Anesthetics

Local anesthetics work primarily as sodium channel blockers. Some of these drugs (notably lidocaine) can be used to treat arrhythmias. To be useful, the local anesthetic must remain in the area of interest. These drugs can diffuse slowly from the tissue of interest and more rapidly in areas of high blood flow. Application of heating modalities prior to injection of local anesthetics decreases their effectiveness. In some cases, the effectiveness of local anesthetic is improved by co-injecting a vasoconstricting agent (epinephrine). In rare cases, accidental injection of lidocaine into a blood vessel during an attempt at infiltration may produce systemic effects. Central nervous system effects include somnolence, confusion, agitation, seizures, and respiratory depression. Cardiac effects consist of arrhythmias, decreased heart rate, and contractility.

Local anesthetics can be administered by several routes, including the typical infiltration of tissues with a hypodermic needle and syringe, topical, and transdermal. Local anesthetics are also used for peripheral nerve or brachial plexus block, especially for upper extremity surgery. These drugs can also be administered via catheter to the epidural or subdural space for anesthesia of the lower extremities (epidural and spinal anesthesia).

Analgesia

Analgesics include opioids, nonsteroidal anti-inflammatory drugs (NSAIDs), and acetaminophen. Opioids bind to specific receptors in the spinal cord and brain to decrease the transmission of pain signals from the periphery to the cortex. NSAIDs are used typically for pain following injury or surgery. With tissue injury or other causes of inflammation, the enzyme phospholipase A2 is activated, forming arachidonic acid. Arachidonic acid is then converted by one of two pathways. The enzyme cyclooxygenase (COX) produces the family of chemicals known as prostaglandins, and thromboxane and the enzyme lipoxygenase produces the various leukotrienes. NSAIDs work by blocking the COX enzyme, which decreases the production of prostaglandins and thromboxane from arachidonic acid. A major adverse effect of NSAIDs has been erosion of the gastric and duodenal mucosa. The lining of the stomach is protected by the local effect of prostaglandins in the stomach. Decreasing the production of prostaglandins by the stomach can lead to serious, even fatal damage. Recently, a second type of the COX enzyme has been discovered. COX1 is present in the stomach, but COX2 is not and appears to mediate much of the prostaglandin production associated with pain and inflammation. New COX2 drugs (Celebrex, Pharmacia, Peapack, NJ and Vioxx, Merck, Whitehouse Station, NJ) have been approved for treating arthritis in individuals at risk for developing gastrointestinal ulceration by NSAIDs.

All true NSAIDs have three basic properties: analgesic, antipyretic, and antithrombotic. In some cases, NSAIDs will need to be avoided in patients with prolonged bleeding times. Acetaminophen does not meet all of the criteria for NSAIDs because it has analgesic and antipyretic properties only. Most NSAIDs and acetaminophen are generally effective against only mild pain, requiring the use of opiate drugs for moderate to severe pain. However, ketorolac tromethamine (Toradol) is one NSAID that can be effective against moderate pain. Although much of the inflammation caused by tissue injury may be attributed to leukotrienes, no lipoxygenase drugs have yet been approved as analgesics. Leukotrienes are intimately involved with airway inflammation, and drugs either decreasing the production of or blocking binding sites for leukotrienes have been approved for asthma.[2]

Opioid analgesics are naturally occurring substances derived from the opium poppy and are very effective against even severe pain. Semisynthetic opioids are produced by modifying naturally occurring compounds. However, natural and semisynthetic opioids have tremendous potential for dependency. Synthetic opioids relieve moderate to severe pain with fewer adverse effects or dependency. Opioids are available in a number of formulations for different routes of administration. Opioids can be administered orally, intramuscularly, intravenously, and transdermally (fentanyl patch).

Opioids bind to a number of specific types of opioid receptors, which tend to be localized to different locations in the brain and spinal cord. In addition, the various types of opioids bind better to different types of opioid receptors. Receptors are located within the substantia gelatinosa, the site of synapse between peripheral nociceptive neurons and second order neurons in the tip of the posterior gray. Binding of opioids to the presynaptic membrane (release site of neurotransmitter from the nociceptive neuron) diminishes the release of neurotransmitter onto the second order neuron and, therefore, decreases the probability of perception of pain at the cortex. In addition, opioids hyperpolarize the postsynaptic membrane on the second order neuron, rendering the release of neurotransmitter by the peripheral nociceptor less effective in producing an action potential in the second order neuron and again, decreasing the probability of relaying a pain message to the cortex. Binding of opioids by receptors in specific regions of the brain excites pain-suppressing neurons. Opioids may also function peripherally by suppressing the release of substance P by peripheral nociceptors. Release of substance P is believed to perpetuate the pain caused by tissue injury and inflammation.

Unfortunately, opioids have a number of adverse effects that vary tremendously in their severity from patient to patient. Opioids are generally sedating and may even produce respiratory depression. Orthostatic hypotension produced by opioids requires the clinician to exercise care in assisting patients with transfers and ambulation. Nausea, vomiting, and constipation are common adverse effects. In fact, opioids are commonly used in preparations designed to decrease gastrointestinal motility. Patients may be prescribed antiemetic drugs as needed when they are taking opioid analgesics.

Patient-Controlled Analgesia

Either opioids or local anesthetics may be used with a programmable pump and either a central line or epidural catheter. Anesthetics cause loss of both sensation and motor function, whereas opioids produce analgesia without loss of motor function. Care must be taken during transfers and ambulation in individuals receiving local anesthetics in an epidural or subdural line due to loss of lower extremity strength.

Patient-controlled analgesia (PCA) is designed to maintain drug levels within the analgesic range. Compared with intramuscular (IM) injections typically given at 3- to 4-hour intervals, PCA will maintain a fairly steady analgesic effect, whereas repeated IM injections allow wide fluctuations in perception of pain just before and after injection. Moreover, peaks in plasma opioid concentration caused by IM injection have a greater potential for causing sedation, nausea, vomiting, orthostatic hypotension, and other adverse effects. A typical protocol for PCA includes a loading dose to achieve initial analgesia rapidly, a provision for demand dosing with lockout intervals over certain time frames such as 1 and 4 hours, and a background infusion rate. The background infusion rate is provided to ensure that plasma opioid concentration does not fall below the therapeutic level, whereas the lockouts provide a safeguard against overdosing. The demand dose is available to the patient as needed, usually by pushing a wired remote button. The patient should be encouraged to use the available demand doses and instructed in the means by which the infusion pumps are controlled in terms of lockout intervals and background infusion. If patients are either too sedated or have too much pain, the PCA pump may require adjustment. For long-term use, access ports with central lines may be used for administering analgesia.

ELECTROTHERAPY

Whereas oral and injectable analgesic drugs require prescription by a physician and administration by a registered nurse, electrotherapeutic means of analgesia can be administered by a number of health care providers. The types of modalities available include transcutaneous electrical nerve stimulation (TENS), interferential current (IFC), and iontophoresis.

TENS, as originally developed, was based on the gate control theory of pain described by Melzack and Wall in 1967.[3] The basis of the gate control theory is that stimulation of larger afferent (sensory) nerves that enter at the same spinal cord level as the nociceptive neurons carrying pain signals diminish perception of pain. Simple, well-known examples of applications of the gate control theory of pain include rubbing a painful area and "running off" the pain.

Nociceptors as well as mechanoreceptors and thermoreceptors have two axons (pseudounipolar neurons) and a cell body that resides in a dorsal root ganglion (trigeminal ganglion for the face). The peripheral axonal process carries information from the periphery encoded as a frequency of action potentials propagated from the distal end to the cell body, which then continues from the cell body along the central axonal process to synaptic terminals in the dorsal gray matter, in particular the substantia gelatinosa. The outer white matter of the spinal cord consists of tracts of axons carrying information either from the brain to the spinal cord (descending tracts) or from the spinal cord to the brain (ascending tracts). The white matter of the spinal cord (as well as the brain) represents myelinated axons, where the fatty myelin substance creates the characteristic color of the outer part of the spinal cord and inner tracts through the brain. The gray matter of the spinal cord lacks the white color due to the relative lack of myelin in an area composed primarily of cell bodies of ascending interneurons that synapse with sensory

neurons, cell bodies of motor neurons that synapse with descending interneurons, and cell bodies of local interneurons that allow the sharing of information within the spinal cord. Thus, the gray matter's color is the result of a sea of cell bodies with some myelinated axons running between them. The substantia gelatinosa has a clear appearance due to the very high proportion of unmyelinated neurons converging in this region.

Much of the sensory information reaching the cortex to provide conscious perception requires a chain of three neurons from the periphery to the cortex. The sensory neuron entering the spinal cord from the dorsal root ganglion is called the first-order neuron. A second order neuron synapses within the gray matter and ascends in the white matter. Second order neurons typically terminate in the thalamus, synapsing with a third-order neuron that carries the information from the thalamus to the cortex. Some sensory systems deviate from this general framework. Well-localized pain linked directly to a specific stimulus is carried in this type of arrangement. Pain that persists due to tissue injury or inflammation is carried through a different pathway in that the second order neuron travels to the reticular activating system, leading to poorly localized pain with a greater persistence and emotional component.

A large number of synapses exist among neurons entering the substantia gelatinosa as well as binding sites for short-acting natural opioids (enkephalins). The gate theory of pain is based on the premise that stimulation of mechanoreceptive neurons with their cell bodies in the same dorsal root ganglion as the nociceptors of interest synapse with interneurons that can "close the gate" to pain information. These "gate-keeping" interneurons are proposed to release neurotransmitter on the synaptic terminals of nociceptors, rendering release of neurotransmitter from the nociceptor more difficult. In addition, enkephalin is likely released onto the post-synaptic membrane of the second order neuron that synapses with the nociceptor. Enkephalin release onto the second order neurons hyperpolarizes the post-synaptic membrane, diminishing the effect of neurotransmitter release by the nociceptor. Release of enkephalin, therefore, both decreases the probability of release of neurotransmitter by the nociceptor onto the second order neuron and decreases the effectiveness of the neurotransmitter released onto second order neurons. As a result, fewer action potentials are developed in the second order neurons and less pain is perceived at the cortical level.

TENS devices are simple electrical stimulators that allow the amplitude, frequency, and duration of biphasic pulses to be adjusted. Lead wires are attached to self-adherent electrodes placed on the skin (Figure 17-1). In addition, several means of modulating the settings for amplitude, frequency, and duration are typically found on

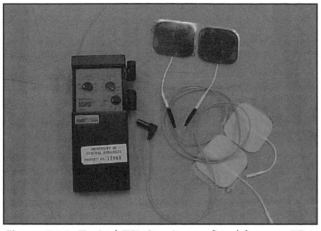

Figure 17-1. Typical TENS unit retrofitted for new FDA standards.

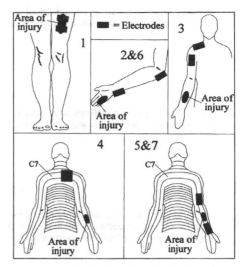

Figure 17-2. Rationales for TENS electrode placement.

commercially available units.[4] For example, a given modulation setting may cause the pulse frequency to cyclically increase and decrease from a set value. Because of the nature of pain carried by the larger lightly myelinated Aδ nociceptive neurons and the unmyelinated C neurons, TENS application is typically directed at diminishing persistent pain associated with the more primitive C neuron and medial spinothalamic tract. Current generated by the TENS device depolarizes mechanoreceptors within the skin, causing inhibition of second order neurons synapsing with nociceptors of the C type of neuron. As such, TENS may be useful for management of persistent pain associated with chronic wounds. A simple means of passing current through the mechanoreceptors associated with the same dorsal root ganglion as the injury is to place electrodes around the site of injury. With a single channel device, electrodes may be placed either medially and laterally to the wound or proximally and distally. A two-channel device allows electrodes to be placed completely around the site of injury. Other approaches include placing the electrodes over the peripheral nerve supplying the area if the nerve is sufficiently superficial (eg, peroneal, medial, ulnar, radial nerves). Electrodes can also be placed over the brachial plexus at Erb's point, between the clavicle and belly of the upper trapezius to manage pain throughout the upper extremity, analogous to the injection of local anesthetic onto the brachial plexus. Some clinicians also attempt to manage pain by placing electrodes paraspinally at the level of the dorsal root ganglion of interest. Configurations used for TENS electrode placements are shown in Figure 17-2.

Conventional TENS uses biphasic pulses at a frequency of approximately 100 Hz, a pulse duration of about 80 ms, and an amplitude great enough that the patient perceives a vibratory stimulus (sensory level of stimulation) but not sufficiently strong to elicit contraction of muscle beneath the skin (motor level of stimulation). Low-frequency

TENS, as the name implies, is performed at a low frequency of 2 to 4 Hz. In addition, low-frequency TENS is characterized by a greater duration (approximately 250 ms) and a greater intensity. The intensity is greater than motor, to the point that the patient can perceive stimulation of nociceptors (noxious level of stimulation). Most patients will perceive an uncomfortable, pricking sensation, and many patients do not tolerate this type of stimulation well, preferring conventional TENS. Low-frequency TENS is not explicable based on the gate control theory of pain. Some have suggested that this pattern of stimulation evokes release of natural opioids. The time frame of the onset of analgesia and persistence of pain relief is consistent with this idea.

During debridement, dressing changes, and any other procedures that create acute pain, conventional TENS is less likely to be effective. Perception of pain occurring during a stimulus is conveyed by Aδ neurons to second order neurons running through the lateral spinothalamic tract to the thalamus and then relayed to the cortex by third order neurons. This pain is, therefore, localizable and graded to the intensity of the stimulus. This type of pain ceases when the stimulus is removed, but pain associated with tissue injury and inflammation and conveyed by C nociceptive neurons may follow at some later time. Another mode of TENS called brief intense may be used for this acute aspect of pain and can be followed by conventional TENS to control the pain that occurs after the painful stimulus is removed. Brief intense TENS is produced by gradually increasing amplitude, duration, and frequency of pulses as tolerated by the patient. Done properly, brief intense TENS produces not just analgesia, but anesthesia. During brief intense TENS, wound debridement may be performed without pain. Following debridement, the TENS device can be reset to conventional set-

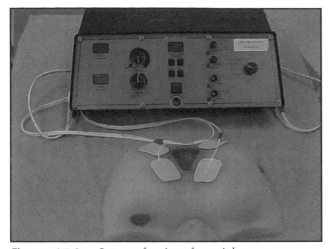

Figure 17-3a. Set-up for interferential current treatment.

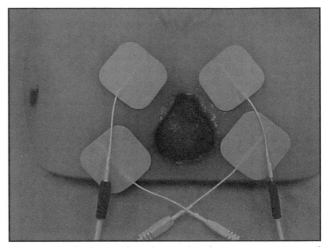

Figure 17-3b. Note the electrode placement pattern of two leads set perpendicular to each other.

tings to manage any pain that might result from tissue injury during debridement.

Interferential current can be used for the same purpose as TENS. Whereas TENS produces current in body tissues through paired electrodes on the skin surface, IFC is actually produced in the tissues by an interference pattern generated by crossing two alternating currents of slightly differing frequency. The difference in the frequency of the two crossing currents produces a cycle of maximum constructive to maximum destructive and back to maximum constructive interference at a rate equal to the difference in frequency of the two alternating currents. Within each cycle, amplitude of the interference current ranges from an amplitude of nearly zero to an amplitude of nearly double the individual alternating currents. Although this cycle is constructed of two currents of 4000 to 5000 Hz, each cycle of interference from minimum to maximum behaves at the tissue level as individual pulses. Each cycle is called a *beat* for the purpose of discussing the physiological effects of IFC. The frequency of beats generated in the tissues is simply the difference in frequency of the two alternating currents. For example, if one current is 4000 Hz and the other is 3990, the beat frequency is 10 Hz and will produce 10 muscle twitches per second if the intensity is great enough. Producing IFC in the tissue requires two channels and four electrodes. Two electrodes from one lead are placed on the skin such that an imaginary line drawn between the two electrodes of the lead intersect a similar imaginary line between the electrodes of the other lead to form an imaginary perpendicular line. When done this way, the current generates the beats in the tissue. The intensity of the IFC varies through the tissue in a cloverleaf pattern. Current intensity is greatest in the tissue between the imaginary lines and reaches a minimum directly below the imaginary lines. To improve the dispersion of current within tissue, a fluctuation of current ampli-

tude causes a shifting of the current distribution such that the "cloverleaf" pattern moves cyclically through the tissue. Due to the way that IFC is generated, specific devices must be used to generate IFC. Recently, several manufacturers have produced portable IFC units that can be carried readily by patients. Set-up for IFC is demonstrated in Figures 17-3a and 17-3b.

To generate analgesia with IFC, beat frequency and amplitude are set as they would be for conventional or low-frequency TENS. However, with IFC, no adjustment for pulse duration is available. Because of the way IFC is generated in the tissues, a much greater quantity of charge is run through the tissue compared with the biphasic pulses of TENS devices. Although this may make little difference in terms of the conventional TENS—gate control type of effect or low-frequency TENS effect—IFC is very useful in generating a brief intense type of effect. Another advantage of IFC compared with traditional biphasic TENS devices is the low skin impedance that results from the much higher frequency transcutaneous current. The lower skin impedance decreases the recruitment of skin nociceptors such that the patient can tolerate enough current to achieve a greater anesthetic effect than can be generated by biphasic pulses of TENS devices. Moreover, IFC is designed to run current through a tissue of interest without the need to place electrodes directly on the tissue of interest. This is particularly beneficial in that current is more likely to stimulate neurons of the correct spinal cord level. Generating an anesthetic effect with IFC is fairly simple. Over the course of 1 to 2 minutes, current is increased gradually as tolerated by the patient until numbness is reported. Over this time, the patient will be able to tolerate increasing amounts of current either in the form of increased beat frequency or amplitude as the current is applied.

Iontophoresis is the use of direct current to drive ionized molecules transdermally. Although many types of compounds have been addressed in the literature for various ailments, modern iontophoresis is typically performed for driving dexamethasone, an anti-inflammatory drug, into tissues to treat chronic musculoskeletal conditions such as tennis elbow. Recently, iontophoresis units have been promoted for pediatric use to "numb" areas as an alternative to infiltration with lidocaine prior to starting lines or suturing lacerations. Application of iontophoresis requires a smaller active, absorbent electrode onto which the solution of ionized medication is suffused. Depending on the electrode size, 2 to 4 mL of solution is used. A larger dispersive electrode is placed on a nearby area. The correct polarity for the medication must be set on the device. Dexamethasone is driven across the skin with a negative electrode and lidocaine requires a positive electrode. Dosage of iontophoresis is quantified in units of mA·min, the product of current in mA and duration in minutes. Although not correct from a physics standpoint (Coulombs would be correct), using this unit allows the clinician to manipulate the two variables to maximize patient tolerance. For example, a dose of 40 mA·min can be generated with an intensity of 4 mA and a duration of 10 minutes or a current of 2 mA and duration of 20 minutes or some other combination of current and duration.

TOPICAL APPLICATION OF LOCAL ANESTHETICS

Another option as opposed to using systemic drugs or electrotherapy is to use local anesthetic applied topically as needed. Several preparations are now available. Both lidocaine and benzocaine are available in a spray. Lidocaine is also available in gel form. For minor acute wounds a combination of lidocaine, neomycin, polymixin B, and bacitracin is available over the counter as Neosporin Plus (Pfizer, Inc., Cambridge, Mass). Another preparation used in the hospital setting is EMLA (eutectic mixture of local anesthetic) cream. EMLA is a combination of 2.5% prilocaine and 2.5% lidocaine in an emulsion with a melting point below room temperature, which keeps both anesthetics in the liquid oil portion. The cream stays in place on the skin and is absorbed sufficiently to avoid the need for infiltration injection of local anesthetics in some circumstances. EMLA is also packaged in a disk within an occlusive dressing with an adhesive tape ring.

Lidocaine has a more rapid onset and prilocaine has a more prolonged effect. In practice, local anesthetic gel or spray is placed on the edges of wounds prior to painful procedures such as debridement, pulsed lavage with concurrent suction or may be done when dressing changes alone are painful.

SUMMARY

Pain management is the responsibility of everyone involved in wound management. It may be provided by analgesic drugs prescribed by a physician, ranging from typical NSAIDs, to ketorolac for moderate pain, to weak or strong opioids for moderate to severe pain. Analgesia can also be provided by electrotherapy using TENS on the brief intense mode during debridement or conventional TENS for background relief. Interferential current has the advantage of being applied to the area surrounding the wound and the greater current passing through the wound. Local anesthetics can be applied to the edges of wounds undergoing debridement as a spray, gel, or cream.

STUDY QUESTIONS

1. Who is authorized to prescribe strong NSAIDs and opioids for pain relief? Why?

2. What are aspects of pain management that may be provided by anyone?

3. What electrotherapeutic devices are available to reduce pain? What is the basic mechanism by which these work?

4. Why is lidocaine used for short procedures and bupivacaine for longer procedures?

5. What is the significance of Erb's point for TENS application?

REFERENCES

1. Ciccone CD. *Pharmacology in Rehabilitation*. 2nd ed. Philadelphia, Pa: FA Davis; 1996.

2. Katzurg BG. *Basic Clinical Pharmacology*. 6th ed. East Norwalk, Conn: Appleton & Lange; 1995.

3. Melzack R, Wall PD. Pain mechanisms: a new theory. *Science*. 1965 Nov 19; 150(699):971-9.

4. Robinson AJ, Snyder-Mackler L. *Clinical Electrophysiology*. 2nd ed. Baltimore, Md: Williams & Wilkins; 1995.

Infection Control

OBJECTIVES

- Describe the microbiology of wounds, including common bacteria-causing wound infection.
- Describe risk factors for wound infection and means of preventing surgical site infection.
- Discuss the indications for culturing wounds and the limitations of culturing.
- Contrast the use of wound biopsy and culture.
- Contrast the processes of sterilization and disinfection.
- Contrast aseptic and sterile techniques.
- Discuss appropriate use of sterile and clean techniques for acute and chronic wounds.
- Discuss indications for systemic medicines for wound infection.
- Discuss indications for topical antimicrobial agents.
- Describe appropriate OSHA regulations for handling potentially infectious material.
- Discuss relevant CDC recommendations for isolation precautions in hospitals, including the evolution of isolation practices.
- List the types of precautions and patients requiring various isolation precautions.

Table 18-1

Host Defense Mechanisms

Cell Mediated	Humoral	Molecular
• T-cell	• Antibodies, especially IgA	• Defensins
• Neutrophils		• Collectins
• Macrophage		

The susceptibility of individuals to infection is determined by a number of factors. Factors include host defense mechanisms, pathogenic properties of microbes, the presence of predisposing factors to infection, and sources of organisms in wounds. Below, common organisms found in wound infections and control of both endogenous and exogenous organisms are discussed.

Host Defense Mechanisms

Both passive and active mechanisms reduce the opportunity for infection, particularly the intact skin. The mechanical barrier provided by skin due to waterproofing is effective for the vast majority of organisms. In addition, growth is diminished by the acidity of skin, the presence of molecular defense molecules called defensins and collectins, and competition with other microbes. The mucosal surfaces are protected additionally by IgA antibodies. If intact skin is breeched by injury, elements of the immune system including neutrophils, macrophages, T cells and antibodies are usually able to prevent infection. Unfortunately, a number of circumstances can lead to infection in different individuals in different ways. First of all, each person's immune system is somewhat different due to the inheritance of unique combinations of cellular and humoral immunity genes inherited from each parent. Secondly, a large number of local and systemic factors may compromise the effectiveness of the immune system (Table 18-1).

Pathogenic Properties of Microbes

A number of bacteria are capable of penetrating the mechanical barrier of the skin and mucosa, in particular those causing sexually transmitted disease. Specific properties conferring virulence are seen in certain bacteria that allow them to escape detection or killing by the immune system. Capsule-forming bacteria include *Streptococcus*

pneumoniae and *Hemophilus influenzae*, which are common culprits in infections of the throat, middle ears, and upper airways. Leukocidins, chemicals toxic to white cells, are produced by *Staphylococcus aureus* and *Clostridium perfringens*. *Pseudomonas aeruginosa* and *Staphylococcus aureus* produce molecules that interfere with lysosomal function. Molecules produced by some bacteria allow rapid spread, especially through fascial planes due to their proteolytic properties. Streptokinase produced in laboratories is used as a thrombolytic agent. Injury-causing molecules on the surface of bacteria are called *endotoxins*. Certain endotoxins are very dangerous, especially those found on the surface of gram-negative bacteria. Bacteremia with gram-negative organisms may produce septic shock and death. Other molecules released from bacteria that may interfere with metabolic processes and cause cell injury are called *exotoxins*.[1]

The presence of bacteria and their chemical products can have a profound effect on healing. At low levels of bacteria, certain aspects of wound healing may occur at a faster rate, but high levels of bacteria inhibit healing. Even at some distance, an abscess can delay healing of another wound. A definitive diagnosis of infection requires the presence of purulent drainage or a spreading inflammation beyond what is expected of normal healing. Quantitatively, a culture obtained by tissue biopsy demonstrating greater than 100,000 organisms per gram or the presence of beta-hemolytic streptococci in even lower concentration indicates infection.[2]

A commonly used rule of thumb is that a wound that heals primarily without discharge is uninfected but is infected if purulent discharge occurs. In such cases, bacteria may not be detected in culture if the purulent drainage consists only of dead bacteria, neutrophils, and tissue debris. However, biopsy cultures of the wound itself, rather than swabs of the drainage, are likely to demonstrate infection; therefore, swab cultures are discouraged. Purulent drainage confined to a suture site (stitch abscess) is not considered infected if healing occurs and the suture sites clear within 72 hours.[3]

Predisposing Factors to Infection

Immunosuppression is a general term for reduced effectiveness of the immune system. Based on the underlying cause, immunosuppression can be divided into two basic categories. *Primary immunodeficiency* is caused by genetic defects in the immune system, resulting in a lack of specific or more general components of the immune system. Specific deficiencies include the lack of IgA antibodies, x-linked agammaglobinemia (Bruton's disease), and thymic dysplasia (DiGeorge's syndrome) in which the thymus and other specific embryologic structures, including the heart, fail to develop normally. A number of more global deficiencies also occur.

Far more common are immunodeficiencies with underlying causes other than genetic, termed *secondary immunodeficiencies.* In the context of wound care, the most important is diabetes mellitus. In particular, neutrophil function is depressed in poorly controlled diabetes mellitus. Other common secondary causes include kidney disease, burns, malnutrition, alcohol and drug abuse, cancer in general, and certain types of cancer of the immune system in particular. Surgery carries with it the risk of infection. A recent study, however, indicated that supplemental oxygen during surgery drastically reduces the risk of operative infection.[4] Other secondary immunodeficiencies include AIDS and administration of immunosuppressive drugs to treat autoimmune diseases (rheumatoid arthritis, lupus, scleroderma, and others) or to prevent transplant rejection.

In addition to opportunistic infections caused by a compromised immune system, alterations in the microenvironment may promote the proliferation of particular types of organisms. Under these altered conditions, facultative infection may occur. This term implies that the infection does not occur unless the environment is facilitated for the organism. This facilitation may occur for a number of reasons. Use of antibiotics that reduce competition for the local microenvironment may allow resistant organisms to proliferate. A classic example is the vaginal yeast infection that occurs frequently after an antibacterial drug is administered for an upper respiratory or urogenital bacterial infection. In addition, altered pH, temperature, or humidity may promote the growth of particular organisms.

Postoperative infections are believed to be due to factors other than simple presence of airborne bacteria. An estimated 30,000 to 60,000 airborne bacteria fall within a 3 to 4 m^2 operating room per hour; however, infection rate has not been shown to be correlated well with the quantity of bacteria present in the air, present in the wound at the time of surgery, or with postoperative infec-

tions. The strongest factor seems to be the duration of the surgical procedure, ranging from 3.6% for procedures of less than 30 minutes to 16.4% for procedures lasting more than 5 hours. Another factor, infection in another area of the body, increases the risk of infection during surgery by three-fold.[5]

In the case of traumatic wounds, time also plays an important role. The number of organisms recovered from traumatic wounds increases rapidly with time. The average time since injury for wounds with fewer than 100 organisms per gram is 2.2 hours compared with 3 hours for wounds with 100 to 100,000. The average time for wounds with greater than 100,000 organisms per gram was 5.17 hours, and only the wounds with greater than 100,000 per gram developed clinical infection in the emergency room series described by Robson et al.[6]

Sources of Organisms in Wounds

A number of normal flora colonizing the skin, sweat glands, hair follicles, and mucosa (resident microbes) can proliferate and become virulent when introduced to the body tissues. Approximately 1,000 organisms per gram of tissue reside in sweat glands and hair follicles. Common resident microbes colonizing the skin include *Staphylococcus epidermidis, Pseudomonas aeruginosa,* and *Staphylococcus aureus.* Transient microbes are introduced by contact with objects or other persons or animals. Intestinal flora may be introduced to wounds by fecal incontinence or poor hygiene. Notable examples of transient microbes include various *Enterococci, Escherichia coli, Proteus, Klebsiella,* and *Lactobacillus* species. Multiple organisms colonizing the mouth and pharynx may be introduced due to poor hygiene or human bites. A tremendous number of bacteria from the environment may contaminate wounds, especially the *Clostridium* species. Bacteria may also enter wounds by direct contact with others, including health care workers, due to improper handwashing (skin-to-skin contact) or by aerosol inhalation. Other means of infection include ingestion of contaminated food or drink and fecal-oral transmission due to improper hygiene or sanitation, which is also a means of food or drink contamination. Some infections may also be caused by arthropod or vertebrate bites. Indirect contact or secondary contamination is caused by contact with contaminated bedding, clothing, instruments, or equipment.

Hospital (or other facility) acquired infections are termed *nosocomial infections.* The most common nosocomial infections are caused by *Staphylococcus aureus, Escherichia coli,* and *Pseudomonas aeruginosa.* The most common organism involved in wound infection is *Staphylococcus aureus.* Wounds may also be infected by facultative gram negative bacteria such as *E coli*, *Proteus*, *Enterobacter*, and *Klebsiella* due to fecal contamination of wounds. Deep wounds are frequently infected by anaerobes such as *Bacteroides*, *Actinomyces*, and *Clostridium* species.

COLONIZATION, CONTAMINATION, AND INFECTION

The ability to control wound infection depends on a thorough understanding of the differences between colonization, contamination, and infection. All wounds, whether acute or chronic, are exposed to microbes. Our ability to reduce the risk of infection is determined by the characteristics of the bacteria and the environment in which the bacteria live. Colonization simply represents a stable population of resident bacteria in low numbers on a surface. As long as the environment remains stable, the surface does not become overrun, and microbes do not invade tissues surrounding the surface. Contamination refers to the introduction of transient microbes to a surface. If a colonized surface such as an open wound experiences contamination, the risk of infection is increased. The aquarium analogy is useful to explain this phenomenon. In a community aquarium, a stable population of fish thrives as long as the environment remains stable. However, the introduction of a new species of fish, which may better compete in the environment, can proliferate at the expense of the other fish, or a change in the environment may cause one of the existing fish to proliferate at the expense of others that do not adapt as well to the new environment. Therefore, contamination or alteration of the wound environment may lead to infection. Infection occurs when tissue is invaded by bacteria that proliferate instead of remaining as a stable population. Operationally, infection is defined as 100,000 (10^5) organisms per gram. A practical definition based on visual inspection of a wound is necrosis of tissue surrounding the wound, which is observable as a deterioration of the wound or darkened dusky or brown areas developing on the wound surface.

A moist, warm environment with necrotic tissue such as an occluded wound is conducive to bacterial overgrowth. The risk of infection is tremendous in an acute wound with large amounts of necrotic tissue available for nourishment of microbes. In particular, burned tissue serves as a tremendous growth medium for bacteria. Partial-thickness wounds can easily degenerate into full-thickness injuries due to bacteria-mediated necrosis of the dermis at the base of a burn injury. Large, contaminated acute wounds, especially those with substantial injuries and tissue necrosis, should be allowed to heal by granulation; suturing or other forms of primary closure of this type of wound produces a cavity that provides an ideal environment for bacterial overgrowth and no opportunity for observation of the wound. Exposure to air, agitation with whirlpool, and filling the wound with absorbent, nonocclusive material such as gauze decrease bacterial count, but an open wound may dry out and slow healing. Occlusive dressings, on the other hand, promote a moist wound environment but provide conditions suitable for bacterial overgrowth. The clinician needs to select nonocclusive wound dressings and appropriate debridement until the bacterial count is low enough to use occlusive dressings. Thorough sharp debridement can rapidly reduce the bacterial count of a wound. Moreover, once sharp debridement is completed, in almost all cases bacterial counts will remain low (<100 per gram).

CULTURING WOUNDS

Two basic reasons are given for performing cultures of wounds. A *quantitative* culture is used to determine the microbial burden. A *qualitative* culture is used to identify which microbes are present and may be followed by sensitivity testing to determine the optimal antimicrobial drug to treat the infection. Although performing routine cultures would seem to have great value in directing wound management efforts, routine swab culture of chronic wounds is not recommended by AHCPR[7] for several reasons and may actually lead to poorer wound management. First, chronic wounds are expected to be colonized; therefore, cultures will grow resident microbes that are unlikely related to any problems with wound healing. Secondly, swabbing the surface of a wound may miss organisms growing beneath the surface, which are our major concern. Therefore, swab cultures may not identify the source (if any) of infection, leading to the use of antimicrobial agents that may further slow healing of the wound and may have adverse effects for the patient either locally or systemically. Moreover, the wrong antimicrobial may be chosen if sensitivity tests are conducted on surface pathogens, rather than those causing infection below the wound surface. Too frequently, the concept that infection interferes with acute wound healing is illogically extrapolated to chronic wounds. The presumption of infection as the cause of a slow healing wound leads to the use of routine cultures and application of topical antibiotic agents, rather than thoroughly investigating the causes of slow healing. Topical agents then further slow wound healing, leading to even harsher handling of the wound.

Culturing may be done by any of a number of personnel, including physicians, nurses, medical technicians, and physical and occupational therapists. When unsure of the preferred technique of a facility, the best option is to ask the medical technician who will be performing the cultures exactly how the swabbing and transport of the culturette should be done. Aerobic and anaerobic culturettes are handled somewhat differently and instructions given with the culturette need to be followed carefully. Some general rules for performing the culture include avoiding swabbing over hard eschar, which will likely have different microbes present than the wound itself due to the vastly different microenvironment. The tip needs to be rotated to cover as much of the swab tip as possible. While swabbing, cover from one edge to the other in a "zigzag" pattern such that 10 points (five on each side) are covered from one end of the wound to the other.

It is generally believed that all chronic wounds, including stage II to IV ulcers, are colonized; and culturing a wound that does not appear to be infected provides no useful information. Moreover, colonization will be minimized through cleansing and debridement of wounds. If purulence or foul odor develops, however, more frequent cleansing or debridement should be done. As discussed, healing of even chronic wounds may be delayed if >100,000 organisms per gram or osteomyelitis exist. The AHCPR has taken the position that swab cultures should not be done routinely for determining if a wound is infected. Instead, the Centers for Disease Control (CDC) recommend either drawing wound fluid through needle aspiration or tissue biopsy for determining if a wound is infected. Because infection is largely dependent on the presence of necrotic tissue, adequate cleansing and debridement will prevent infection in most cases. The AHCPR guidelines recommend a 2-week trial of topical antibiotics if a clean ulcer is not healing or if exudate continues despite optimal care for 2 to 4 weeks and to evaluate bone for osteomyelitis (X-ray).[7]

ANTIMICROBIAL METHODS

Several important definitions must be understood to practice good infection control. These terms include sterilization, disinfection, and antisepsis. Sterilization refers to total destruction of all microbial life, including spores and viruses. Antisepsis is a reduction in the number of organisms present on skin or tissues. A related term, disinfection is defined as a reduction of number of organisms present on inanimate objects.

Antimicrobial methods may be divided into physical and chemical methods. Certain types are more appropriate for sterilization, others for antisepsis or disinfection. Factors to be considered for any method include how long the process is applied, the temperature and pressure at which the process is applied, the quantity or concentration of heat or chemical, the nature of the item receiving the process, the type and quantity of microbe, including spores, and whether the items are contaminated with body fluids that may act as a protective layer for the microbe. Physical methods include heat—both dry and moist—pressure combined with heat, cold, desiccation, radiation, ultrasound, filtration, and hypertonicity. In general, physical methods are useful for sterilization, whereas chemicals are frequently used for antisepsis and disinfection. However, a combination of physical and chemical methods may be used for any of the three types of antimicrobial methods.

Sterilization

Heat can be used for either sterilization or disinfection. However, heat is not suitable for many items and certainly not for antisepsis. A combination of time and temperature is necessary to destroy all microbes. In addition, contamination of items with body fluids, which can form an insulating coat on the microbes, increases the heat load necessary to achieve sterilization. In the case of instruments contaminated with body fluids, thorough cleaning and chemical disinfection may be required prior to sterilization with heat. Dry heat is less effective on some types of microbes, especially on items contaminated with body fluids. Moist heat (either steam or boiling) is more effective at removing proteinaceous material from instruments. The addition of pressure by sterilizing in an autoclave is effective at destroying spores that may survive dry or even moist heat. Of particular concern is destruction of viruses that may withstand boiling. Safe guidelines promoted in the literature include autoclaving for 20 minutes at 250°F (121°C) and 15 psi, boiling for 30 minutes (longer at higher elevations), or dry heat (baking) for 1 hour at 356°F (180°C). Appropriate packaging, including pressure sensitive tape, should be used for autoclaving. Due to the heat and pressure of the autoclave, no sealed containers should be used. Items that cannot tolerate normal autoclave temperatures may be treated at a lower temperature for a longer time or may require chemical disinfection.[1]

Another approach for heat-sensitive items such as catheters is gas sterilization. Ethylene oxide is a chemical oxidizing agent, which is highly effective but also difficult to use. Radiation is sometimes used to sterilize items. X-rays or gamma rays (ionizing radiation) induce tremendous genetic damage that in large enough doses is capable of sterilizing instruments as well as foods and drugs. Ultrasound is highly effective at removing adherent materials from the surface of metal. The cleansed materials may then be further disinfected and sterilized.

Disinfection

Three levels of disinfection are commonly described. High-level disinfection destroys all microorganisms and viruses. Intermediate-level disinfection destroys all microbes except spore-forming, and some nonlipid and small viruses. The third type, low-level disinfection, provides little action against spore-forming bacteria, mycobacteria, and some fungi and small viruses. Certain items can be suitably disinfected with heat. For example, laundering clothing and bedding at high temperatures with suitable detergents is generally sufficient. In the case of chemical disinfection, the interaction of disinfectants and microbes must be considered. The effectiveness of chemical disinfectants is dependent on the concentration of the chemical, the pH, and presence of body fluids on the items to be disinfected; therefore, instructions need to be followed carefully. Moreover, instruments and other items should be washed thoroughly before disinfection to remove proteinaceous material that may protect microbes from the disinfectant. High-level disinfection needs to be used when concern exists regarding spore-forming bacteria or viruses. Disinfection is useful for treating items that come in contact with intact skin. Instruments that will contact wounds, especially if used for debridement, must be sterilized. Sterile dressings and gloves should be used on acute wounds or on individuals with immunodeficiencies, whereas clean dressings and gloves may be used on chronic wounds of individuals with relatively normal immunity. On the other hand, dressings or gloves should not be left in the open for extended periods to accumulate surface contamination. These materials should be kept in closed containers, protected from airborne contamination or splashing.

The chemical chosen for disinfection should be chosen for the particular situation. A large number of high-level disinfectants are available commercially. Their effectiveness is determined by the factors described previously, in particular concentration, temperature, and the presence of body fluids. Surfaces should be scrubbed with detergent to remove body fluids. Surfactant and chelating agents in the detergent increase the effectiveness of removing proteinaceous contaminants. In addition, the disinfectant should be left on the surface for the prescribed time to be effective. High-level disinfectants need to be rinsed thoroughly to avoid injury to the patient. Surfaces of whirlpool tubs usually receive high-level disinfection, although they are obviously left open to airborne contamination and are subject to contaminants present in tap water used to fill the whirlpool tub. Other types of hydrotherapy such as pulsatile lavage are performed with sterilized solutions, usually prepackaged sterile saline.

Disinfectants include several types of agents, including soaps/detergents, alcohols, heavy metals, oxidants, chlorine, iodine compounds, and other agents. Phenolics are used commercially in home disinfectants (eg, Lysol [Reckitt Benckiser, Wayne, NJ]). Phenolics include the disinfectant originally used by Lister, carbolic acid, as well as phenol, xylenols, cresol, and orthophenylphenol. Similar to alcohols, these agents are effective tuberculocides but not sporicides. In particular, chlorine compounds are used in hydrotherapy. Sodium hypochlorite, the active ingredient of laundry bleach, has a short half-life

and is inactivated readily by organic material. Sustained release forms of chlorine, such as Chlorazene (chloramine-T) (Ferno-Washington, Inc., Wilmington, Ohio) are frequently used to disinfect water used for hydrotherapy in a whirlpool tank. Although they are indicated for skin preparation and hand scrubbing prior to surgery, sustained-release forms of iodine, such as povidone-iodine, have also been used to disinfect water used for hydrotherapy.

Antisepsis

Like disinfection, chemical antimicrobial methods are the mainstay of antisepsis. Chemicals used for antisepsis are called *antiseptics*. Physical means are generally not suitable for antisepsis due to the potential damage to skin or body tissues. Moreover, many chemicals that are highly effective for disinfection are too damaging to be used as antiseptics. Antiseptics reduce the number of microbes on the body surface. However, microbes may still be harbored in hair follicles and the ostia of sweat and sebaceous glands. Research indicates that a reduction of approximately 95% may be obtained with good technique. Soaps and detergents act as disinfectants by removing surface microbes. In addition, they damage cell membranes by dissolving phospholipids. Many soaps and detergents have antimicrobial agents added, such as acetic acid and benzoic acid for handwashing. Chlorhexidine gluconate and hexachlorophene (Phisohex, Sanofil Pharmaceuticals, New York, NY) are commonly used as antiseptics for handwashing or topical bacterial infections. In particular, hexachlorophene is neurotoxic, and both chlorhexidine gluconate and hexachlorophene should be thoroughly rinsed from the skin. These agents are used occasionally as whirlpool disinfectants, although they have questionable value at the dilutions used and may be ineffective against a number of organisms at their full strengths. Ethyl and isopropyl alcohol in 70% solutions are effective disinfectants for bacteria and are tuberculocidal but not sporicidal. Aerosolized ethyl alcohol foams and isopropyl alcohol gels are available for handwashing to rapidly reducing the counts of transient bacteria. Alcohol and iodine solutions are used for antiseptic scrubs to further reduce microbial counts. Even with surgical scrubbing, microbial counts are still unacceptably high, requiring the use of sterile gloves. Antiseptics are also used in sprays as air fresheners containing ingredients such as alcohol, triethylene glycol, and benzethonium chloride.

Salts of heavy metals are available commercially as antiseptics. Mercury chloride is commonly used for first aid on acute wounds (Merthiolate, Mercurochrome) and silver nitrate has been used as an ophthalmic antiseptic for neonates. Silver nitrate left on skin or open wounds is highly toxic. It causes severe drying and necrosis of tissue and is not recommended for use on open wounds. Hydrogen peroxide is a commonly used, commercially available agent proposed to work as an oxidizing agent, particularly for anaerobes, and produces effervescence due to the reaction with tissue catalase, providing a mild debriding function. Iodine compounds are used for antisepsis as well as disinfection. Iodine is formulated as a slow release polymer such as Betadine (Purdue-Frederick, Norwalk, Conn) to produce continual release of iodine on the skin surface or combined with alcohol (tincture of iodine). Iodine compounds are approved by the FDA for surface antisepsis as either a skin scrub or surgical prep but are not approved for use in open wounds. Iodine compounds have been clearly shown to interfere with the processes of wound healing. In addition, high concentrations of iodine can cause iodine burns or lead to systemic iodine toxicity, manifested as neuropathy, cardiovascular, renal, and hepatic toxicity. Heavy metals, halogens, iodine, and bromine are bacteriocidal, virucidal, and tuberculocidal but not sporicidal. Acids such as acetic acid and boric acid are effective against a number of common bacteria. In particular, acetic acid is commonly used for treating wounds infected by *Pseudomonas aeruginosa*, and Dakin's solution is used to destroy *Staphylococcus* and *Streptococcus* species.

Recently, ultraviolet lamps have been approved for antiseptic use. Like X-rays and gamma rays, ultraviolet produces severe genetic damage. The dose necessary for antisepsis is relatively small, requiring exposure for several seconds with minimal risk to growing tissue in the wound when used appropriately. Paper and gauze may be used to filter substances to decrease contamination with microbes. Paper is frequently used for face masks, and gauze is frequently placed as a covering over wounds. Paper and gauze need to be kept dry to be effective as filters. Wet gauze, in particular, can transmit microbes into a wound. Moist dressings are usually covered by a dry gauze or paper material to prevent transmission of microbes from the air into the wounds. Additionally, high-efficiency particulate air (HEPA) filters are used to decrease microbes as well as allergens from the air. Ionizers may also be used to remove particulate material from the air; however, the ionized particles settle on surfaces and require dusting, vacuuming, or mopping to remove them.

Other Antimicrobial Methods

Cold as a technique is primarily bacteriostatic, rather than bacteriocidal. Cold reduces the rate of growth of microbes. Allowing temperature to increase to room temperature causes bacterial growth to resume and spores to germinate. Refreezing will simply slow the growth of a larger number of bacteria. *Desiccation* (drying) is frequently used in the preparation of foods and drugs. Desiccation combined with vacuum is called *lyophilization*. Spores or encased microbes may be found in desiccated body fluids found in the environment including

floors, dressings, clothing, and other items in the environment. Airborne dust may carry these microbes into wounds where a warm, moist, and frequently occluded environment may aid in the proliferation of the microbe. Hypertonicity is generally used for preserving food rather than wound management.

CONTROL OF ENDOGENOUS ORGANISMS

Endogenous organisms refer to those already present on the person. Several means are available to control endogenous organisms. A common means of preventing bacterial access to the wound is by skin preparation with chlorhexidine/alcohol or iodine/alcohol. Cleansing wounds with mechanical irrigation such as pulsatile lavage with concurrent suction is useful for traumatic wounds with gross contamination. Generally, if given the choice of topical and systemic antimicrobial drugs, systemic drugs are preferred. The depth of penetration of topical agents is often insufficient. The concern with bacteria in the wound is not surface colonization but invasion of tissue below the wound surface where topical agents are unlikely to reach. Protecting wounds on the sacrum and ischial tuberosities from feces is another important aspect of managing colonization and preventing infection.

CONTROL OF EXOGENOUS ORGANISMS

Microbes present on a surface other than the body are termed exogenous organisms. Control is usually achieved by sterilization of invasive instruments and disinfection of equipment such as hydrotherapy tanks and turbines. Although we tend to focus on transient microbes, resident microbes—while not generally pathogenic—can cause infection in immune compromised individuals or when deposited into a patient's tissue. Moreover, microbes may also be transmitted from patients to therapists.

Although not completely effective in removing microbes from the skin, care needs to be taken during handwashing to minimize what is left on the skin of the clinician. One must distinguish between handwashing, which is done to minimize the number of transient organisms on the hands, and scrubbing, which is done to minimize both transient and resident organisms present on the hands. Handwashing is a vigorous and brief rubbing of hand surfaces together with lathered hands, followed by rinsing with flowing water. Scrubbing is a specific sequence of cleaning for up to 10 minutes and is required to enter a sterile field, which also requires a cap, sterile gown, mask, and shoe covers. Handwashing involves soap or detergent, sometimes combined with mild antimicrobial

<hr>

Table 18-2

HANDWASHING TECHNIQUE

- Turn on the faucet with foot or knee control, or a clean paper towel
- Operate soap control with foot control or use a clean paper towel
- Wash thoroughly for 30 seconds
- Rinse thoroughly under flowing water, but do not make contact with the faucet or sink
- If contact is made, handwashing must be restarted
- Allow water to run toward elbows; do not allow water from arm to run down to hands
- Dry with clean paper towels and then turn off water with paper towels
- Clean examination gloves may be worn under sterile gloves for added protection
- Handwashing is to be done before and after each patient
- Disposable soap containers are preferred to refillable containers; bar soap should not be used
- Avoid being splashed at the sink

<hr>

agents. Scrubbing is done with a combination of iodine and alcohol or other harsh antimicrobial agents (Table 18-2).

Proper handwashing technique avoids touching the sink with the hands. Water controls and nonrefillable soap dispensers that use knee or foot controls are preferable to controls that require the use of hands. Care must be taken during handwashing to prevent contamination with *Pseudomonas* and other microbes from contact with the sink, handles, faucet, or from using solutions diluted with nonsterile water. If not available, use clean paper towels to touch faucet controls. A scrub cannot be performed without knee or foot controls. A scrub must be followed by drying with a sterile towel. Proper handwashing may be followed by drying with paper towels, but contact with the outside of the towel dispenser must be avoided. Proper handwashing techniques are depicted in Figures 18-1a through 18-1i.

Absolute sterile technique is not justifiable for all patients. Even for surgical procedures, varying levels of sterile technique are practiced. In particular, much greater precautions are taken for orthopedic surgery than for other types. For most wound care, clean technique and use of universal precautions are sufficient. Universal precautions include wearing gloves for anticipated contact with blood, secretions, mucous membranes, nonintact skin, and moist body substances for all patients. Handwashing between patients is essential and gloves must be changed before treating another patient. With any type of patient contact, the hands should be washed for 10 seconds with soap and friction to remove transient microbial flora, and then rinsed with running water. In certain contexts, the term *standard precautions* may be used in the place of universal precautions.

Each institution should have policies and procedures in place related to infection control. Each clinician, as well as students under supervision, is responsible for following body substance isolation (BSI) precautions. Universal precautions refer to operating under the assumption that any contact carries the risk of transmitting microbes. Clean technique dictates that during treatment of multiple ulcers on the same patient, the clinician should attend to the most contaminated ulcer last (eg, in the perianal region). In contrast, with normal sterile technique, the clinician would change sterilized gloves for each wound on the patient. The following body substance isolation precautions (universal precautions) are suggested by the AHCPR. They may need to be modified to make them appropriate to the setting in which the patient is seen as well as the patient's condition (Table 18-3).

Additional barriers such as gowns, plastic aprons, masks, or goggles must be worn when moist body substances (secretions, blood, or body fluids) are likely to soil the clothing or skin, or splash in the face. Protective eyewear, masks (or a face shield that covers the eyes and face), gloves, and in some cases protective gowns and caps should be used for pressure ulcer irrigation when there is reasonable expectation that wound secretions might be aerosolized. In any case, the mucous membranes of the eyes, nose, and mouth should always be protected with a minimum of a face mask and goggles. A face shield provides additional protection. The day-to-day assumption that body fluids will not be splashed on the clinician is a breach of good protective practice. The clinician may never experience a facial splash; however, one cannot predict with complete confidence that any given wound will never splash. The cost of disposable masks and reusable goggles is small compared to the possible outcome of infectious material contacting the eyes, nose, or mouth.

Even in the case in which the clinician uses clean technique, sterile instruments should be used to debride ulcers. Clean dressings, rather than sterile ones, may be used on

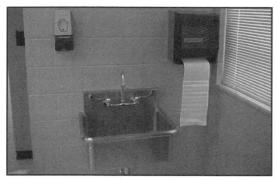

Figure 18-1a. Handwashing: soap dispenser, sink, and paper towel dispenser.

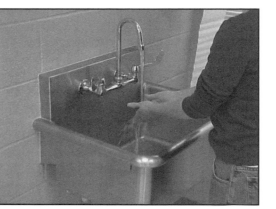

Figure 18-1b. Wetting hands.

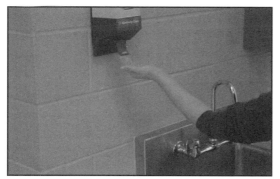

Figure 18-1c. Obtaining soap.

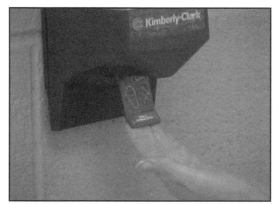

Figure 18-1d. Close-up of nonrefillable soap dispenser.

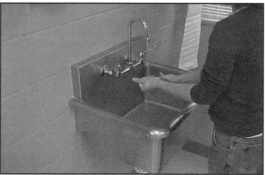

Figure 18-1e. Lathering.

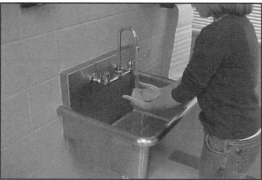

Figure 18-1f. Rinsing.

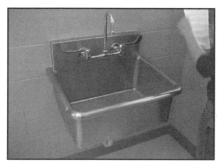

Figure 18-1g. Drying hands.

setting. Disposal of contaminated dressings in the home should be done in a manner consistent with local regulations. In some areas, this may allow the disposal of all items in the regular trash or may require the use of biohazard containers.

TOPICAL ANTIMICROBIAL AGENTS

A large number of antimicrobial agents have been used on open wounds. Most of these, however, are designed for preparation of the skin preoperatively and for immediate use on acute wounds. They are not designed, indicated, or

pressure ulcers and other chronic wounds as long as dressing procedures comply with institutional infection-control guidelines. Clean dressings may also be used in the home

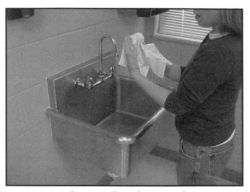

Figure 18-1h. Handwashing technique.

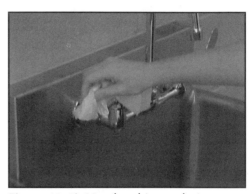

Figure 18-1i. Handwashing technique.

Table 18-3

AHCPR RECOMMENDATIONS FOR BODY SUBSTANCE ISOLATION PRECAUTIONS

- Use clean gloves for each patient
- When treating multiple ulcers on the same patient, attend to the most contaminated ulcer last (change gloves if **any** fear of cross-contamination)
- Use sterile instruments for debridement
- Use clean dressings
- Follow local regulations for disposal of contaminated dressings

approved for use on chronic wounds. These agents are often misused or overused. Although they may be useful temporarily, they must be used prudently with the specific goal of preventing or treating infection. However, because infection and eschar are slow healing, these agents are used often in an illogical attempt to speed healing. Considering that these agents are toxic to bacteria, fungi, protozoa, and even many viruses, the clinician should also consider what these agents do to fibroblasts and epithelial cells. If the immediate goal is related to ridding the wound of unacceptable numbers of microbes, then a limited course may be prudent. One must keep in mind that the concern is for organisms that have achieved a true tissue level, not simply bacteria colonizing the surface of a wound.

Many topical agents lack the penetration necessary to be effective when applied topically. Silver sulfadiazine, in particular, is sufficiently water soluble to be effective. Once a wound is debrided, clean, and stable, these agents will only retard wound healing. AHCPR guidelines state specifically that antiseptics should not be placed in wounds (these agents are discussed individually later). AHCPR recommends a 2-week trial of topical antibiotics for clean ulcers that are not healing or are continuing to produce exudate after 2 to 4 weeks of optimal care. If an antibiotic is selected for topical use, the AHCPR recommends using an agent that is effective against gram-nega-

tive, gram-positive, and anaerobic organisms. Triple antibiotic and silver sulfadiazine are mentioned specifically. The AHCPR guidelines recommend against use of topical antiseptics such as povidone-iodine, iodophor, sodium hypochlorite, Dakin's solution, hydrogen peroxide, and acetic acid in wound tissue. Moreover, systemic antibiotic therapy for patients with bacteremia, sepsis, advancing cellulitis, or osteomyelitis should be used. AHCPR guidelines suggest that systemic antibiotics are not required for pressure ulcers with only clinical signs of local infection. The American Diabetes Association recommends against the use of any topical antiseptics or antibiotics and recommends aggressive sharp debridement and systemic antibiotics.[8]

As previously discussed, povidone-iodine is a compound designed to produce sustained release of iodine. It is very beneficial in reducing risk of infection as a surgical preparation and temporary use on acute wounds. However, it is not recommended for use in chronic wounds. It may be used to prevent cross-contamination of hydrotherapy equipment. At a concentration of 0.001%, it is noncytotoxic for fibroblasts. However, it is often used on gauze-packed wounds in concentrations much higher than this and has never received approval to be used in wounds, but only for prepping skin for surgery or as a surgical hand scrub solution. Hypochlorite (household bleach) and the less cytotoxic chloramine (chlorazene) are used routinely to prevent cross-contamination of hydrotherapy equipment. Unless a patient has more than one wound in a whirlpool tank or other container, the use of these chlorine compounds is questionable. Dakin's solution is a combination of sodium hypochlorite and boric acid that is effective against *Staphylococcus* and *Streptococcus* species. It was an important development in treating acute wound infections and likely prevented a number of wartime amputations. However, it is frequently prescribed for use on chronic wounds that are not infected. It is highly cytotoxic unless diluted and the AHCPR guidelines state explicitly that Dakin's solution should not be used on chronic wounds.

Acetic acid, the active ingredient of vinegar, in a 0.25% solution is highly effective against *Pseudomonas*, but is caustic and damages healthy tissue. The AHCPR guidelines also make specific mention of acetic acid in terms of harming healing tissue. Acetic acid may be useful for a short course of several days in wounds infected by *Pseudomonas aeruginosa.* Hydrogen peroxide is a tremendously overrated antimicrobial agent. Although it is a household staple for treatment of minor acute wounds, it has little antimicrobial action compared with other available agents. It is sometimes used for its mechanical effect of effervescence. The enzyme catalase in blood converts H_2O_2 to H_2O and O_2, but this provides minor debridement value, which could be performed in other ways. Silver nitrate is very effective against gram-negative bacteria, especially in a single application following contamination, but it is more useful as a hemostatic agent. It is very caustic and will discolor the skin (black). Its caustic nature allows the skilled clinician to use it to burn off excessive granulation tissue or to open curled-over wound margins (epiboly). Mercurochrome has useful antimicrobial action on small, partially healed, superficial wounds or for a small number of applications to minor acute wounds.

Neosporin is a combination of three antibacterial drugs (neomycin, polymixin B, and bacitracin) and is highly effective against most gram-negative and gram-positive bacteria found on skin. It is, therefore, indicated for most minor acute wounds. Moreover, its petroleum base allows moisture retention to prevent scab formation. Polysporin only contains two of the three antimicrobials present in Neosporin (missing neomycin). It also has a petroleum base, and it is commonly used on facial wounds, including burns. Polysporin is also available in a powder, which is often poured into open wounds. Triple antibiotic is a solution of three antimicrobials: neomycin, polymixin B, and gramicidin. It is useful topically on a temporary basis for either a deep acute wound, such as a gunshot wound, or as a short topical course for a nonhealing chronic wound suspected to be infected.

Silver sulfadiazine inhibits DNA synthesis of microbes and is a broad spectrum antimicrobial with a cream formulation applied topically. It is especially useful for burns, has a soothing effect, and prevents gauze bandages from adhering to wounds. Although it may have adverse effects on fibroblasts and keratinocytes, it is highly effective in reestablishing bacterial balance. Therefore, it should be discontinued once bacterial balance is achieved. Silver sulfadiazine has also been implicated in Stevens-Johnson syndrome, an immune reaction that results in epidermal and mucosal blistering. This condition is potentially but rarely lethal. Stevens-Johnson syndrome has also been linked to a number of other antibiotics in addition to silver sulfadiazine.

SYSTEMIC ANTIMICROBIAL AGENTS

Many systemic antimicrobial drugs exist to treat infection. Entire texts are written to describe them. For chronic wounds, antibiotics are often not useful. Systemic antibiotics do not reach therapeutic levels in chronic granulation tissue but are important in the cases of acute wounds with advancing cellulitis. The purpose of this section of this chapter is to provide some background information for the clinician working with a patient for whom these drugs have been prescribed by a physician. As with any type of drug, antimicrobial agents have a therapeutic index that must be considered. Therapeutic index is the ratio of the median toxic dose (TD_{50}) to the median effective dose (ED_{50}) ($TI = TD_{50}/ED_{50}$). Ideally, all antimicrobial drugs would have selective toxicity such that they would only harm bacteria (or protozoa or fungi), not the patient. Another consideration is that some antibacterial drugs are bacteriostatic, whereas others are bacteriocidal. Under most conditions, simply rendering bacterial replication difficult is sufficient (bacteriostatic agents). However, certain conditions dictate using drugs that kill existing bacteria (bacteriocidal agents). Strategies currently available for management of infection include inhibition of cell wall synthesis, damaging bacterial cell membranes, inhibition of bacterial protein synthesis, inhibition of bacterial DNA/RNA function, and modification of energy metabolism. As research continues on bacterial genomes, many researchers expect to have newer and more specific strategies available in the future.

The earliest and still very important category is the cell wall active agents (beta lactams). These drugs prevent synthesis of cell walls around all bacteria but are not effective on mycoplasma, which lack a cell wall. Drugs in this category include penicillins (amoxicillin, oxacillin, methicillin, ampicillin, piperacillin, nafcillin, etc), cephalosporins, vancomycin, bacitracin, monobactams, and carbapenems. Polymixin acts at the cell membrane, rather than the cell wall, and along with bacitracin is more suitable for topical use than systemic use due to toxicity. Penicillins were the first antibiotics. These drugs were initially isolated from *Penicillium* molds that contaminated bacterial cultures and inhibited the culture's growth.

Unfortunately, some bacteria have an enzyme called *beta-lactamase* that alters the structure of the active part of the penicillin molecule and confers resistance. One drug developed to overcome the problem is Augmentin (GlaxoSmithKline, Pittsburgh, Pa), a combination of the penicillin amoxicillin and a beta-lactamase inhibitor (clavulanate). Allergies to these drugs are common and can be severe.

Cephalosporins have an action similar to penicillins and may be used as an alternative drug if penicillin is ineffective. These drugs are classified as first, second, third generations with an increasingly broader spectrum. Unfortunately, these drugs also have been linked to allergic reactions similar to penicillins. Like the penicillins, these drugs are easily identified by their names. Cephalosporins usually have ceph, cef, or kef in the name with the exception of some of the trade names such as Ceclor, Suprax, and Fortaz.

Vancomycin is frequently reserved as a "last resort" for resistant species or given empirically until sensitivity testing is completed in the lab. One particular organism has received much publicity recently. Termed VRE for vancomycin-resistant *Enterococcus*, this bacterium is spread easily by contact between health care providers and patients due to breakdowns in universal precautions. Vancomycin, as well as several other -mycin antibiotics, is nephrotoxic and ototoxic.

Bacitracin and polymixin B are commonly used together topically. Bacitracin inhibits cell walls and polymixins damage cell membranes. Several preparations are available over the counter containing both (eg, Polysporin). Preparations containing both plus neomycin are also available for topical use (eg, Neosporin). Bacitracin and polymixins are broad spectrum and useful topically but too toxic for systemic use.

Bacterial protein synthesis inhibitors include the antibiotic groups *aminoglycosides*, *macrolides*, and *tetracyclines*. Aminoglycosides are broad spectrum aerobic gram-negative antibiotics. They bind to bacterial ribosomes to disrupt protein synthesis. However, like vancomycin they are ototoxic and nephrotoxic. Several are in common use and have names that end in -mycin. Exceptions to the mycin name include vancomycin and macrolides listed below. Popular examples include gentamycin, streptomycin, neomycin (used topically), and tobramycin, which is also available in a form that can be inhaled for infections commonly seen in cystic fibrosis.

Macrolides interfere with enzyme systems responsible for bacterial protein synthesis. Unfortunately, these also may interfere with the breakdown of certain other drugs. One popular antihistamine has been removed from the market due to interaction with erythromycin. Available types include the erythromycins, azithromycin (Zithromax, Pfizer, Cambridge, Mass), and clarithromycin

(Biaxin, Abbott Laboratories, Abbott Park, Ill). Tetracyclines interfere with ribosomal function and are broad spectrum agents. They are commonly used for chlamydial and rickettsial diseases (typhus, Rocky Mountain spotted fever, Q fever) and for Lyme disease. However, serious adverse effects limit use, the drug interacts with calcium, discolors teeth in children and pregnant women, and impairs growth and development of teeth and bones.

Antibacterials that inhibit DNA/RNA include quinalones, which inhibit coiling of DNA, such as ciprofloxacin (Cipro, Bayer Pharmaceuticals, West Haven, Conn), and sulfonamides, which disrupt folic acid synthesis. Silver sulfadiazine, which is used topically for burns and other acute wounds, is a broad spectrum topical agent and is mentioned here due to its mechanism of action. These drugs are sometimes combined with trimethoprim (Bactrim, Roche Laboratories, Nutley, NJ). However, these drugs are also associated with allergic reactions, including Stevens-Johnson syndrome, and some severe hematological disorders.

Metronidazole (Flagyl, Rhone-Poulenc Rorer, Collegeville, Pa) is frequently used for anaerobic infections with penetrating injury and rupture of the gastrointestinal tract, but is associated with peripheral neuropathy, seizures, and leukopenia. The same drug is also used for certain protozoal infections and used topically as a gel for rosacea.

Fungal infections are unusual in wounds. In general, fungal infections are usually either facultative or opportunistic. Facultative refers to the need for special conditions (eg, decreased competition, or altered pH or moisture). Generally, an opportunistic infection occurs under conditions of decreased immunity in which normally benign organisms or viruses cause infections. Several agents are available for treating either systemic or surface fungal infections.

STERILE TECHNIQUES

No matter how well done, no technique can be sterile. We can strive for conditions that are as close as reasonably possible, but even in an operating room we cannot guarantee sterility. With the presence of any air movement, clothing that is not sterilized, and any particulate matter, deposition of a small number of microbes onto what we would consider sterile is virtually assured. However, the cleaner our procedures are, the lower the risk of infection becomes. *Sterile* refers to the complete absence of viable microbes, often in conditions such as surgery. A sterile field is an area in which no viable microbes exist. In contrast, *unsterile* can refer to a condition that may result from a number of causes. An item is considered unsterile if it has not been appropriately sterilized, if it has come in contact

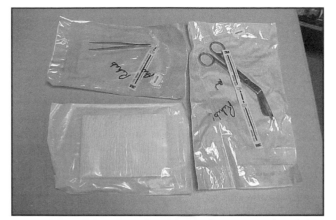

Figure 18-2a. Variety of sterile packages: sterilized forceps, scissors, and disposable towel.

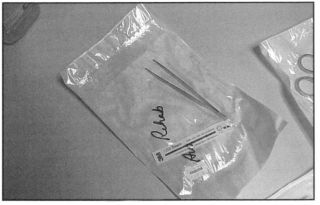

Figure 18-2b. Close-up to show indicator strip inside the forceps package.

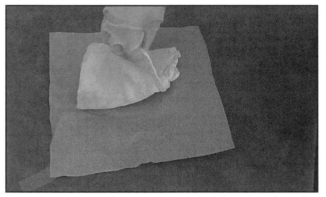

Figure 18-3a. Sterile towel. Removal from package by its corner.

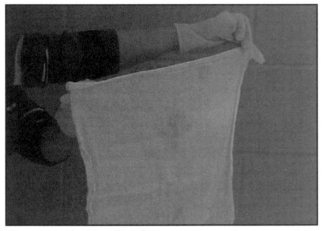

Figure 18-3b. Handling by two corners. By convention, none of the corners or edges within 1 inch are considered sterile.

with an item that is no longer considered sterile, has entered a field that is not sterile, or if it has exceeded its shelf-life. Very few packages of materials have expiration dates on them, and exceeding listed shelf-life is highly unlikely given the rate at which most supplies are used. Packages of sterilized equipment typical of those obtained from a central sterile supply are shown in Figures 18-2a and 18-2b. Shelf-life is the length of time that an item that has been sterilized and packaged is considered to still be sterile if the package is unopened. *Contamination* is the process in which an item, surface, or field has come in contact with anything that is not sterile.

Some general rules may be followed to maintain a field as close to sterile as possible. First, only sterile materials should be used in a sterile field. A sterile towel (Figures 18-3a and 18-3b) may be used to create a sterile field, but only one side of a sterile towel will be sterile; and because the corner of the sterile towel is handled to create the sterile field, a 1-inch border around the towel is considered to be unsterile. When a sterile towel is used to dry a patient from a sterile whirlpool, the sterile side is used; the other side may be touched with clean, unsterile hands. Any wet sur-

face will be contaminated, as water carries contaminants through to the sterile side of the towel. Packages placed on a clean surface are considered to be contaminated on the outside, but the inside of the sterilized package may be used as a sterile field (Figures 18-4a and 18-4b). However, wet paper packages used for circumstances such as wet-to-dry dressings are not sterile fields but are usually acceptable for a short time, normally within the range of less than 1 minute before water soaks through and allows contamination to be carried from below the towel (Figure 18-5).

Sterile gowns are used infrequently outside the operating room or burn unit. These gowns are considered sterile only down to the waist in the front; the forearms (up to the elbow) are considered sterile, but from the elbow to the shoulder is not considered sterile. The logic behind the declaration of sterile and nonsterile areas within the extremity is due to the inability to see behind oneself and the possibility of bumping an object. For these same rea-

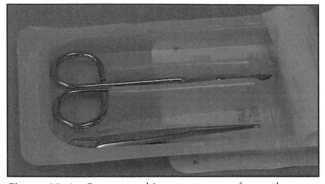

Figure 18-4a. Proper and improper use of a package as a sterile field. Inside of the package is considered sterile and may be used as a sterile field.

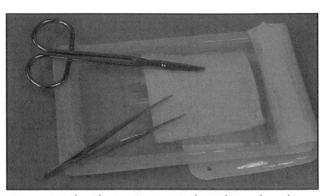

Figure 18-4b. Placing items on the edges of packages contaminates them.

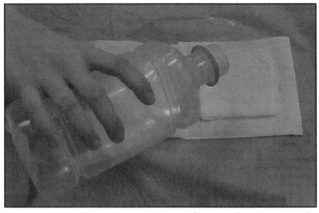

Figure 18-5. Excessive wetting of a sterile 4 x 4 inch leads to contamination due to soaking through the package.

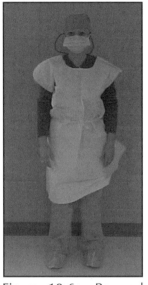

Figure 18-6a. Personal protective equipment: surgical cap, gown, gloves, shoe covers, and goggles.

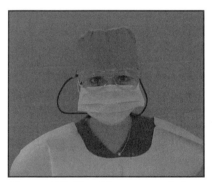

Figure 18-6b. Close-up of face protection.

sons, one should never face the back of another if working with others in a sterile field; being back-to-back or front-to-front is acceptable. Communication with the other individuals, however, is the best way to prevent contamination of others. Also, using the same simple rules, sterile gloved hands must be kept within prescribed sterile areas of the gown and not allowed to hang below the waist. When using sterile materials on a sterile, draped table, sim-

ilar rules apply. Tables draped with a sterile field are considered sterile only on the top surface; sides are not.

In many cases only sterile or, depending on the situation, clean gloves are necessary to protect the wound from contamination and the clinician from body fluids. However, the costs of dealing with accidental body fluid contamination are so great that the extra costs of time and materials for personal protective equipment are minimal in comparison. Of greatest importance is the use of either goggles and masks or face shields to protect the clinician's face, eyes, and mucous membranes from any possible body fluid contamination. Also, depending on the extent of the wounds and the patient's immune status, gowns, caps, and shoe covers should be used to protect the clinician's clothing, hair, and shoes from contact with the patient or patient's body fluids.[9] Personal protective equipment is shown in Figures 18-6a and 18-6b.

Several rules regarding containers must be enforced. For the most part, these rules follow common sense as we consider the potential for secondary contamination versus the potential for airborne contamination. The foremost rule to remember is that the edges of any container are unsterile unless the container has been sterilized and has just been opened from a package. Following this rule, cap edges and tops are considered to be unsterile. Caps must not be removed with sterile or clean gloves that have been or will be in contact with the wound or regloving must be done. When removing caps from containers, the cap is laid inside-up, but not within the sterile field. We are generally willing to accept some degree of airborne contamination but not surface contamination that results if the cap is laid inside-down.

Tubes from which contents are squeezed require either a second person to squeeze the tube as the contents are needed or the contents must be squeezed onto a sterile surface such as a 4 x 4 gauze sponge before gloving. We need to assume that the outside of the tube is unsterile. If a second person is squeezing the tube onto the clinician's gloved finger to apply to the wound or surrounding skin, the clinician must be careful to avoid touching any part of the tube, including the tip.

The inside of any sterile package can be considered sterile if peeled open properly. Opening the package completely to avoid reaching over an unsterile area of the package is a safer approach in one sense, but on the other hand, the longer a package is open to the atmosphere, the greater the risk of airborne contamination. Using this approach, tools such as scissors and forceps may be placed back in the package or on a sterile towel. When using this technique, one must avoid allowing the instrument to contact the edges of the packages where they were opened. It is very tempting to lay an instrument over the edge of a package to improve the ease of picking it up; however, doing so contaminates the handles of instruments.

When working under either sterile or clean conditions, the clinician must cover all hair including facial hair, as well as removing all dangling earrings, bracelets, and necklaces. Although many individuals seem comfortable in covering rings and wristwatches with gloves, prudent practice dictates removing them before handwashing and donning either sterile or clean gloves and then washing hands again before putting jewelry back on.

Following the rules of sterile fields can be difficult but is important in minimizing risks to both the patient and clinician. One of the simplest means to facilitate good practice is to have nonsterile personnel available for help as needed to avoid breaking sterile field or having to reglove.

Gloving

As a minimum, clean examination gloves should be worn both to protect the clinician from the patient's body fluids and to protect the patient's body fluid from contaminants on the clinician's hands. Donning sterile gloves requires special techniques, which are sometimes obvious from following package instructions, but not all manufacturers include instructions. The two basic rules are that the inside of the gloves is considered unsterile and the outside of the gloves is considered sterile. Therefore, the hands may only make contact with the inside of the gloves and only the outside of a glove is allowed to touch another glove. Furthermore, the inside of the package is sterile until touched by hands.

Based on these rules, the clinician peels the package open and makes certain that all other needed packages are open before gloving and that the clinician's hands will not need to go outside of sterile field again (eg, to take a patient out of a whirlpool). The package is oriented so the words "right" and "left" or "R" and "L" are upright.

The inside package is folded so that what becomes the outside of the wrapper can be grasped without touching the inside of the package. The inside package can then be pulled open using this folded-over part of the wrapper in the center. Avoid touching the inner surface of this wrapper and pull hard enough to keep the wrapper open. The wrapper will re-close if not pulled far enough. The following sequence is based on the concepts discussed above.

The inside of gloves is considered unsterile so hands may touch insides of gloves but not outside, and the outside of one glove may touch outside of the other but not skin or the inside of the glove. Reaching carefully, place the fingers into the glove for the nondominant hand in a scooping manner. With the dominant hand, pull on the inside surface of the glove until fingers are in, but do not try to pull the first glove all of the way on. Next, using the gloved nondominant hand, scoop underneath the fold in the glove for the dominant hand so that the glove on the nondominant hand only makes contact with the outside of the glove on the dominant hand. The partially gloved nondominant hand is used to pull the glove fully onto the dominant hand, but only touching the outside of the two gloves to each other. At this point, the dominant hand is completely gloved and the nondominant hand is partially gloved. To finish gloving the nondominant hand, place the fingers of the gloved dominant hand inside the folded cuff of the other glove, and pull the glove all of the way onto the nondominant hand, only touching outside of the glove.

When gloves are removed, the outsides of the gloves should only touch the outside of the other glove, not the

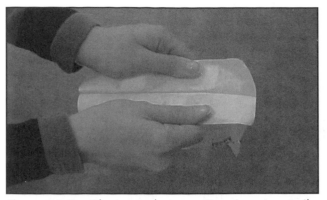

Figure 18-7a. Gloving technique. Opening any sterile package should be done in this manner to avoid touching inside the package.

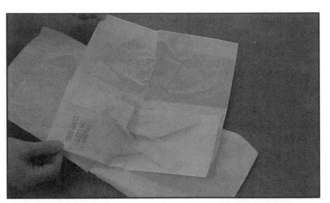

Figure 18-7b. Opening package to reveal first glove.

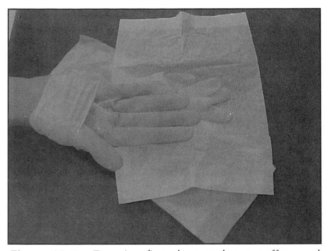

Figure 18-7c. Donning first glove to leave cuff turned over.

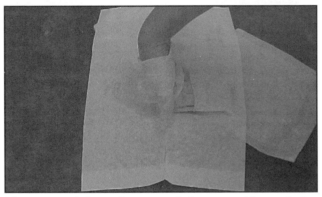

Figure 18-7d. Scooping second glove, touching only the outside of the second glove with the outside of the first glove.

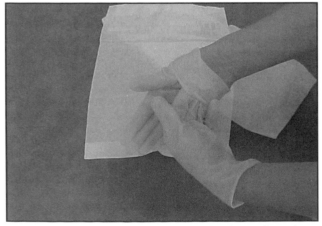

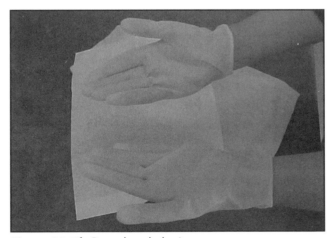

Figure 18-7f. Completed gloving.

Figure 18-7e. Pulling down the cuff of the first glove with the second glove, touching only the outside of the first glove.

skin; carefully pull gloves off inside-out so that hands only contact the inside surface of gloves. Wash your hands as soon as possible after gloves are removed. Do not write notes, restock supplies, or do anything else before doing

so to avoid secondary contamination from the gloves onto other objects. Techniques for donning and doffing sterile gloves are demonstrated in Figures 18-7a through 18-7f.

Latex, in particular, is a major concern in wound management. Both the clinician and patient need to be considered. Due to the institution of universal precautions, a large number of both patients and clinicians have been exposed and sensitized to latex.[10] Latex allergy is potentially fatal and must be taken seriously. The most common problem with latex is a nonimmunologic, irritant dermati-

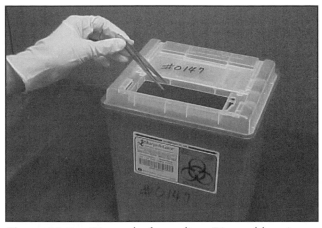

Figure 18-8a. Disposal of supplies. Disposable scissors are placed in an approved sharps container.

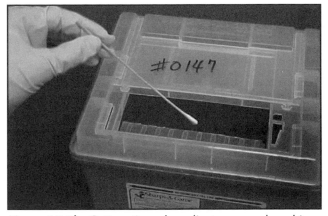

Figure 18-8b. Cotton-tipped applicators are placed in a sharps container due to the possibility of breaking and creating a sharp edge.

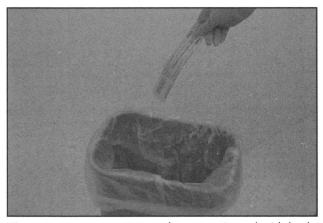

Figure 18-8c. Items not grossly contaminated with body fluids are placed in a regular trash can.

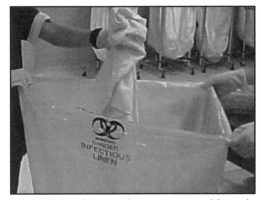

Figure 18-8d. Typical contaminated laundry bag.

tis. Type IV immune reactions in the form of contact dermatitis are much more common than a type I allergic/anaphylactic reaction.[11] About 7% to 12% of health care workers who are exposed to latex on a regular basis have positive skin tests to proteins present in latex gloves. All patients with spina bifida are automatically treated as if they are latex-sensitive, although the actual percentage is believed to be between 28% to 67%. Moreover, clinicians must be familiar with objects other than gloves containing latex that may contaminate surfaces that contact the latex-sensitive person. For this reason, latex and nonlatex exam gloves should be kept apart and hands should be washed after using latex gloves to avoid contaminating others with latex proteins. Moreover, it has been suggested that powder-free gloves are less likely to expose individuals to latex proteins by minimizing airborne latex exposure.

WASTE DISPOSAL

Waste disposal is generally the last item that occurs following patient care, although some waste disposal may be necessary during procedures. In many facilities, clinicians

may be observed to dispose of all waste in red biohazard containers. Noncontaminated waste placed in biohazard containers needlessly costs each facility thousands of dollars each year for special disposal. Careful consideration allows the clinician to be selective in disposal of materials. The quantity of outer packages that are grossly contaminated during procedures can be minimized by handling only the contents or judicious use of sterile fields. Certainly, any grossly contaminated items and sharp instruments must be placed in appropriate biohazard containers, whereas packages that do not contact body fluids directly should be placed in regular waste containers. Contaminated dressings, gauze, gloves, and similar items should be placed in a red, marked biohazard bag. Waste containers are depicted in Figures 18-8a through 18-8e.

Sharp instruments such as needles, scalpel blades, forceps, and scissors that could puncture a biohazard bag should also be placed in puncture-resistant, rigid "sharps" containers (see Figure 18-8a). Cotton-tipped applicators placed in a plastic bag have the potential for being broken. When these items are broken, they almost always create a jagged edge that can pierce a plastic bag and injure another person. Therefore, cotton-tipped applicators should also be placed in a sharps container. Personnel should never attempt to retrieve items that have been placed accidentally or deliberately in any waste containers, whether regular, biohazard, or sharps. In addition to trash, soiled reusable articles and linen should be placed in containers that are securely sealed to prevent leaking. Double bagging is not necessary unless the outside of the bag is visibly soiled.

OCCUPATIONAL SAFETY AND HEALTH AGENCY REGULATIONS

The Occupational Safety and Health Agency (OSHA) created regulations for occupational exposure to blood-borne pathogens, which became effective on March 6, 1992. Specific definitions and regulations are given in the paragraphs below.[12]

OSHA Definitions

Blood means human blood, human blood components, and products made from human blood.

Bloodborne pathogens means pathogenic microorganisms that are present in human blood and can cause disease in humans. These pathogens include, but are not limited to, hepatitis B virus (HBV) and human immunodeficiency virus (HIV).

Contaminated means the presence or the reasonably anticipated presence of blood or other potentially infectious materials on an item or surface.

Contaminated laundry means laundry that has been soiled with blood or other potentially infectious materials or may contain sharps.

Contaminated sharps means any contaminated object that can penetrate the skin including, but not limited to, needles, scalpels, broken glass, broken capillary tubes, and exposed ends of dental wires.

Decontamination means the use of physical or chemical means to remove, inactivate, or destroy bloodborne pathogens on a surface or item to the point where they are no longer capable of transmitting infectious particles and the surface or item is rendered safe for handling, use, or disposal.

Exposure incident means a specific eye, mouth, other mucous membrane, nonintact skin, or parenteral contact with blood or other potentially infectious materials that results from the performance of an employee's duties.

Handwashing facilities means a facility providing an adequate supply of running potable water, soap, and single-use towels or hot air drying machines.

Occupational exposure means reasonably anticipated skin, eye, mucous membrane, or parenteral contact with blood or other potentially infectious materials that may result from the performance of an employee's duties.

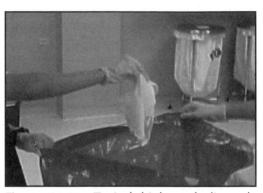

Figure 18-8e. Typical biohazard disposal bag.

Other potentially infectious materials means (1) the following human body fluids: semen, vaginal secretions, cerebrospinal fluid, synovial fluid, pleural fluid, pericardial fluid, peritoneal fluid, amniotic fluid, saliva in dental procedures, any body fluid that is visibly contaminated with blood, and all body fluids in situations where it is difficult or impossible to differentiate between body fluids; (2) any unfixed tissue or organ (other than intact skin) from a human (living or dead); and (3) HIV-containing cell or tissue cultures, organ cultures, and (4) HIV- or HBV-containing culture medium or other solutions; and blood, organs, or other tissues from experimental animals infected with HIV or HBV.

Parenteral means piercing mucous membranes or the skin barrier through such events as needlesticks, human bites, cuts, and abrasions.

Personal protective equipment is specialized clothing or equipment worn by an employee for protection against a hazard. General work clothes (eg, uniforms, pants, shirts, or blouses) not intended to function as protection against a hazard are not considered to be personal protective equipment.

Regulated waste means liquid or semiliquid blood or other potentially infectious materials; contaminated items that would release blood or other potentially infectious materials in a liquid or semiliquid state if compressed; items that are caked with dried blood or other potentially infectious materials and are capable of releasing these materials during handling; contaminated sharps; and pathological and microbiological wastes containing blood or other potentially infectious materials.

Source individual means any individual, living or dead, whose blood or other potentially infectious materials may be a source of occupational exposure to the employee. Examples include, but are not limited to, hospital and clinic patients; clients in institutions for the developmentally disabled; trauma victims; clients of drug and alcohol treatment facilities; residents of hospices and nursing homes; human remains; and individuals who donate or sell blood or blood components.

Sterilize means the use of a physical or chemical procedure to destroy all microbial life including highly resistant bacterial endospores.

Universal precautions is an approach to infection control. According to the concept of universal precautions, all human blood and certain human body fluids are treated as if known to be infectious for HIV, HBV, and other blood-borne pathogens.

The concept of universal precautions is defined under these regulations in which any potential source of blood-borne pathogens is handled to minimize risks. The regulations state: "Universal precautions shall be observed to prevent contact with blood or other potentially infectious materials. Under circumstances in which differentiation between body fluid types is difficult or impossible, all body fluids shall be considered potentially infectious materials." In addition, the regulations place responsibility on both the personnel and administration of facilities to analyze their individual circumstances to minimize risk through three basic means—engineering controls, work practice controls, and personal protective equipment.

Engineering controls refer to the development and implementation of devices to isolate or remove the risk of exposure. Examples include sharps disposal containers and self-sheathing needles.

Work practice controls means controls that reduce the likelihood of exposure by altering the manner in which a task is performed (eg, prohibiting recapping of needles by a two-handed technique).

This term refers to the means in which the tasks that could expose an individual are altered. An example is prohibition of recapping needles with two-handed technique. Facilities are also obligated to periodically examine engineering controls and maintain or replace them on a regular schedule. Important work practice controls dictated by OSHA include a specific statement that all procedures involving blood or other potentially infectious materials are to be done to minimize splashing or spraying.

A second work practice statement is that eating, drinking, smoking, applying cosmetics or lip balm, and handling contact lenses are prohibited in work areas where exposure is likely to occur. Thirdly, food and drink are not allowed to be kept in refrigerators, shelves, and other areas where blood or other potentially infectious materials are present.

For conditions that engineering and work practice controls cannot completely eliminate or minimize exposure, personal protective equipment (PPE) is required by the OSHA regulations. For such conditions, employers are obligated to provide PPE at no cost to employees. According to OSHA, appropriate PPE may consist of gloves, gowns, laboratory coats, face shields or masks and eye protection, mouthpieces, resuscitation bags, pocket masks, or other ventilation devices. OSHA defines *appropriate* in such a way that the personal protective equipment does not permit blood or other potentially infectious materials to pass through to or reach the employee's work clothes, street clothes, undergarments, skin, eyes, mouth, or other mucous membranes. This is qualified by stating that blood and other potentially infectious material does not pass through the PPE under normal conditions of use and for the duration of time during which PPE is used. Employers are responsible for ensuring that employees use appropriate personal protective equipment with the exception of extraordinary circumstances in which the PPE, in the opinion of the employee, might cause more harm than benefit. Under these circumstances an analysis of the circumstances is to be undertaken to determine whether policy or procedure changes are necessary to prevent such problems from recurring.

Employers are responsible for having PPE appropriate for any personnel requiring it, including any necessary sizes or accommodating allergies (eg, providing hypoallergenic gloves). Employers are also responsible for cleaning, laundering, disposal, repair, or replacement of PPE as needed to maintain its effectiveness at no cost to the employee. To prevent spread of pathogens contaminating the PPE, all PPE must be removed and left within the work area. Facilities will typically place disposal containers within the appropriate work area rather than in common areas such as gyms or hallways, and durable PPE is left in a designated area within the work area and not carried out into common areas. OSHA states that after use, all PPE is to be placed in an appropriately designated area or container for storage, washing, decontamination, or disposal.

Gloves are to be worn whenever employees anticipate potential for hand, mucous membrane, or nonintact skin contact with blood or other potentially infectious materials or the potential for handling or touching contaminated items or surfaces exists. Disposable gloves are to be replaced as soon as practical when contaminated or as soon as feasible if they are torn, punctured, or when their ability to function as a barrier is compromised and they are not allowed to be reused. Utility gloves, primarily used for cleaning tasks, may be decontaminated and reused, but must be discarded if they exhibit signs of deterioration.

Whenever splashes, sprays, or droplets of blood or potentially infectious materials and contamination of the eyes, nose, or mouth can be anticipated, masks in combination with eye protection devices must be worn. Eye protection devices include goggles, glasses with solid side shields, and chin-length face shields. Although not part of OSHA regulations, clinicians working with wounds should use eye, nose, and mouth protection at all times, with a preference for a full face shield to prevent ricochet off other areas of the face or the potential for nonintact skin elsewhere on the face.

Gowns, aprons, or other protective body clothing such as lab coats are required in situations of potential exposure. The type is not specified, but the regulations state that the characteristics of the clothing depends upon the task and degree of exposure anticipated. Any garments penetrated by blood or other potentially infectious materials must be removed immediately or as soon as feasible. For routine wound care, disposable paper gowns or washable gowns are sufficient.

OSHA regulations call for surgical caps or hoods and/or shoe covers or boots to be worn in instances when gross contamination can reasonably be anticipated, with specific examples of autopsies and orthopedic surgery. Although not mentioned in the OSHA regulations, shoe covers should be worn in high-traffic wound care areas, especially with patients with heavily draining lower extremity wounds likely to contaminate the floor. The floor should be disinfected as needed, and shoe covers should be changed between patients or when leaving the work area. In addition, head covers should also be used during pulsatile lavage or any time splashing can be reasonably anticipated.

OSHA regulations state that employers shall ensure that employees wash their hands immediately or as soon as feasible after removal of gloves or other personal protective equipment. Moreover, employers are obligated to provide readily accessible handwashing facilities, but in cases in which provision of handwashing facilities is not feasible, employers must provide antiseptic hand cleanser and clean cloth, paper towels, or disposable antiseptic towelettes. OSHA regulations state that when this alternative is used, handwashing with soap and running water must be done as soon as feasible. Employers must also ensure that employees wash hands and any other skin with soap and water, or flush mucous membranes with water immediately or as soon as feasible following contact of such body areas with blood or other potentially infectious materials.

Regulations exist for both reusable and disposable sharps. For reusable sharps, the regulations call for them to be placed immediately or as soon as possible after use in appropriate containers until properly reprocessed. By OSHA regulations, a container is considered to be appropriate if it is puncture resistant, it is labeled or color-coded, and leakproof on the sides and bottom. Single-use contaminated sharps are to be discarded immediately or as soon as feasible in closable, puncture-resistant, leakproof (sides and bottom), labeled, or color-coded containers. OSHA calls for placement of containers such that during use, containers are easily accessible and located as close as is feasible to the immediate area where sharps are used. The containers are to be kept upright throughout use, replaced routinely, and are not be allowed to be overfilled. Sharps containers must be closed immediately prior to removal or replacement to prevent spillage or protrusion of contents during handling, storage, or transport, and placed in a secondary container that is closable and made to contain all contents and prevent leakage if leakage is possible. Secondary containers must also be labeled or color-coded according to OSHA standards. Reusable containers, typically used for reusable sharps, are not to be opened, emptied, or cleaned manually or in any other manner that would expose employees to the risk of percutaneous injury. Note that the requirement for sharps containers are for containers that are puncture resistant. Protrusion of the contents through the walls of puncture-resistant containers will not occur under normal use. However, mishandling of these containers could result in puncture. Also note that the primary container is to be leakproof on the bottom and sides. These containers can leak if moved from an upright orientation or if overfilled. Personnel using or handling these containers should be trained to avoid spilling or puncturing the containers.

Employers are responsible for ensuring that worksites are maintained in a clean and sanitary condition. Because of variation in the type of activities and patient populations, appropriate written schedules for cleaning and methods of decontamination are to be determined and implemented based upon characteristics of the worksite, type of surface to be cleaned, type of soil present, and tasks or procedures being performed in the area. Regardless of the cleaning schedule, however, all equipment and environmental and working surfaces are to be cleaned and decontaminated after contact with blood or other potentially infectious materials. Contaminated work surfaces are to be decontaminated with an appropriate disinfectant after completion of procedures. Decontamination is to be done immediately or as soon as feasible if surfaces are overtly contaminated or after any spill of blood or other potentially infectious materials.

OSHA regulations state that handling of contaminated laundry should be minimized and bagged or contained at the location where it was used. To minimize handling, contaminated laundry is not to be sorted or rinsed in the location of use. Contaminated laundry is to be placed and transported in bags or containers labeled or color-coded appropriately. In cases in which universal precautions are used in the handling of all soiled laundry, any labeling or color-coding that permits recognition by all employees is acceptable. As discussed with sharps containers and any other biohazard container, any time that soak-through or leakage from the bag or container is likely, laundry is to be placed and transported in leak-proof bags or containers. Employers are also responsible to ensure that employees who have contact with contaminated laundry wear protective gloves and other appropriate personal protective equipment.

Employers are obligated to offer the hepatitis B vaccine and vaccination series to all employees who have occupational exposure. Employers are also responsible for post-exposure evaluation and follow-up to all employees who have had an exposure incident. Evaluations are to be made available at no cost to the employee, available at a reasonable time and place, and performed by or under the supervision of a licensed physician or by or under the supervision of another licensed health care professional and provided according to recommendations of the US Public Health Service, and all laboratory tests are to be conducted by an accredited laboratory at no cost to the employee.

Contaminated waste is placed in containers that are readily recognized by any employees. Labels are to be fluorescent orange, orange-red, or predominantly so, with lettering and symbols in a contrasting color and affixed as close as feasible to the container by string, wire, adhesive, or other method that prevents their loss or unintentional removal. Red bags or red containers may be substituted for labels.

OSHA regulations require that employers provide and ensure participation by all employees with occupational exposure in a training program provided at no cost to the employee and during working hours. Training is to be provided at the time of initial assignment to tasks where occupational exposure may take place and at least annually. Employers are also to provide additional training as needed if changes in tasks or how tasks are performed affect the employee's occupational exposure. The training program must at the minimum address the following elements:

1. where the regulations can be accessed and an explanation of the regulations

2. the epidemiology and symptoms of bloodborne diseases

3. the modes of transmission of bloodborne pathogens

4. the employer's exposure control plan

5. tasks and other activities that may involve exposure to blood and other potentially infectious materials

6. use and limitations of methods to prevent or reduce exposure including appropriate engineering controls, work practices, and personal protective equipment

7. types, proper use, location, removal, handling, decontamination, and disposal of personal protective equipment

8. the basis for selection of personal protective equipment

9. information on the hepatitis B vaccine and the appropriate actions to take and persons to contact in an emergency involving blood or other potentially infectious materials

10. methods for reporting any incident involving bloodborne pathogens and the medical follow-up that will be made available

11. information on the post-exposure evaluation and follow-up that is required of the employer

12. signs, labels, and any color coding required for biohazardous materials

13. an opportunity for interaction with the person conducting the training session

OSHA requires that the instructor providing the training is knowledgeable in the subject matter covered by the elements contained in the training program as well as how it relates to the specific workplace for which the training is done.

This information is usually provided as an annual inservice during work hours with a post-test examination and roster to provide accountability of the training and new employee orientation. Usually other information such as emergencies and fire are bundled with these training sessions. Cardiopulmonary resuscitation and airway management are provided in-house through the American Heart Association with a two-year renewal cycle.

SUMMARY

Working with wounds creates the opportunity for wounds to be contaminated and for wounds to contaminate clinicians and others working in the facility, including those who empty waste containers or transport or clean laundry. Control of infection in wounds requires an understanding of the terms colonization, infection, contamination, resident microbes, and transient microbes. Acute wounds contaminated with any microbes are at risk for infection and, therefore, are treated harshly with aggressive debridement, irrigation, and application of topical antibiotics and on occasion systemic antibiotics. Chronic wounds, on the other hand, are colonized by a number of species of microbes in a limited number. Contamination of an open wound presents the opportunity for a new microbe to grow out of control, causing infection. The terms sterilization, antisepsis, and disinfection were introduced. Sterilization removes all microbes and is necessary whenever invasive procedures or sharp debridement are performed. Routine wound care requires clean technique, but following general principles of sterile technique reduces the risk of contamination. Individuals with compromised immune systems require greater care to minimize the introduction of new microbes to the wound. OSHA standards require both work practice and engineering controls to minimize risk of exposure to bloodborne pathogens and use of personal protective equipment when these controls cannot eliminate the risk. PPE includes protection of the eyes, nose, and mouth with goggles, glasses, face masks, or face shields as appropriate; gloves at any time of exposure to body fluids; and gowns, caps, and shoe covers when appropriate. Universal precautions dictate assuming that any body fluids contain bloodborne pathogens. Both the employer and employee are obligated to follow OSHA regulations as described. Annual review of OSHA regulations is required.

Study Questions

1. What is the difference between colonization and infection? What role does contamination play?

2. List common causes of immunosuppression. How is management of these patients different?

3. Describe the differences between sterilization, disinfection, and antisepsis. When is use of antiseptic agents in wounds appropriate?

4. During what aspects of wound management is the use of gloves required? Of gowns? Of shoe covers? Of caps?

5. Under what type of wound care must sterile instruments be used?

6. For what type of wound care are caps, face masks, sterile gowns, and gloves necessary?

7. What types of items should be disposed of in a red or biohazard-labeled bag? What items should be placed in a biohazard-labeled, puncture-resistant container? What items should go in the regular trash?

References

1. Burton GRW, Engelkirk PG. *Microbiology for the HealthSciences*. 5th ed. Philadelphia, Pa: Lippincott-Raven Publishers; 1996.

2. Robson MC. Wound infection. A failure of wound healing caused by an imbalance of bacteria. *Surg Clin North Am.* 1997;77:637-650.

3. Ad Hoc Committee of the Committee on Trauma, Division of Medical Sciences, National Research Council: Report: Postoperative wound infections; the influence of ultraviolet radiation of the operating room and the influence of other factors. *Ann Surg.* 1964;160 (Suppl 1).

4. Greif R, Akca O, Horn E-P. Kurz A, Sessler DI. Supplemental perioperative oxygen to reduce the incidence of surgical-wound infection. *New Eng J of Med.* 2000;342:161-167.

5. Guideline for the Prevention of Surgical Site Infection. Available at: *http:// www.cdc.gov. ncidod/ hip/SSI /SSI_guideline.htm.*

6. Robson MC, Duke WF, Krizek TJ. Rapid bacterial screening in the treatment of civilian wounds. *Journal of Surgical Research.* 1973;14:426-430.

7. Bergstrom N, Bennett MA, Carlson CE, et al. Treatment of Pressure Ulcers. Clinical Practice Guideline, No. 15. Rockville, MD: US Department of Health and Human Services. Public Health Service, Agency for Health Care Policy and Research. AHCPR Publication No. 95-0652; December 1994.

8. American Diabetes Association: Consensus Development Conference on Diabetic Foot Wound Care (Consensus Statement). *Diabetes Care.* 22:1354-1360, 1999.

9. Guideline for Isolation Precautions in Hospitals. Available at: *http://www.cdc.gov/ncidod/hip/isolat/isolat.htm.*

10. Sussman GL, Beezhold DH. Allergy to latex rubber. *Ann Intern Med.* 1995;122:43-46.

11. Sussman GL, Liss GM, Deal K, et al. Incidence of latex sensitization among latex glove wearers. *J Allergy Clin Immunol.* 1998; 101: 171-178.

12. OSHA Regulations (Standards - 29 CFR) Bloodborne Pathogens. 1910.1030. Available at *http://www.osha-slc.gov/OshStd_data/1910_1030.html.*

Burn Management

- Discuss common causes of thermal injury; relate them to age and occupation.
- Describe systems available to classify severity of burn injury.
- Describe means of distinguishing among different severities of burn injury.
- Describe the means of quantifying the extent of burn injury.
- Discuss first aid for burn injury.
- Describe typical medical management of severe thermal injury.
- Describe types of skin grafting/replacement available.
- Discuss how skin grafting affects exercise programs.
- Discuss appropriate exercises for individuals with thermal injuries.
- Discuss scar management following thermal injury.

RISK FACTORS AND POPULATIONS

Burn injuries are tremendously common; nearly everyone experiences them on occasion. Fortunately, most of these are inconsequential with a short period of discomfort. Although most are self-treated and not reported, an estimated 2.5 million burn injuries per year require some degree of medical attention, with 70,000 of these requiring hospitalization. A disproportionate number—approximately 35% of serious burn injuries—involve children. Many serious burn injuries occur either on the job or in motor vehicle and other crash injuries; however, 75% to 85% occur in the home, particularly in the kitchen and bathroom, with hot foods and liquids spilled in the kitchen being the largest single source of burns to children. Individuals with peripheral neuropathy secondary to diabetes mellitus are also at great risk due to lack of sensation and may experience scalds from not being able to adequately determine the temperature of bath water or injuries from placing feet too close to a fireplace. One such individual severely burned his legs and feet by wearing black rubber boots while riding a garden tractor on a hot day.

The two primary age groups at risk for death from burn injury are very young children up to 5 years old and those who are older than 65 who lack the ability to escape life-threatening situations and are less able to tolerate physical stress of the post-burn injury period. Up to the age of approximately 5 years old, burns consist mainly of scald injury with an estimated 70% of these scald injuries being preventable. These injuries include kitchen injuries from cooking; unattended hot food, liquids, and appliances; bathroom injuries from hot water; chemicals; and in older homes, electric grooming appliances in the absence of ground-fault interrupter circuits. Other areas of concern in the home include lamps with dangling cords, radiators, space heaters, and hot mist vaporizers. Unattended matches and lighters in the hands of small children are also a major concern.

In the older child (5 to 12 years), experimentation with heat-producing products, power lines, and above-ground transformers become major sources of risk of burn injury. In teenage years, with greater involvement in household and working experience, preparing food, gasoline, car repairs, occupational accidents, and sun become more prominent as causes of burn injury. In adults, gasoline, smoking, electric accidents, and occupational accidents become more common causes of injury. Finally, in the adult older than 65 years of age, falling asleep while smoking, scalds, burning yard waste, ignition of clothing, tripping and falling on hot pipes, heaters, and radiators become important causes.

EVALUATION OF BURN INJURIES

A brief review of salient points of skin anatomy is necessary to explain evaluation of thermal injuries to the skin. The epidermis is the avascular layer of the skin, composed of four strata (five on the palms and soles). The deepest stratum, the *stratum basale*, is the regenerative layer. The interface of the dermis and epidermis forms an undulating, wavelike surface; the area of the dermis that extends up into these waves is the *papillary dermis*, and the thicker region of the dermis beneath this is the *reticular dermis*. Melanocytes are present in the stratum basale, and necrosis down to this layer carries the risk of pigment loss from the skin. Of the sensory receptors located in the dermis, the Pacinian corpuscle is located most deeply. The other characteristic is the presence of hair follicles, an appendage of the epidermis, diving deeply into surrounding reticular dermis.

An injury limited to the epidermis will not damage blood vessels or living cells, but injury to the epidermis may produce some inflammation of the vascular layer below. A deeper wound would next affect the papillary dermis. Injury to the papillary dermis will cause inflammation with leakage of fluid from the capillaries of the papillary dermis into the space between the dermis and epidermis, causing blistering and redness. Because of the presence of sensory receptors, exquisite pain will result. Severe injury to the papillary dermis that extends partially into the reticular dermis will coagulate blood vessels in the papillary dermis but leave blood flow in the reticular dermis and hair follicles intact. Cell death through the reticular dermis causes anesthesia and coagulation of the blood vessels throughout the skin. Blood may be trapped in coagulated vessels visible from the surface of the skin, but the skin will not blanch and refill. A wound that does not extend through the entire reticular dermis will allow blanching and refill of the skin. In addition, if the deep reticular dermis remains viable, vibration and pressure sensations will be intact from the Pacinian corpuscles located deep in the dermis.

Two classifications of severity of burn injury are in common use. The older terms—first, second, and third degree—are common among lay people and continue to be used by many health care providers. The preferred terminology, which is based on the depth of injury, uses the terms *superficial*, *superficial partial-thickness*, *deep partial-thickness*, and *full-thickness*. Some sources describe a severe electrical injury with substantial subcutaneous involvement as a fourth-degree burn. Table 19-1 summarizes characteristics of the different classes.

For most of the classifications, clinicians should be able to translate terms. A first-degree burn is equivalent to a superficial burn. A second-degree burn is equivalent to a

Table 19-1

CLASSIFICATION SYSTEM OF BURN INJURIES

Degree	Cause	Appearance	Color	Pain Level	Healing Time
First/superficial	Sunburn, scald, flash flame	Dry, no blisters	Pink	Painful	2 to 5 days with peeling, no scarring
Second/ superficial partial-thickness	Contact with hot liquids or solids, flash flame, chemical	Moist blisters	Pink to cherry red	Painful	5 to 21 days, no grafting
Deep, partial-thickness No corresponding degree		Dry, and leathery Hairs (if any) resist tugging	Mixed white, waxy, pearly, or deep khaki Blanches with pressure	Some pain	If no infection, then 21 to 35 days If infected, converts to full-thickness
Third/full-thickness	Contact with hot liquids or solids, flame, chemical, or electrical	Dry, leathery	Mixed white, waxy, pearly, or deep khaki, mahogany, charred	No pain in area but painful in surrounding areas of partial and superficial thickness	Large areas may need months with skin grafting, small areas need weeks with or without grafting

superficial partial-thickness burn, and a third-degree burn is the same as a full-thickness burn. A deep partial-thickness burn, also called a *deep dermal wound*, does not have an equivalent degree and is difficult for beginners to distinguish from a full-thickness burn.

Sunburn is an example of a superficial-thickness or first-degree burn. The skin is reddened and painful due to irritation of the papillary dermis by the injury to the epidermis. Later, itching may become problematic. Because injury is limited to the epidermis, no treatment is needed unless a large surface area is involved. Within a few days, the damaged epidermis exfoliates and the epidermis regenerates without scarring. Usual causes include sunburn, brief contact with small quantities of hot liquid, or mildly hot objects.

Superficial partial-thickness or second-degree burns (Figure 19-1) represent some damage to the vascularized dermis. Inflammation of the dermis causes leakage of blood vessels, producing blisters and pain. Controversy remains on the issue of whether to deliberately rupture blisters. These blisters, which may range in size from millimeters to centimeters in diameter, prevent contamination of the dermis below and loss of water vapor from the wound. However, these blisters may rupture spontaneous-

ly and become contaminated under uncontrolled conditions. Chemicals within the blister fluid may also slow healing of the wound. Blisters may be debrided with surrounding necrotic tissue and covered with a broad spectrum antibiotic such as silver sulfadiazine or polymixin and bacitracin, which is often used on the face. As the inflammatory process proceeds, blister formation may increase in the injured area over 3 to 5 days with new blister formation and increasing size of blisters. This depth of burn is typically caused by scalds, brief contact with hot objects, and brief contact with flame. If the blisters rupture, the wound will appear moist and red. Healing occurs spontaneously within 2 weeks without scarring, but some loss of skin pigment may occur.

Deep partial-thickness burns (Figure 19-2) are the most difficult to distinguish, especially early on. They may be a variety of colors, ranging from tan to white and red. Slow capillary refill will be present compared with more superficial injuries. Sensory testing will reveal preservation of pressure sensation to a pin prick but not a normal sharp sensation. Because of the depth of the hair follicle within the skin, hair follicles are still viable in deep partial-thickness injuries. Therefore, one may be able to distinguish deep partial-thickness injuries from full-thickness by

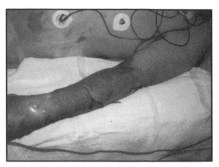

Figure 19-1. Partial-thickness burn caused by flames from an explosion. Courtesy of Arkansas Children's Hospital, Little Rock, Ark. (Also shown in Color Atlas following page 274.)

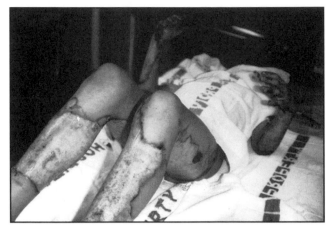

Figure 19-2. Deep partial-thickness burn injury with areas of full-thickness injury. Courtesy of Arkansas Children's Hospital, Little Rock, Ark. (Also shown in Color Atlas following page 274.)

pulling on available hairs. If the injury is caused by flames, however, hairs may not be available for evaluation of the depth. In full-thickness wounds, hairs slide out easily, but resistance to pull occurs with deep partial-thickness wounds. Staging cannot be done accurately for a few days post-burn with this severity of injury. Continued insult, including infection, causes further necrosis of deep dermis, and deep partial-thickness burns may become full-thickness injuries.

In all types of injury, new epithelial cells will be thinly layered and dry and, therefore, easily damaged. Regenerating skin must be protected from mechanical trauma, elevated temperature, and sun exposure. The coagulated tissue may form eschar with tremendous swelling and possible vascular compromise. Therefore, capillary refill of distal tissues must be checked. In the case of circumferential eschar with swelling in deep partial-thickness and full-thickness burns, an incision through eschar to relieve pressure on subcutaneous tissues, called an escharotomy, will need to be performed (Figure 19-3). Depending on the location, an escharotomy may be needed even if the wound is not circumferential if pressure becomes high in a limb compartment. With deep partial-thickness injuries, spontaneous healing by regeneration of epithelial cells from around hair follicles, sweat glands, and edges of the wound is possible; however, scarring is likely to occur. Contraction of the scar may be unacceptable for functional or cosmetic reasons; therefore, this depth of injury may require skin grafting. In deep partial-thickness and full-thickness injuries, moisturizers are needed to prevent excess drying secondary to damage to sebaceous glands.

Full-thickness burn injuries (Figures 19-4a and 19-4b) destroy all epidermis and dermis. No regeneration of epithelial cells can occur except at wound edges. Full-thickness burns may also initially be red, but the blood is merely trapped in the necrotic tissue and the wound will not blanch and refill when a gloved finger pushes on the wound and releases, whereas a deep partial-thickness

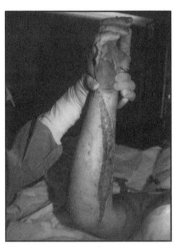

Figure 19-3. Escharotomy to relieve pressure within the forearm and distal arm. Courtesy of Arkansas Children's Hospital, Little Rock, Ark. (Also shown in Color Atlas following page 274.)

wound with remaining blood flow to dermis will have sluggish capillary refill. These wounds are also characterized by tough, dry eschar and may require escharotomy. Full-thickness burns are caused by prolonged contact with hot objects, scalding with very hot liquid, and particularly by ignition of clothing. Although some smaller wounds may close due to granulation tissue and epithelialization from the edges, wound contraction associated with healing by secondary intention of full-thickness wounds more than a few centimeters across is likely to cause functional impairments; therefore, grafting is generally done on all full-thickness burn injuries. Even grafts may contract without appropriate intervention.

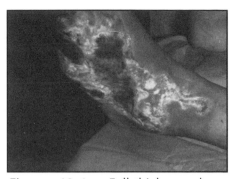

Figure 19-4a. Full-thickness burn caused by a contact burn: before debridement. Courtesy of Arkansas Children's Hospital, Little Rock, Ark. (Also shown in Color Atlas following page 274.)

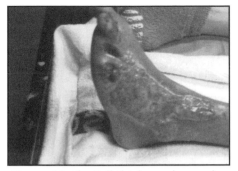

Figure 19-4b. Full-thickness burn after debridement. Note the loss of the fourth and fifth toes to the burn injury. Courtesy of Arkansas Children's Hospital, Little Rock, Ark. (Also shown in Color Atlas following page 274.)

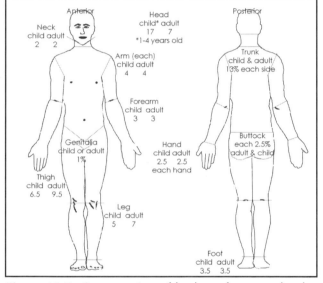

Figure 19-5. Computation of body surface area by the Lund and Browder method.

Subdermal burns are unusual and require tremendous transfer of heat. They may occur when a person is exposed to prolonged heat, such as being trapped in a fire, but most often are caused by electrical injury. These wounds are very extensive and will frequently require more than a simple skin graft, such as a flap containing subcutaneous tissue to cover the defect. These wounds will likely not experience much swelling, but they are associated with a high risk of death from cardiac and respiratory arrest. Shattering of bone and coagulation of large blood vessels may also cause amputation of a limb either during the injury or later by a surgeon. These injuries produce both entry and exit wounds with damage in between. Damage occurs where resistance is greatest along the path. Current travels easily through blood vessels but may produce coagulation, thereby destroying the circulation to a limb. Bones are severely damaged due to their greater resistance to cur-

rent than other tissues. The heat produced by a current equals I^2R (current squared times resistance). Particularly severe exit wounds may occur in individuals touching high-voltage power lines while standing on a metal ladder.

Most burn injuries will be combinations of depths, except for superficial thickness. Progressing away from the area exposed to the greatest amount of heat, a less severe depth of injury is observed from the site of injury. Definite determination of the stage of injury may require 3 to 4 days due to evolution of the wound and presence of eschar. A concept frequently used to explain this phenomenon is to classify areas of the injury into three zones: the zone of coagulation, the zone of stasis, and the zone of hyperemia. The zone of coagulation represents the area that received the most severe injury and irreversible cell injury. The zone of stasis represents an area of less severe insult with reversible cell injury characterized by sluggish blood flow. This region surrounds the zone of coagulation, and cell death may occur in this zone in the presence of further insult. Surrounding the zone of stasis is the zone of hyperemia. This area is inflamed but is expected to recover completely, even without further care. A deep partial-thickness wound is an example of a zone of coagulation that extends to the reticular dermis. The remainder of the reticular dermis would likely be in the zone of stasis. Further injury to the reticular dermis would convert the deep partial-thickness injury into a full-thickness injury.

Body Surface Area

Two methods of computing extent of burned body surface are in common use. Both are used to quantify extent in terms of percentage of body surface area. The Lund and Browder method uses charts with percentages of body surface area assigned to certain body parts based on careful research of typical body proportions. Diagrams for adults and children are shown in Figure 19-5. The adult chart may be used for children 7 years of age to adult. The child's version is used for newborns up to the age of 7. Certain body parts are not assigned a number directly, but a letter. A legend below the chart corresponding to the letters assigns values for the head and lower extremities on both the adult and child versions. Although this method is fairly accurate and takes into account changes in body proportions with age, the Lund and Browder method takes some time to compute.

The rule of nines (Figure 19-6) was developed to rapidly estimate percentage of involved body surface area for triage purposes. Areas of the body are divided into segments with 9% of body surface area, except for the trunk (18% for the front and 18% for the back), and the perineum is assigned 1% to total 100%. Each upper extremity is given 9% (4.5% for the anterior and posterior surfaces). The anterior surface of each lower extremity is given 9%, as is the posterior surface; the front of the head and back of the head are each given 4.5% for a total of 9%. The head is 9%, each upper extremity is 9%, each lower extremity is 18%, the trunk is 36%, and adding 1% for the perineum yields 100%. This system is not as accurate as the Lund and Browder method but is rapidly computable. Moreover, this system does not account for changing body proportions with age as well as the Lund and Browder system. Only a child's and an adult's rule of nines chart is available, and the simplicity of adding nines is also lost for the child. The need for this system is not as important as it once was due to decreasing mortality with improved treatment of burn injury.

Because the percentage of burned surface area alone is not a sufficient predictor of need for medical attention, the burn index was developed. The burn index takes into account both body surface area involved and severity of burns. Burn index is computed as: BI = (% BSA with partial-thickness burn x 0.5 point) + (% BSA with full-thickness x 1 point), where BSA stands for body surface area. For example, if 30% of the BSA has superficial or deep partial-thickness burns and 10% has full-thickness: BI = 30 x 0.5 + 10 = 25. A second example is a situation in which 10% has partial thickness and 15% has full thickness. Burn index in this case is: BI = 10 x 0.5 + 15 = 20. Burn index is used to compute risk of mortality but does not take into account the person's pre-existing medical condition. Prognosis must also take the patient's age and general state of health into account. A frequently used rule of thumb is to subtract the patient's age and the percentage of body surface area burned from 100 to determine the probability of survival.

FIRST AID FOR BURNS

First aid for burns should be taught at an early age to everyone. The first thing that should be done is to stop the burning process as quickly as possible to minimize burn injury and to remove the person from the source of heat. Should clothing become ignited, the person must follow

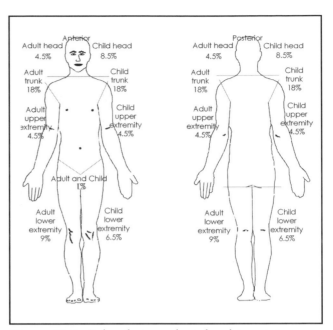

Figure 19-6. Rule of nines chart for determining percentage of body surface area: adult and child.

the basic rules of "stop, drop, and roll" to extinguish any flames. Other than high-voltage electric shock, ignition of clothing produces the most severe burn injuries. After any flames are extinguished, all burned clothing must be removed. Smoldering clothing continues to transfer heat to the body. In some cases, clothing may adhere to the skin. If so, what is not adherent should be cut, if possible. Cool water, not cold water or ice, should be poured over the burned area for 3 to 5 minutes. Cold water is also capable of increasing the injury produced by heat. In the case of a chemical injury, the area should be flushed continuously with cool water for 30 to 40 minutes. However, one must be careful not to flush chemicals onto uncontaminated parts of the body. If the person is wearing contact lenses, they should be removed before flushing. In the case of chemical injury, the label, if available, should be read and instructions should be followed. Otherwise, a poison control center must be contacted and instructions followed if the substance can be described.

Jewelry, belts, or other constricting garments should be removed as soon as possible; swelling occurs rapidly and can be severe. Ointments, butter, or anything that is not sterile should not be applied to the burn to prevent infection of the damaged tissue. Burns should then be covered with a soft, clean, dry dressing, bandage, or sheet, and the person should be kept warm while emergency personnel are en route. Medical attention should be summoned as soon as possible.

For minor burns, an antiseptic spray or cream with local anesthetic may be applied to the wound along with a sterile dressing to protect the wound. If the wound does not appear to heal, or if it appears to weep or have a foul odor, the injured individual should seek medical attention.

In the case of an electrical injury, the person in contact with electricity should not be touched until the source of current is disconnected. At that time, the primary concern is circulation and breathing. With high-voltage injuries, cardiopulmonary resuscitation may be required. Other life-threatening complications that may occur with any type of wound include hypovolemic shock due to fluid loss through wounds, osmotic effect of dead tissue, and loss of plasma proteins from damaged blood vessels. Injury to the airways and lungs due to heat and inhaled toxins is immediately life-threatening and may cause death prior to intervention. Even with immediate survival, airway injury may cause death days later due to development of ARDS (acute respiratory distress syndrome). Other delayed causes of mortality include burn infection, renal failure secondary to hypovolemic shock, and immune suppression. Burn infections are likely due to the presence of necrotic tissue and the lack of circulation to mount an immune response. Bacteremia, especially with gram-negative species, may produce septic shock.

BURN INTERVENTIONS

Treatment of the burned person may include some or all of the following depending on the extent and severity of burns. Medical management includes emergency care, pain management, surgical debridement, and grafting. Physical therapists and other health care providers may be involved in further debridement, dressing changes, exercise, positioning and splinting, and scar management.

Persons with small, partial-thickness wounds may require no emergency medical procedures, only pain medications and either brief inpatient or outpatient care for debridement, dressing changes, exercises, positioning, splinting, and scar management.

Medical Management

Major burns due to a combination of severity or body surface area are life-threatening and may have complications requiring emergency care. Other aspects of medical management include pain management, surgical debridement, and grafting. Life-threatening complications of burn injuries include hypovolemic shock due to fluid loss through wounds, osmotic effect of dead tissue, loss of plasma proteins from damaged blood vessels, injury to airways and lungs due to heat and inhaled toxins that may lead to the development of ARDS, and burn infection. Burn infection may be caused by loss of the first barrier to infection, the presence of necrotic tissue, decreased blood flow to the burned area, and immune suppression. Following burn infection, bacteremia, especially if gram-negative organisms are involved, may produce septic shock and death. In particular, fungal infections are problematic.

Those with large, full-thickness wounds will receive emergency care, including an intravenous line, copious quantities of intravenous fluid, immediate cleaning, weighing and debridement as tolerated, with surgical debridement as soon as the patient is medically stable. These patients will also receive nutritional support and will have an elevated room temperature to compensate for his or her hypermetabolic state. These patients are hospitalized approximately 1 day for each percent of body surface area burned plus 5 days for each grafting procedure, barring serious complications. Many individuals are hospitalized for months and may be intubated several times during the course of hospitalization. Wound infections will also add to the length of stay.[1]

Grafting

Large full-thickness burns can only regenerate from the edges; therefore, reepithelialization is too slow to be feasible. Moreover, repair by secondary intention is more likely to lead to unacceptable wound contraction and loss of function. Persons with large full-thickness burns will need skin grafts to cover their wounds. The types of grafts available include an autograft taken from unburned areas of the patient's own skin (donor site). The thighs, buttocks, and trunk are the most common, but the site depends on the size of the wound and what areas are not burned. An allograft is skin derived from another person, usually a cadaver. A patient receiving such a graft may need immunosuppressive drugs to prevent rejection. A xenograft is taken from another species, usually a pig. Artificial skin and cultured skin may be used when not enough viable skin is available for grafting. Over several weeks, a small area of skin can be grown into a large sheet under culture conditions. Artificial skin with both epidermal and dermal components has recently been approved by the FDA.

Removal of skin is done under anesthesia with a device called a *dermatome*. Either a full-thickness or split-thickness may be cut. A full-thickness graft removes the entire thickness of the reticular dermis and is required for areas such as the face, neck, and flexor surfaces (eg, the elbow and axilla). Split-thickness grafts are cut approximately 0.017 inches in thickness and may be either placed as a sheet or meshed before attaching them. One or more partial-thickness sheets are taped or stapled to the recipient site. The recipient site must be clear of necrotic tissue and care taken to avoid accumulation of blood or serum under the graft. A sheet graft initially adheres to a site by a fibrin clot. Later, blood vessels invade the sheet and either anastomose with existing vessels in the sheet or form new vessels in the sheet. The advantage of a sheet is a cosmetically better result, but accumulation of fluid under the graft or infection will cause failure of the graft to take. A meshed split-thickness graft can be stretched to cover as much as three times the size of the donor site, which increases the efficiency of wound coverage. Applying a split-thickness, meshed graft converts a single large wound into multiple small wounds with a short distance for cells to migrate to

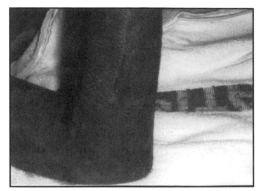

Figure 19-7. Healed split-thickness graft of the forearm and distal arm. Courtesy of Arkansas Children's Hospital, Little Rock, Ark. (Also shown in Color Atlas following page 274.)

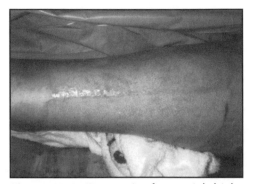

Figure 19-8. Donor site for partial-thickness grafting. Note healing, which will allow this area to be repeatedly harvested for partial-thickness grafting. Courtesy of Arkansas Children's Hospital, Little Rock, Ark. (Also shown in Color Atlas following page 274.)

fill the wound. In addition to the greater coverage of a meshed graft, fluid will not accumulate beneath and cause graft failure. Unfortunately, the cosmetic appearance of a healed split-thickness graft is usually undesirable, leaving a characteristic diamond pattern on the healed skin (Figure 19-7).

Full-thickness donor sites can then be covered with a split-thickness graft to heal the donor site. Split-thickness grafts can be harvested repeatedly after 10 to 14 days to cover more areas (Figure 19-8). This process allows autografting to cover large areas. Several reasons exist for failure of skin grafts to take. As discussed, grafts first adhere to the recipient site by fibrin clot, and within several days blood vessels invade the graft and collagen fibers form between the graft and underlying tissue. Inadequate excision or debridement of necrotic tissue from the underlying tissue, inadequate contact of the graft due to accumulation of blood or serum, infection or excessive mobility of the graft on the site are the primary reasons for grafts to fail. In many facilities, stretching and active exercise of the grafted areas are discontinued for 3 to 5 days for upper extremity and trunk grafts, and 7 to 10 days for lower extremity grafts. Other facilities allow active movement within the range of motion within the limit of staple pain on the day following grafting.

Debridement and Cleansing

Debridement and cleansing may be the responsibility of physical therapy, occupational therapy, or burn technicians, and may involve whirlpool therapy. The type and extent of debridement or cleansing depend on the severity of the wound in terms of the depth of injury and the percentage of body surface area burned. Small, partial-thickness wounds may be cleaned and debrided on a daily or twice per day (BID) basis. Large full-thickness wounds may be surgically debrided to the extent possible immediately upon arrival in a burn center. During hydrotherapy or other cleansing, water temperature should not exceed

body temperature; excess heat can exacerbate damage to reversibly damaged cells. Breaking of blisters of superficial partial-thickness wounds continues to be controversial. The fluid in these blisters is considered sterile, so rupturing the blisters exposes necrotic tissue to environmental flora and increase of risk of infection. On the other hand, rupturing blisters and removing necrotic tissue decreases risk of infection; moreover, certain mediators of inflammation within the blister fluid have been proposed to slow wound healing. Eventually, with debridement, all blisters will rupture as surrounding skin peels off into the blister.

Dressing changes can follow the use of a whirlpool or basin, and sterile saline to continue debridement and remove topical medications and remaining contaminants. Silver sulfadiazine may be covered with a dressing or left uncovered. A simple bandage roll may suffice to protect the silver sulfadiazine from being removed by normal contact of the extremity during activity. In the case of superficial partial-thickness burns with blisters, fanfolding the bandage roll or placing multiple gauze sponges over the blisters may be necessary to absorb drainage should the blisters rupture. Once necrotic tissue is debrided, the risk of infection is substantially decreased, as is the need for silver sulfadiazine. Wounds should be at least briefly evaluated every time dressing is changed, as wounds may evolve over a period of 3 to 4 days after the injury.

Range of Motion, Positioning, and Splinting

Exercise, positioning, and splinting are performed to avoid contractures and edema.[2] It is generally held that the position of comfort is the position of contracture; therefore, when only one side of a limb is burned, the simple solution is to splint or position it so that the burned surface is put on a stretch. The second consideration is the propensity of given body segments to develop contractures. The most likely areas are the hand, axilla, neck, elbow, and foot. Contractures on the face may occur at the

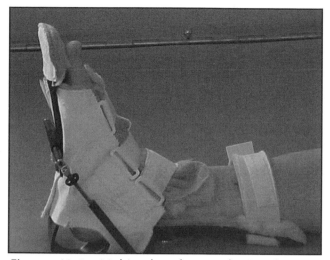

Figure 19-9. Multipodus foot orthosis phase II (Restorative Care of America, St. Petersburg, Fla) for preventing contracture of the ankle.

epicanthus, the commissures of the mouth, and the lower lip. Burns to the anterior or lateral neck will cause flexion or lateral deviations of the head. Patients need to be positioned with the neck extended and rotated to the opposite side of any scar formation. This position may be accomplished by the use of two mattresses on the bed with the body supported by the upper mattress and the head by the lower. Contracture of the anterior axillary fold will primarily limit shoulder abduction, whereas scarring of the posterior axillary fold will limit shoulder flexion. Patients will need to have the shoulders placed in abduction and/or flexion with burns to these areas to reduce the risk of contractures. The affected upper extremities may be placed in a tubular stocking and suspended from the overhead frame or IV poles to achieve the desired position. Burns involving both the neck and axilla on the same side are particularly troublesome. Stretching the axilla places the skin of the neck on slack, and stretching the neck requires the axilla to be placed on slack. Obviously, the patient should not be placed permanently in either position. A schedule should be developed to accommodate the positioning needs for both body segments.

The hand is at risk for a number of deformities. Formerly, the functional position of the hand was promoted for cases in which it was determined that the hand would become contracted. This position is considered to be thumb opposition, slight wrist extension, and slight finger flexion to promote grasp and allow the patient to reach the mouth for feeding and grooming. The palm is very adherent and taut. Left untreated, burn injury can produce finger flexion and opposition contractures. A burn of the palm will require a full-thickness graft to decrease the risk of contracture. The skin of the dorsum of the hand can accommodate substantial swelling, which in turn can pro-

duce a variety of deformities of the fingers. Untreated swelling of the dorsum of the hand produces a claw hand deformity with metacarpal-phalangeal extension and proximal and distal intraphalangeal joint flexion. Injury to the relatively superficial extensor tendons of the hand can also produce boutonnière, swan neck, or mallet finger deformities.

Burns of the lower extremities may produce contractures into hip abduction and flexion and knee flexion, but the foot is at greatest risk of loss of function. The foot can develop either a contracture into dorsiflexion or plantar flexion, depending on the surface injured. Plantar flexion contractures are common problems when both sides are involved and the patient is bed-bound. The weight of the foot compounded by sheets and blankets over the feet place the foot in a plantar flexed position. Simple low temperature thermoplastic splints placed on the foot are generally inadequate to overcome the forces of plantar flexion, and more sophisticated and expensive devices are needed to prevent loss of dorsiflexion (Figure 19-9).

As a general rule, if a patient is burned on both a flexor and extensor surface, one may choose to splint or position the joint in extension because of the greater ease of stretching tissue back into flexion than stretching back into extension. Frequent range of motion into both directions becomes even more imperative in this situation to minimize shortening in either direction. If possible, one should position the patient's body segments to avoid dependence of the burned area and promotion of edema. In addition, skin creases above and below the burned area should be evaluated. As scarring and wound contraction proceed, the reservoir of skin elasticity is taken up in all directions from the site of injury. However, skin elasticity is not equal in all directions of the body. Langer's lines are a graphical means of discussing this phenomenon. Along the extremities, the skin is more extensible in a proximal-distal direction than in a medial-lateral direction. On the trunk, head, and neck, the skin is more extensible in the cephalic-caudal direction than medially and laterally. Some of these Langer's lines are curved or oblique, especially at the transitions between body segments. Skin is more extensible between adjacent Langer's lines than along them. Because the skin has more tension along these lines than between them, a round wound preferentially contracts perpendicular to these lines, resulting in an oval scar with an appearance of being elongated along a Langer's line instead of a round scar. Another manifestation of this pulling up of the slack in the skin is the loss of extensibility at adjacent skin creases. If a burn occurs over three adjacent skin creases such as the wrist, elbow, and shoulder, the middle joint is most affected by loss of extensibility; and in the case in which two adjacent surfaces are injured, the more proximal joint is more likely to lose extensibility.

Exercise

Although prevention of contracture needs to be the primary goal of therapy, strength and cardiovascular condition need to be maintained as much as possible. For smaller wounds treated in the whirlpool tank for debridement, active range of motion exercises can be done at the same time. Many patients who otherwise could not tolerate active movement of a hand or other body part can do so in the turbulent water. The patient needs to start moving the affected segment early. As the wound evolves and nerves regenerate, the patient may become increasingly unwilling to move affected parts of the body. Because of the potential for loss of extensibility throughout a limb due to scarring, active range of motion of other joints in the same extremity must also be encouraged, in spite of pain.

The type of exercise used to promote range of motion may range from passive range of motion in which the movement is performed without any assistance of the patient to active-assisted range of motion in which the patient assists with movement guided by another person. If the clinician is familiar with them, PNF (proprioceptive neuromuscular facilitation) patterns can be used to more efficiently stretch several joints at once with movement in three planes simultaneously. Active range of motion is performed by the patient, but the patient may receive verbal or tactile cues to guide the motion. A person who is unresponsive can only receive passive range of motion. However, the force placed on the healing skin cannot be gauged well by the person performing the movement, and the movement can be excessive.

During range of motion exercise, the clinician needs to monitor for skin blanching, complaints of pain, excessive force needed to move a body segment, and signs of apprehension from the patient. Generally, these signs will occur at the same point in the stress-strain relationship of the skin when the burned skin is stretched into the linear portion of the stress-strain relationship and slack has been taken out of the skin. The type and location of the pain reported by the patient also guides the force applied. Pain in the area of limited skin movement accompanied by tightness and blanching indicates the need to reduce force. A pain caused by movement, especially compression of the tender skin overlying a moving body segment, is not an indication to stop exercise. Finally, if a patient demonstrates optimally expected range of motion but the skin over the area blanches, the patient will continue to need therapy until the body segment can be moved independently through the range of motion without blanching.[3] Moreover, the patient receives little benefit to neuromusculoskeletal function by allowing another person to move the patient's limbs and trunk.

Active range of motion exercises are least likely to harm healing tissue and grafts but may be too difficult for a given individual to accomplish, especially one with an altered nutritional status, diminished strength, severe pain, and already limited range of motion. Active-assisted range of motion is often an intermediate step in the progression to active range of motion exercises. When the patient is near the end of safe range of motion, the patient will decrease the assistance in moving the limb, letting the clinician or caregiver know that appropriate range of motion has been achieved.

Active range of motion exercises are generally indicated if edema needs to be reduced in a particular body segment, if tendons are exposed, and during the first week after a skin graft. The muscle pumping effect assists in the removal of excessive fluid from the body part, and a conscious, alert patient is less likely to exceed a safe range of motion for a given body segment than a clinician might. Active-assisted range of motion exercise is typically indicated for a person with sufficient strength and coordination to follow verbal and tactile cues but already has elevated metabolic demands such that active exercise may increase cardiovascular demands excessively. If existing scar tissue needs to be stretched or if stretching of an area of an escharotomy or skin graft adherence is needed, the type of motion may need to be increased to active-assisted range of motion. Passive range of motion becomes necessary in certain cases that are rather obvious, such as peripheral nerve injury or other loss of motor input to the limb, including the use of general anesthesia. Passive range of motion may also be indicated for areas that need more extensive tissue elongation or an area of escharotomy. In addition, if the patient cannot tolerate active-assisted range of motion due to excess metabolic demands, passive range of motion may be necessary for a number of days. Passive range of motion exercises should not be performed in the cases of finger burns with an indeterminate depth due to risk of tendon injury, in areas of heterotopic ossification, exposed tendons, or in extremely resistive or combative patients.

Range of motion exercises may be done while the patient is in full dressings, during dressing changes so the clinician can see the skin's response to the motion, or during anesthesia. If the burn wounds are covered, active range of motion exercises are preferred to avoid excessive force that cannot be adequately monitored. More forceful, passive range of motion can be performed more readily while the patient is under anesthesia. Advantages include the ability to more accurately determine the available range of motion and identify soft tissue restrictions, rather than limitations due to weakness or pain during active motion. Moreover, because the patient cannot feel the tissue mobilization, more thorough stretching can be performed. Disadvantages of performing passive range of motion during anesthesia include the potential for excessive movement that may result in joint dislocation, fractures, tearing of compromised ligaments and tendons, and tissue separation.

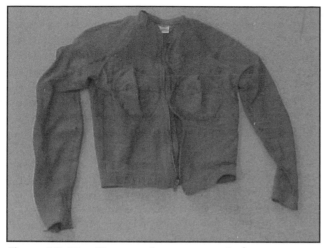

Figure 19-10a. Compression garment: jacket.

To recover lost range of motion, prolonged low-load stretch is preferred. This can be accomplished with the use of a dynamic splint, which uses springs or similar devices to move an extremity toward the desired position, or a CPM (continuous passive movement) machine. A CPM moves the affected extremity through a range of motion that can be specified in terms of its starting and stopping angle and the speed through which the extremity is moved. Gravity-assisted range of motion can be accomplished by positioning a patient such that gravity pulls the desired body segment in the desired direction. For example, a person with decreased knee extension may lie in prone with a weight attached to the foot. In this type of therapy, the clinician needs to monitor for blanching and skin dryness to prevent cracking of the relatively weak and brittle scar tissue of a healed burn injury.

Strength training is needed to avoid loss of lean body mass due to negative nitrogen balance. With increased demands for protein and calories to repair a wound, the resultant hypermetabolic state can lead to wasting of muscles. The patient can be instructed in simple exercises that combine range of motion and strength. Avoid exercises that place frictional or shearing forces on grafted skin and donor sites.

Cardiovascular exercise is needed to maintain or improve cardiopulmonary function. Upright positioning progressing to ambulation and other cardiopulmonary training is needed to improve hematocrit and plasma volume. While working to achieve improved orthostatic tolerance, the clinician should monitor vital signs, especially if the patient experienced extensive burns or has been medically unstable. The patient may not initially be able to tolerate an upright position for ambulation. The clinician may need to wrap the lower extremities in elasticized bandages to maintain central venous pressure in upright position secondary to fluid loss. The patient may need to start with sitting up, dangling legs, or a tilt table protocol to develop sufficient orthostatic tolerance for cardiopul-

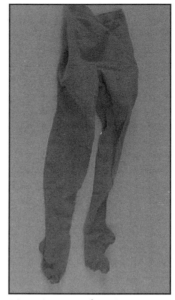

Figure 19-10b. Compression garment: leggings.

monary training. If the patient lacks the mobility to reposition, a tilt table may be necessary to provide upright positioning.

Burns may have destroyed large numbers of sweat glands, diminishing a patient's ability to dissipate heat. During exercise, avoid overheating the patient. Have a fan available and provide rest and water breaks during the activity. Upper extremity ergometry is particularly useful for burn rehabilitation for several reasons: movement of the upper extremity ergometer encourages upper extremity range of motion; because the patient is in a seated position, he or she can take frequent rest breaks as needed; and with the lower extremities wrapped, the patient is better able to tolerate upright positioning in addition to the cardiovascular training that can be provided.

Scar Management

Burn wounds, more so than other types, are likely to result in proliferative scarring. Pressure garments are typically used to minimize overrepair. Examples of pressure garments are shown in Figures 19-10a through 19-10c. Garments are specially measured and custom-made to exert equal 35 mmHg pressure on recovering skin. Rather than elasticized garments, clear acrylic masks are used to exert pressure on the face to minimize scarring. Early use (within 6 months of injury) will give better results. These pressure garments have been useful up to 2 years if the scar is still actively in the remodeling stage and highly vascularized. Pressure garments must be worn 23 hours per day and only taken off for bathing. Garments are available for any body part with delivery of a custom garment in 24 to 48 hours. At the time of this writing, the mechanism by which pressure affects scar formation is not fully under-

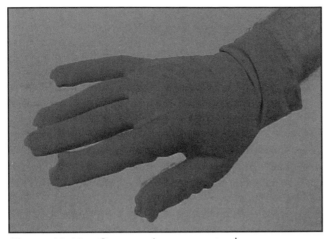

Figure 19-10c. Compression garment: glove.

stood. Some literature is suggestive of a hypoxic effect on fibroblasts, diminishing collagen formation. Another theory suggests a mechanical effect that prevents the formation of whorls of collagen and promotion of flatter ribbons of collagen fibers. Some recent research reports have questioned whether sustained pressure is actually effective in reducing hypertrophic scarring. Other treatments include friction massage and ultrasound to the scars, neither of which is feasible with large areas of burns. Other options for scar management include the use of either silicone or glycerin sheets. The mechanism by which either type affects scar remodeling is not known but does not appear to be related to the chemical properties of either type of sheet.

Summary

Burns are common injuries, although most are minor and self-treated. Major burns are severe injuries requiring intensive care and rehabilitation. Typical causes of burns for different age groups are described. The depth of injury is expressed by the first-, second-, and third-degree system, but in the medical community the terms superficial, superficial partial thickness, deep partial thickness, and full thickness are preferred. Severe thermal or electrical burn can produce subcutaneous injury. The evaluation of depth of injury is based on knowledge of the properties of different layers of the skin. Reddening, blistering, capillary refill, and sensory evaluation can help determine the depth. Burn injuries may evolve over the course of a few days, making the diagnosis difficult. The extent of surface area burned is performed using either the Lund and Browder system, or for rapid computation, the rule of nines may be used. Percent body surface area burned is not sufficient; depth of injury, comorbidity, and age must also be taken into account. Therapy includes wound debridement, dressing changes, exercise, positioning, and splint-

ing. Debridement and dressing changes for large full-thickness injuries are usually performed by technicians in burn centers, but less severe injuries may be managed in a physical therapy inpatient or outpatient clinic. Grafting, exercise, positioning, and splinting are performed to minimize loss of elasticity of the skin. If possible, the injured area is kept on stretch, but both surfaces may be injured and clinical decisions to minimize loss of function must be made. Critical areas include the neck, axilla, elbow, and foot. The appropriate use of active, active-assisted, and passive range of motion are described. In addition, exercises must be directed at maintaining muscle mass and cardiovascular function.

Study Questions

1. Where do most burn injuries occur? What age group is most susceptible? What type of injury typically occurs in this age group?

2. Contrast the Lund and Browder and rule of nines methods.

3. Why are both of these methods inadequate to describe the severity of a burn injury?

4. List complications of burn injuries that frequently cause mortality.

5. How can one distinguish between deep partial-thickness and full-thickness burn injuries?

6. What is the expected outcome of superficial partial-thickness wounds?

7. Under what circumstances are full-thickness grafts required?

8. Why do full-thickness wounds need to be grafted?

9. Why must patients not be allowed to stay in their preferred position following burn injuries?

10. How can patients with burns be mobilized if their blood pressure falls with standing?

11. What option is available for providing gravitational stress to an immobile patient with burns?

12. What concerns exist about thermoregulation after a burn injury? What can be done?

References

1. Committee on Trauma. *American College of Surgeons: Guidelines for Operation of Burn Units.* Chicago, Ill: American College of Surgeons; 1999.

2. Richard RL, Staley MJ. *Burn Care and Rehabilitation: Principles and Practice.* Philadelphia, Pa: FA Davis; 1994.

3. Staley MJ, Richard R. Burns. In: O' Sullivan SB, Schmitz TJ, eds. *Physical Rehabilitation. Assessment and Treatment.* 4th ed. Philadelphia, Pa: FA Davis; 2001.

20 Plan of Care

OBJECTIVES

- Discuss the relationship between physical impairments and plan of care.
- Discuss the relationships among impairments, functional limitations, and plan of care.
- Modify a plan of care based on impairments, functional limitations, disability for prevention, and healing of wounds.
- Set goals and determine appropriate outcomes for patients with various sets of abilities and disabilities, lifestyles, and resources.
- Discuss modifications of interventions necessary for the elderly patient.
- Describe prevention of skin injury in elderly persons.
- Discuss means of optimizing wound management in children.
- Determine when referral to other health care providers is appropriate.
- Determine appropriate topics and means of providing patient education.

TERMINOLOGY OF THE DISABILITY MODEL

In years past, goals were set for a patient based upon remediation of a documented impairment. For example, a deficit in range of motion would be remediated in terms of increased range of motion. Over time, however, the remediation of an impairment for the sake of remediation was questioned. Physical therapists were nudged in the direction of writing functional goals. As an example, shoulder range of motion would be improved to allow the patient to perform a task necessary to the individual's function in home, work, or community, such as dressing, operating machinery, or caring for children. Plans of care became a hodge-podge of impairment and function-driven goals to be attained. Many clinicians either consciously or unconsciously began to incorporate the model of disablement into developing a plan of care. In November of 1997, the American Physical Therapy Association first published the *Guide to Physical Therapist Practice*.[1] A second edition was published in January of 2001.[2] This document is based on the model of disablement and directs the thought process of the clinician through impairment, functional limitation, and disability.[3,4]

A given patient may be seen by a clinician at any one point on the continuum from impairment, functional limitation, or disability. As defined in the guide, *impairment* is a loss or abnormality of physiological, psychological, or anatomical structure or function; *functional limitation* is a restriction of the ability to perform at the level of the whole person, a physical action, activity, or task in an efficient, typically expected, or competent manner; and *disability* is defined as the inability to engage in age-specific, gender-specific, or sex-specific roles in a particular context and physical environment. Placed in the context of the patient-clinician interaction, remediation of an impairment is not based on the impairment itself but to overcome functional limitations and prevent disability. Interaction may also occur to allow the patient to adapt to functional limitations to prevent or minimize disability, or to retrain the patient for new roles following disability.

In terms of wound management, the plan of care should not be focused on the "hole in the patient," but on the "whole of the patient." The outcome of the plan of care is ultimately to prevent or minimize functional limitations and disability secondary to integumentary impairments and to prevent secondary impairments. Secondary impairments result either directly or indirectly from another impairment. For example, the person placed on bed rest because of a neuropathic ulcer may develop cardiopulmonary complications due to bed rest. Diminished cardiopulmonary function or cardiopulmonary disease would be a secondary impairment. Use of total contact casting or other means of keeping the patient ambulatory is an example of preventing secondary impairments. This is an excellent example of how two interventions—bed rest and total contact casting—may address the same impairment, but one intervention is superior due to the prevention of a secondary impairment.

Commonly, wounds represent secondary impairments. Cardiopulmonary, musculoskeletal, or neuromuscular impairments resulting in immobility may cause integumentary impairments (wounds). For example, an individual with a spinal cord injury is at high risk for development of pressure ulcers. An important role of the clinician is to prevent these secondary integumentary impairments by identifying how the skin is placed at risk due to cardiopulmonary, musculoskeletal, or neuromuscular impairments. The clinician then devises a plan of care to remediate the impairments that create the risk to the skin and prevent the secondary impairment manifesting itself as a wound.

COMPONENTS OF THE PLAN OF CARE

The plan of care is developed through the systematic process of examination, evaluation, diagnosis, and prognosis. Specific impairments are identified based on physical examination, risks of functional limitations, and disability by evaluating the impact of the impairments on the patient's roles, lifestyle, home, resources, and available assistance. The clinician is responsible for taking a thorough history that may include general demographic information, social history, occupation/employment, growth and development, and living environment. In addition, the history of the current condition, current and prior functional status and activity level, current medications, past history of the current condition, past medical and surgical history, family history, health status, and social habits are considered in determining a diagnosis, which is defined in the guide as a cluster of signs and symptoms, syndromes, or categories.

In contrast to the pathology-driven diagnostic categories used by physicians, the diagnoses described in the guide are impairment-driven. Based on the history and diagnosis, a prognosis is developed. Prognosis as defined in the guide includes the predicted optimal level of improvement in function and amount of time needed to reach that level. Prognosis may also include a prediction of levels of improvement that may be reached at various intervals during the course of therapy.

The plan of care describes the interventions to be used, as well as the goals and outcomes of the interventions. In this model, goals refer specifically to remediation of impairments and outcomes related to minimizing functional limitations, optimizing health status, and preventing disability. The hope of clinicians is to prevent disability. Although not addressed specifically in the guide, outcomes may be limited to minimizing disability, rather than preventing it. The plan of care may also include development of a maintenance program, education, and periodic reassessment of the maintenance program.

PROCEDURAL INTERVENTIONS

Actions required of the clinician include identifying the cause of wounds and how to prevent recurrence, identifying factors that interfere with healing, appropriately selecting and applying wound care products, appropriate debridement (if required), and selection of adjunctive therapies as indicated.

Healing is most effective if the wound microenvironment is optimized. This optimization includes maintaining an appropriate moisture level. A dry wound must be moistened, and a heavily draining wound needs to be managed to either absorb excessive moisture or to decrease the cause of the copious drainage. Macromolecules produced in the wound, including glycosaminoglycans, fibronectin, collagen, and growth factors need to be retained in the wound while acceptable levels of nonpathogenic organisms and protection from pathogens in the environment are achieved. An appropriate microenvironment is usually accomplished through the use of occlusive dressings that retain fluid in the wound while either absorbing or allowing evaporation of excessive moisture. Maintaining wound temperature near core body temperature (98.6°F, 38°C) produces optimal fibroblast replication.

Wound moisture is particularly critical to allow the migration of epithelial cells, movement of enzymes, growth factors, and structural molecules through the wound. However, excessive moisture can cause damage to the intact surrounding skin, causing maceration and damaging the source of epithelial cells needed to resurface the wound. Incontinence creates an even greater problem because of the acidity of urine and feces. Allowing the wound to dry out was once encouraged as a means of preventing infection. However, it became clear that dry wound beds impede wound healing. Desiccated fibrin and blood act as a dressing to retain moisture below and keep out pathogens. Unfortunately, scab formation slows epithelial cell migration as epithelial cells are forced to migrate deeply and through a dry environment. Scab formation is mainly an issue for wounds greater than a few millimeters in diameter. For narrow, especially linear, wounds requiring minimal epithelial cell migration, scab formation is a minor issue.

For superficial wounds, reepithelialization can occur from appendages and wound edges, but for deep wounds involving the full thickness of dermis, epithelialization proceeds from the edges only, and full-thickness wounds greater than a few centimeter in diameter may require operative repair. Full-thickness or deeper wounds fill with granulation tissue before reepithelialization. A moist wound bed assists in migration and proliferation of fibroblasts as well as epithelialization.

A second consideration is the issue of bacterial balance. Bacterial balance requires an understanding of infection, contamination, and colonization. All chronic open wounds are colonized by microbes, but wounds do not necessarily need to be handled with strict sterile techniques. However, this does not mean that the clinician may be careless in maintaining cleanliness of the wound. Further contamination of a wound increases the risk of infection. *Contamination* refers to the introduction of new microbes into the wound. Although the immune system and the balance of microbes keep pathogens from running wild in the wound, introduction of new bacteria or changes in the environment of the wound may allow one type of bacterium to multiply rapidly and injure cells in the wound. Certain microbes may begin to digest the interstitial space and spread subcutaneously, forming tunnels, sinus tracts, and abscesses as well as infecting and spreading through the interstitial space, producing cellulitis. Microbes may also gain access to the circulation or lymphatic system, causing sepsis, osteomyelitis, endocarditis, meningitis, and septic arthritis.

Infection occurs when tissue is invaded by bacteria rather than simple colonization of the wound surface. Infection is operationally defined as 100,000 organisms per gram of tissue; a more practical definition involves the necrosis of tissue surrounding the wound, often manifested as brownish or dusky discoloration or spots in the tissue bed. Although occlusion promotes growth of cells needed for healing a wound, occlusion will also promote the growth of certain types of bacteria in the wound and, therefore, infected wounds should not be occluded. Grossly contaminated wounds and wounds suspected to be infected should be allowed, at least initially, to heal by secondary intent until the wound is clean and stable. Any cavity in the tissue provides an environment conducive to bacterial overgrowth and prevents observation of the wound. Exposure to air and agitation with whirlpool or other types of hydrotherapy decrease bacterial count, but allowing the wound to dry out slows healing. Therefore, the clinician must be ready and willing to drastically alter the treatment plan depending on whether the goal is prevention/treatment of infection or promotion of granulation and epithelialization. Occlusive dressings are indicated when healing is to be promoted and the wound is not infected. Nonocclusive dressings such as gauze are indicated in wounds that are infected or are at high risk for infection such as grossly contaminated wounds. Nonocclusive dressings should be used until the bacterial count is low enough to use occlusive dressings.

The third consideration is the management of drainage. One aspect that is often neglected is the drainage caused by rough handling of wounds by the clinician or caregiver. By minimizing wound handling, inflammation is reduced. Inflammation is caused by debridement, excess agitation, and frequent dressing changes, leading to edema and serous drainage. Another means of reducing drainage is to debride necrotic tissue more rapidly. Protracted debridement with daily or even BID rough handling of the wound and the persistence of necrotic tissue promote inflammation and lead to drainage. Debridement is discussed more thoroughly in Chapters 12 and 13. A number of dressings are available to absorb a wide range of drainage. Gauze, alginate, foam dressings, and hydrocolloid fillers can absorb moderate to maximum drainage over a range of time spans, ranging from a few hours to a few days. Hydrocolloid sheets and semipermeable films are used to retain moisture within the wound. Hydrocolloid sheets additionally absorb some excess drainage, whereas semipermeable film and foam dressings allow some evaporation of excessive drainage. Purulent drainage, however, is a clear sign to stop occluding the wound. Purulence should be absorbed with either gauze or alginate. Although aggressive sharp debridement is preferred, wounds may be filled with antibiotic-soaked gauze if other factors indicate. Another problem caused by chronic inflammation due to rough handling is the leakage of fibrinogen into the wound bed. Fibrinogen may be converted to fibrin on the wound surface, causing a hard yellow eschar to form on the wound surface. This type of eschar is particularly difficult to debride.

In a dry wound, moisture can be both retained and added by using amorphous hydrogel on the wound bed and an occlusive dressing to retain the moisture. When retaining moisture in a wound, some moisture may run over the surrounding skin causing maceration. A moisture barrier cream or skin sealant can be effective in preventing maceration. Dressings are described more thoroughly in Chapter 15 and moisture barriers and skin sealants are discussed in Chapter 16.

FORMULATING THE PLAN OF CARE

The plan of care needs to flow from the items discussed above. Given two patients with identical characteristics, two different plans of care are likely to be needed. Variances in the plan of care should be viewed as accommodations to the unique combinations of patient characteristics, including physical condition, cultural beliefs and behaviors, resources, and lifestyle. The plan of care needs to represent the optimum combination of appropriate wound care and the reality of how the plan interacts with the patient.

Treatment planning may follow four basic decision points with accommodations for circumstances other than characteristics of the wound. The four basic decision points are:
1. Presence, suspicion, or reasonable assumption of impending infection

2. Type of debridement suited to the patient and the wound
3. Depth of tissue loss
4. Management of drainage and surrounding skin

Presence, Suspicion, or Reasonable Assumption of Impending Infection

In the cases in which infection is known to be present, infection is suspected, or one may reasonably suspect that infection will occur, treatment decisions are directed primarily toward managing infection. Interventions directed toward eliminating infection may, in fact, slow wound healing. However, infection is sufficiently serious to warrant precedence over other aspects of wound management. Other aspects are not ignored; rather, potential conflicts in management of the different aspects of the wound are resolved by allowing certain aspects to take precedence.

Infection can be managed in a number of ways. Critically important to bear in mind is the relationship between the presence of necrotic tissue and infection. Necrotic tissue provides a foothold for pathogenic bacteria that otherwise would remain under control on a relatively clean wound surface. Based on this principal, infection can be managed by sharp debridement or other means of rapid debridement. The National Pressure Ulcer Advisory Panel recommends sharp debridement of pressure ulcers with impending infection. The American Diabetes Association recommends aggressive sharp debridement of neuropathic ulcers. Some wounds may be managed by nonspecific debridement such as wet-to-dry dressings, pulsatile lavage, irrigation, or other forms of hydrotherapy. In particular, acute wounds at risk of infection because of gross contamination, such as gunshot wounds, motor vehicle, agricultural and industrial accidents, may be treated with the application of antibiotics or surface antiseptics for a small number of days. The National Pressure Ulcer Advisory Panel recommends only a brief trial of surface treatment for pressure ulcers that fail to respond to optimal care. The American Diabetes Association, on the other hand, does not recommend surface treatment at all, instead calling for sharp debridement and parenteral antibiotics specifically selected for the identified pathogen. Acute wounds, especially wounds that have not received care for several hours, will need aggressive lavage, debridement, and possibly treatment with antibiotics.

Type of Debridement Needed

The second point is the need for debridement. Several factors come into play. These factors include economics of the health care setting, patient satisfaction, patient/caregiver skill, and clinician skill. Debridement is necessary for any wound with necrotic tissue. The type of debridement, however, needs to be determined based on a number of institutional, personal, and wound characteristics. In the acute care setting in which discharge is dependent upon the wound becoming clean and stable, rapid debridement is necessary. Some clinicians may choose to perform non-specific mechanical types of debridement, often using hydrotherapy. Clinicians with the skill to perform sharp debridement can achieve a clean, stable wound rapidly. In many cases, especially with neuropathic ulcers, sharp debridement can be achieved in a single visit. The wound may need to be monitored and some further minor debridement may be necessary if discharge is pending completion of a round of intravenous antibiotic treatment. In many cases, however, the patient is now discharged to home with home health visits to complete a course of intravenous antibiotics. If clinician skill or patient preference dictates against sharp debridement, pulsatile lavage with concurrent suction may be a reasonable alternative. Whirlpool therapy, however, is generally not a reasonable alternative. Exceptions include wounds with a large surface area requiring low-level agitation and minor burns on extremities that require the cleansing of residues (eg, silver sulfadiazine).

Soaking a wound to loosen necrotic tissue and using serial instrumental debridement once or twice a day to cut loosened necrotic tissue is a common practice but offers no advantage over sharp debridement or pulsatile lavage with concurrent suction. Whirlpool agitation is generally ineffective at debriding areas of subcutaneous involvement with undermining, tunneling, and sinus tracts. Tips for pulsatile lavage devices can readily reach these areas. Venous insufficiency is exacerbated by placing the limb in a dependent position with the thigh compressed against the edge of the tank and warm water increasing blood flow to the affected leg. The elevated temperature of typical whirlpool therapy increases the demand for blood flow without increasing flow in cases of arterial insufficiency and increases the risk of further tissue injury in thermal injuries and skin with diminished sensation. Moreover, fragile skin, especially in the elderly, can be damaged by the agitation and maceration caused by soaking the extremity for 20 minutes.

In settings in which timeframe is not critical or the quality of life is not dependent on rapid debridement of the wound, autolytic and chemical debridement are reasonable. However, the patient or a caregiver must be able to determine if wound infection occurs. Infection demands immediate sharp debridement. In an outpatient or home health situation, a patient may express preference for autolytic or chemical debridement because of pain management or psychosocial factors. In a long-term care setting in which rapid debridement will not impact quality of life, the patient and clinician may agree to a more protracted but less invasive debridement procedure. For exam-

ple, a bedfast individual with an open heel ulcer will not become ambulatory simply because of sharp debridement of the wound. On the other hand, a person who needs to be ambulatory and could be if not for a foot wound may decide on sharp debridement and either total contact casting or alternatives discussed in Chapter 8 to become ambulatory sooner.

Depth of Tissue Loss

The third decision point is the presence of subcutaneous tissue loss, including undermining, tunneling, and sinus tracts. When infection is present or debridement is ongoing, these tissue defects are typically filled with gauze material. Wet-to-wet or wet-to-dry dressings with or without antibiotic solution are typically used to fill these. Packing strips with or without iodine may be used for tunnels and sinus tracts. Packing strips come in various widths and may need to be fan-folded as they are placed in a tunnel or sinus tract. Although the cotton material may cause inflammation of the tissue in the wound, absorption of infectious drainage and preventing occlusion that promotes growth of bacteria takes precedence. Undermined areas and simple areas of subcutaneous loss are likewise filled with either 4 x 4 or 2 x 2 gauze sponges until the risk of infection is minimized. Once the wound is stable, non-irritating filling materials should be substituted. Alginates, hydrofibers, and combinations with collagen are good choices for filling these subcutaneous defects. Alginates and hydrofibers are available in both sheets and ribbons/ropes. These materials maintain their tensile strength while absorbing drainage and can be readily removed from the wound, even tunnels and sinus tracts. Collagen present in the material is absorbed by the wound and may speed healing. A suitable secondary dressing needs to be placed over the wound based on the drainage and desired frequency of dressing change.

Management of Drainage

The fourth decision point is based on drainage and manipulation of the desired frequency of dressing change. With subcutaneous tissue loss, both a primary and secondary dressings are chosen. For a simpler full-thickness or partial-thickness wound, a primary dressing may be sufficient. The type of dressing chosen must be based on multiple factors, again based on the order of precedence: infection, debridement, subcutaneous involvement, and drainage. If a wound is infected and filled with gauze, a nonocclusive secondary dressing needs to be employed. Typical choices include bandage rolls, self-adherent gauze bandages, and abdominal pads attached with tape by window paning. Bandage rolls may be used on any body part and can be fan-folded to increase absorption. Abdominal pads can be gently pulled back and retaped from one cor-

Figure 20-1a. The plan of care begins with data gathering. The examination consists of a history and physical examination with a review of systems and special tests used to rule in or rule out suspected causes of the wound. Following data gathering, the clinician undergoes a mental processing of the data. This process is called the evaluation. Based on the data, the clinician develops the impairment-driven diagnosis according to the processes described in the *Guide to Physical Therapist Practice*. Although not necessary for every patient,

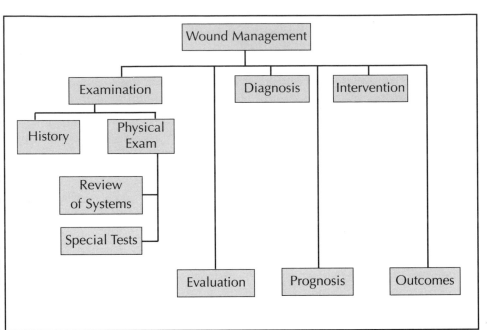

the clinician may also seek to confirm or refute a pathology-driven diagnosis. The prognosis is developed based on the diagnosis and unique combination of circumstances of the patient derived from the history and physical examination. Interventions are devised based on the examination, diagnosis, prognosis, and patient preferences and resources. Appropriate outcomes are derived in consultation with the patient, family, caregivers, and other involved clinicians.

ner (or more if necessary) to inspect a wound. These absorbent materials may on occasion be used over materials such as alginates or hydrofibers to absorb copious drainage for a few days as inflammation resolves. Ideally, an occlusive dressing is used over a nongauze wound filler; however, initially the drainage may overwhelm most occlusive dressings.

When occlusion of the wound is appropriate, the quantity of drainage and characteristics of the patient and dressings must be considered. A desiccated wound can be rehydrated with amorphous hydrogel covered with a simple dressing such as a semipermeable film. A light drainage from a partial-thickness or full-thickness wound without subcutaneous involvement may be covered with a semipermeable film. Hydrocolloids are the most occlusive wound dressing and are ideal for wounds that are clean and stable and, therefore, only need to be protected. Ideally, the hydrocolloid dressing is left in place for 5 days or more. Depending on the drainage and extent of subcutaneous involvement, alginate, hydrofiber, or foam may be needed beneath the hydrocolloid sheet. The hydrocolloid dressing is changed at the desired interval of 5 to 7 days or earlier if the dressing becomes white and swollen. Leaving an overhydrated occlusive dressing in place too long risks maceration of surrounding tissue.

Hydrogel sheets are popular dressings for abrasions, and chemical and radiation burns due to their soothing effect. They can macerate surrounding skin, however, and they can desiccate, allowing the wound bed to desiccate as well if left in place too long.

Foam dressing materials are good choices when a wound is ready for occlusion but drainage is too heavy for hydrocolloid sheets. For a heavily draining wound with subcutaneous involvement, foam sheets can be placed into a wound as a primary dressing with a hydrocolloid secondary dressing. Composite dressings constructed of contact material surrounded with absorbent material and a waterproof exterior can also be used on this type of wound. Composite foam and film dressings may also be useful but may not last as many days as desired by the clinician. The decision points are summarized in Figures 20-1a through 20-1g.

In addition to the characteristics of the dressing materials, the patient characteristics and wound location must be considered. A bulky dressing should not be placed on an area where it will catch onto clothing and shoes or other items in the environment. If the person will be showering, a film, foam, or hydrogel dressing will not stay in place. Hydrocolloid sheets are waterproof on the outside and if kept out of direct spray can last several days even with showering.

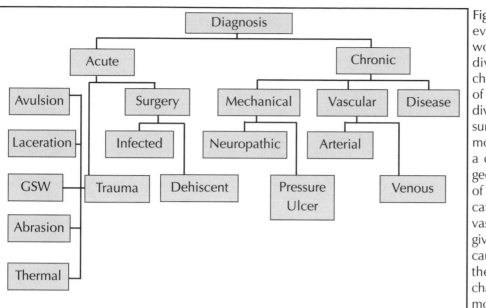

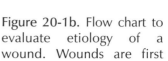

Figure 20-1b. Flow chart to evaluate etiology of a wound. Wounds are first divided into acute and chronic. Within the category of acute wounds, causes are divided into traumatic and surgical wounds of the type most likely to be referred to a clinician other than a surgeon. Within the category of chronic wounds, the subcategories of mechanical, vascular, and disease are given. Although many other causes of wounds exist, for the purpose of this flow chart, only the most common are demonstrated.

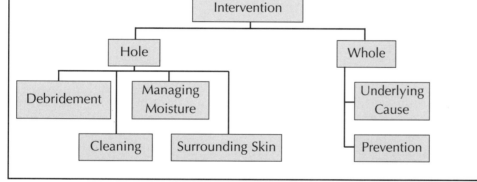

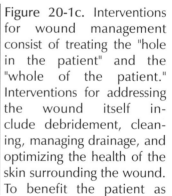

Figure 20-1c. Interventions for wound management consist of treating the "hole in the patient" and the "whole of the patient." Interventions for addressing the wound itself include debridement, cleaning, managing drainage, and optimizing the health of the skin surrounding the wound. To benefit the patient as a whole, the underlying cause of the wound is addressed and preventive measures are taken to prevent either recurrence of the wound or the development of new wounds elsewhere.

MODIFICATIONS FOR THE CARE OF AGING SKIN

Foremost, the choice of wound products to be used on the skin of the elderly must take into account the fragile nature of the skin. Moreover, because of decreased inflammation, and greater risk of malnutrition and dehydration, the clinician must assume a longer period for healing. Therefore, dressings that need to be changed frequently or have strong adhesive need to be used with care or avoided. Tape of any kind must be used judiciously. In particular, silk and plastic tape should not be used. Alternatives such as stretch netting should be considered. When occlusive dressings are chosen, hydrocolloids and semipermeable films should be used only if nonadherent foam or hydrogel sheets are not practical. If films or hydrocolloid sheets are to be used, skin protectant needs to be placed on the surrounding skin. In addition, the absorbency of the dressing needs to be optimized. Although thin hydrocolloid sheets permit better visualization of the wound, thicker hydrocolloid sheets may be necessary to prolong time between changes. Filling the wound with an absorbent material such as alginate or hydrofiber can also prolong wearing time of hydrocolloid and semipermeable film dressings. When these dressings are removed, care must be taken to avoid injury to the skin. The skin should not be pulled with the dressing as it is removed. Gentle peeling of hydrocolloid sheets or stretching of a semipermeable film tangentially to the skin surface as the skin is held in place may reduce the risk of injury.

Cleansing of wounds needs to be done as gently as possible. Pulsatile lavage with suction may be done at a lower impact pressure or replaced by gentle irrigation as necessary. Mechanical damage and maceration can result from vigorous whirlpool therapy for cleansing or nonselective

Figure 20-1d. Flow chart outlining the reasons and methods for debridement by the four basic means: mechanical, autolytic, chemical, and sharp debridement.

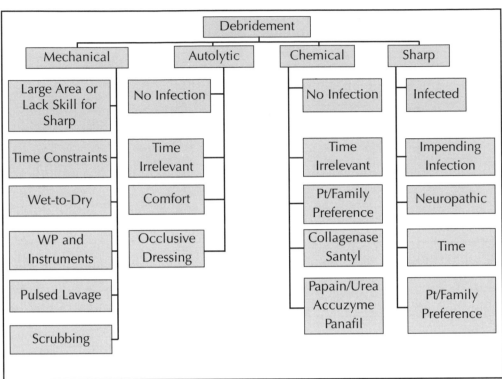

Figure 20-1e. Flow chart for managing drainage. The first division is into clean wounds and infected wounds, with only nonocclusive dressings or alginates as options. Clean wounds are categorized by the quantity of drainage. Selected examples of wounds typically observed to have different levels of drainage and types of primary dressings appropriate for the drainage are listed.

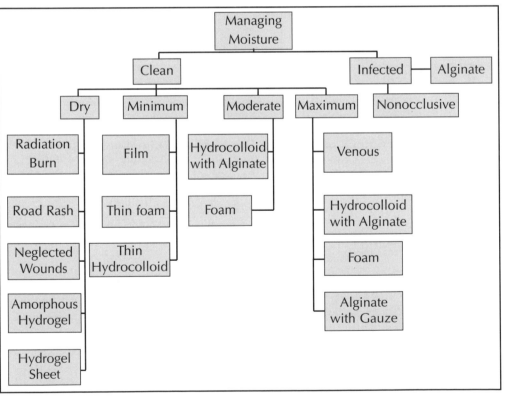

debridement. For many elderly patients, the clinician must consider the risks and benefits of different types of debridement. Frequently, orders are received for whirlpool and wet-to-dry dressings on the wounds of the elderly. Additives to the whirlpools or topical agents placed on the wound may cause severe injury to the wound or surrounding skin.

Frequently, elderly patients with wounds are in the terminal stage of an illness and may not benefit from the full scale of options available from the clinician. The clinician

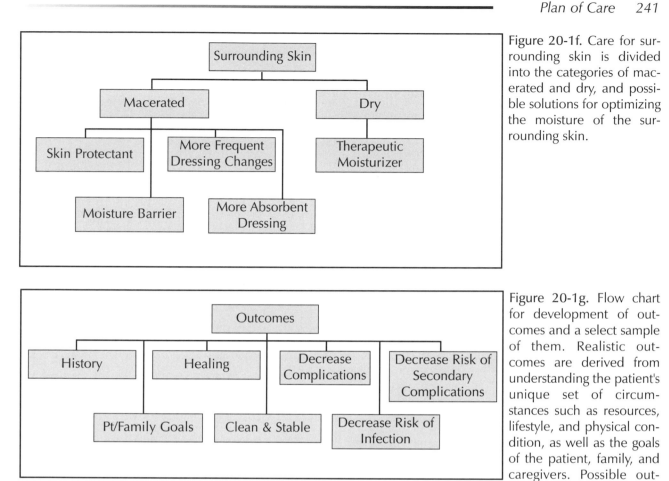

Figure 20-1f. Care for surrounding skin is divided into the categories of macerated and dry, and possible solutions for optimizing the moisture of the surrounding skin.

Figure 20-1g. Flow chart for development of outcomes and a select sample of them. Realistic outcomes are derived from understanding the patient's unique set of circumstances such as resources, lifestyle, and physical condition, as well as the goals of the patient, family, and caregivers. Possible outcomes range from complete healing to reducing the risk of secondary complications that would likely exacerbate the condition of a patient with terminal disease.

must determine what benefits the patient will receive from any given intervention. Often, wound healing is not achievable due to the nutritional or cardiopulmonary status of the patient, and goals are limited to reducing the risk of infection and managing drainage and odor of the wound. In such cases, sharp debridement provides no benefit unless the wound is infected or infection is imminent. In these cases, treatment optimizing autolytic debridement is appropriate.

PREVENTION OF SKIN INJURY IN THE ELDERLY

In addition to selecting wound care products carefully, a number of other forms of skin protection should be considered. The skin of the elderly tends to become dry, brittle, and may fissure and tear with minor trauma. Therapeutic moisturizers may be necessary, especially during the winter or in low-humidity environments. Bed frames and rails should be inspected for sharp edges and padded as needed.

OPTIMIZING WOUND HEALING IN CHILDREN

Compared with adults, children have a better outcome from laceration repair. Lacerations in children are irrigated less frequently than those of adults (53% vs 77%) and more frequently scrubbed (50% vs 45%). However, children are less likely to have wound infections (2.1% vs 4.1%) and have a better cosmetic outcome than adults.[5] Comparing the characteristics of wounds of children and adults, wounds are much more likely to occur on the head (86% vs 38%), to be linear, shorter, less likely to be contaminated, and more commonly caused by blunt trauma compared with adults. The greater prevalence of children's wounds on the highly vascular head may be responsible for the lower infection rate, rather than some intrinsic difference in wound healing between children and adults.[6]

Although children are believed to have a greater ability to heal than adults, several factors relevant to children may slow healing. Children, especially neonates, have a greater surface area to body mass ratio and more difficulty in regulating body temperature than adults, which may impair healing. Young children, like elders, are at greater risk of malnutrition, especially in the presence of digestive disease or prematurity. Premature neonates have more fragile skin than full-term infants and, as such, are more susceptible to wounds due to weaker intracellular attachments. Due to the tremendous instrumentation required in the neonatal intensive care unit, premature infants are at great risk for injury during handling. Moreover, multiple lines and equipment in conjunction with a lack of voluntary movement may place the neonate at risk of pressure ulcers from this instrumentation. In particular, infants are susceptible to occipital pressure ulcers due to their disproportionate head size.[7] Risk factors for children in intensive care include age less than 36 months, ventricular septal defect (study involved children receiving open heart surgery), intubation longer than 7 days, and being in intensive care longer than 8 days.[8] Infants are also at risk of skin injury secondary to persistent contact with urine and feces on the perineal skin.

CASE MANAGEMENT

Each clinician has an ethical obligation to provide optimum care within the clinician's range of knowledge, skills, and abilities. As part of this, the clinician is ethically obligated to refer a patient to a clinician with the appropriate knowledge, skills, and abilities to provide optimal benefit for the patient. In the case of arterial insufficiency, the patient obviously needs the services of a vascular surgeon. If a wound becomes infected or infection cannot be controlled by sharp debridement, referral to an orthopedic or general surgeon becomes necessary. If a wound requires more extensive debridement than can be managed without an operating or special procedures room, requires general anesthesia, or the patient has tunneling or sinus tracts that will need to be opened, referral to a surgeon is needed. If a clinician lacks skill at sharp debridement, at least this aspect of care needs to be turned over to a person who is skillful; if the clinician wishes to continue to see patients likely to need sharp debridement, he or she should undergo appropriate training. Other potential referrals include complicated cases of nutritional risk; management of incontinence; need for splints, adaptive or assistive devices, orthoses, prostheses; mobility or activities of daily living training; psychological counseling; assistance in obtaining financial resources and caregivers, vocational training; or creating a plan of care within constraints imposed by payers.

PATIENT EDUCATION

The *Guide to Physical Therapist Practice* specifically addresses patient education as one of the components of the therapist's interaction with a patient/client, in addition to procedural interventions, documentation, communication, and coordination of patient care. Each patient has a unique educational and lifetime learning background and level of self-efficacy. Some individuals are in a position of directly supervising and performing the bulk of their care, whereas others are completely dependent on others in developing and carrying out a plan of care.

The clinician must, therefore, interview the patient, family, and caregivers to ascertain their level of understanding of the process by which the wound developed and how to facilitate its healing. Topics for discussion include the etiology of the wound, rudimentary principles of wound healing, the purposes and mechanisms of action of any interventions, and expected outcomes. Most individuals will not be able to process all of this information at once and will need periodic reinforcement, including opportunities for the patient to discuss progress during each visit and to ask questions. The clinician should also periodically assess the patient's or caregiver's cognitive (knowledge), psychomotor (ability to apply the knowledge), and affective (attitudes toward the process) learning.

SUMMARY

The plan of care is a blueprint for interventions provided based upon the history and physical examination of the patient, a diagnosis of the cause of the wound healing, the prognosis for healing, and modified based on a unique set of circumstances related to the patient's ability to follow through with the plan. Decision points include the need to treat infection, the need for debridement, filling subcutaneous defects, and managing drainage to optimize wound moisture while simultaneously maintaining the integrity of the surrounding skin. The skin of the elderly and neonate are at greater risk of injury due to anatomical and physiological differences. Elderly skin has less contact area, decreased thickness and blood flow, and is vulnerable to tearing and bleeding. A number of risk factors for injury are present in neonates, especially premature infants. Decreased ability to regulate heat, potential for malnourishment, inability to reposition, and the presence of multiple lines and devices increases risk of injury and slows healing. Both infants and the elderly need to be handled gently to avoid skin injury.

STUDY QUESTIONS

1. How does the care setting affect the plan of care?
2. How might an immobile terminally ill patient's plan of care differ from an ambulatory person's plan of care for a foot wound?

3. What two critical functions do dressings serve in managing wound drainage?

4. What are critical reasons for performing sharp debridement? Under what circumstances would sharp debridement not be performed?

5. What patient characteristics need to be considered in choosing a dressing that the patient will need to change at home?

6. Explain the greater risk of tearing and bleeding that occurs in the skin of the elderly.

7. Describe steps that can be taken to minimize damage to the skin of the infant and elderly patient.

8. List risk factors for skin injury and slow wound healing commonly present in premature infants.

REFERENCES

1. American Physical Therapy Association. Guide to physical therapist practice. *Physical Therapy*. 1997;77:1177-1619.

2. American Physical Therapy Association. Guide to physical therapist practice, 2nd edition. *Physical Therapy*. 2001;81:1-768.

3. American Physical Therapy Association. Physical disability. Special issue. *Physical Therapy*. 1994;74:375-506.

4. Verbugge L, Jette A. The disablement process. *Soc Sci Med*. 1994;38:1-14.

5. Hollander JE, Singer AJ, Valentine S. Comparison of wound care practices in pediatric and adult lacerations repaired in the emergency department. *Pediatr Emerg Care*. 1998;14:15-18.

6. Pieper B, Templin T, Dobal M, Jacox A. Prevalence and types of wounds among children receiving care in the home. *Ostomy Wound Management*. 2000;46:36-42.

7. Malloy-McDonald MB. Skin care for high-risk neonates. *Journal of Wound, Ostomy, & Continence Nursing*. 1995;22:177-182.

8. Neidig JRE, Kleiber C, Oppliger RA. Risk factors associated with pressure ulcers in the pediatric patient following open heart surgery. *Prog Cardiovasc Nurs*. 1989;4:99-106.

Documentation

21

OBJECTIVES

- Describe elements of the medical, family medical, social, work, and home history to document in an initial evaluation.
- Provide rationales for selecting elements of a physical examination to confirm, rule out, or perform a differential diagnosis based on a patient's history.
- Provide a rational basis for developing a diagnosis for a patient.
- Develop a prognosis based on a patient's history and physical examination.
- Develop a rational plan of care based on a patient's history, physical examination, limitation of resources including availability of caregivers, and geographical and work schedules of individuals.
- Discuss standards of care for optimizing outcomes of patient education and intervention.
- Discuss appropriate use of imaging techniques for documenting wound management.

THE NEED FOR DOCUMENTATION

The old axiom has been "If it isn't documented, it wasn't done." We have now evolved to optimizing documentation of patient care to maximize reimbursement. Regardless of the motivation for documentation, the important aspect is that documentation provides a clear road map of where we expect patient care to go, any detours, and the final destination. Many facilities use forms for documenting wound management. Some are universal forms; others use forms specific for different types of wounds (eg, a form for burn injuries, another for pressure ulcers, another for venous insufficiency ulcers). The advantage of using forms specific to a given type of wound is that the information requested on the form is more likely to be relevant to the patient, and the clinician will not forget to ask certain questions or perform certain tests based on the clinician's initial impression of the type of wound. The disadvantage is that the clinician may not know the true cause of a wound and does not reach an accurate diagnosis until the form has been completed, especially for a wound that presents a difficult differential diagnosis.

Proper documentation can be difficult if a logical sequence is not followed. In this chapter, documentation following the *Guide to Physical Therapist Practice*[1] is described. This system is based on continuous development and testing of hypotheses of causal and contributing factors that have led to the patient's current state of health. The clinician must then select tests to confirm, refute, or modify hypotheses regarding these causal and contributing factors. As the clinician takes a verbal history or reads a history from a form, the process of developing hypotheses is already occurring. Frequently, a referring clinician has provided a diagnosis for the patient's condition. This diagnosis may be a good starting point but must not be the sole focus of the patient history or physical examination. The clinician must be particularly wary of less common ailments that may masquerade as common ailments. The clinician must also be looking and listening for factors that may contribute to the patient's condition. For example, a patient may be referred with a diagnosis of cellulitis superior to the medial malleolus with open wounds that have remained open for 2 years. Immediately, the clinician is suspicious of venous insufficiency, so the questions start down the road of confirming contributing factors for venous insufficiency. If the patient reports a history of diabetes, the clinician will immediately begin asking questions related to neuropathy and arterial insufficiency. In both of these cases, the clinician will perform an examination of the peripheral circulation to rule out arterial insufficiency, a contraindication for compression.

ELEMENTS OF THE HISTORY

For facilities other than acute care hospitals, a standardized history form becomes increasingly important. Hospital-based facilities will have a history and physical examination section that should contain all relevant information. Information critical to the treatment plan for the wound, however, should be kept in a centralized area of the chart so an individual taking over care of the patient will not be required to read an entire chart. In addition, the hospital chart provides lab values and lists medications. This information can supplement what is on the history. For example, a history of congestive heart failure or rheumatoid arthritis may not be explicitly documented in the history and physical, but medications listed in the chart may cue the clinician to inquire about these conditions.

In an outpatient facility, the standardized history form can be useful if done carefully. Often, simply asking a patient to fill out the form is not sufficient. Key items should be confirmed verbally with the patient and, if possible, with a family member or caregiver. A list of prescription drugs, over-the-counter remedies, and herbal remedies should be listed. Often, patients will not remember all of the medications by name. Asking patients to bring in or show all of their medications will improve the accuracy of the drug review (Figure 21-1). In particular, questions related to diabetes are critical, and anyone who reports a history of diabetes mellitus should be asked about glycemic control, including current blood glucose and HbA1c to determine short- and long-term glycemic control.

Questions about standing and walking are particularly important for lower extremity ulcers. A person with wounds consistent with venous insufficiency needs to be asked about standing. A person with apparent neuropathic ulcers needs to be asked about walking, shoes, and other items discussed in Chapter 8. Also, the patient should be asked about any symptoms that accompany walking that may be suggestive of intermittent claudication. Questions about lifestyle, general health, vision, balance, and available care at home are important in developing a treatment plan that can be followed by the patient and any caregivers.

ELEMENTS OF THE PHYSICAL EXAMINATION

The physical examination performed during the initial visit will be much more comprehensive than that of subsequent visits. In particular, general health and mobility, and

SAMPLE HISTORY FORM

List present conditions being managed by a licensed health care provider (physician, physical therapist, occupational therapist, speech therapist, audiologist, podiatrist, nurse, osteopath, psychologist, or other).

_____

_____

List current medications including prescriptions, over-the-counter medications, herbal or other self-administered remedies, and any dietary modifications. Obtain and review use of all of your medication bottles prior to filling out this part of the form.

_____

_____

List any surgical procedures and the condition for which they were performed.

_____

_____

List previous medical conditions, treatments received for them, and the outcomes of treatment.

_____

_____

Family History (circle all that apply):

Heart disease   Diseases of arteries or veins   Stroke   Diabetes   Respiratory disease

Have you been told that you have heart, lung, blood vessel, endocrine, digestive, kidney, skin, or any other disease?
            yes   no

If so specify _____

Do you presently have any of the following symptoms (circle all that apply):

Chest pain	yes	no	
Shortness of breath	yes	no	
Dizziness or feeling faint	yes	no	
Difficulty sleeping while lying flat in bed (need to raise head to breathe)	yes	no	
Swelling of the legs, ankles, or feet	yes	no	
Palpitations or abnormal heart rhythm	yes	no	
Pain or cramping of legs with activity that is relieved by rest	yes	no	
Loss of sensation of any part of the body	yes	no	specify_____
Coldness of any part of the body	yes	no	specify_____
Frequent urination	yes	no	
Getting up at night to urinate	yes	no	
Elevated blood sugar	yes	no	don't know
Night sweats	yes	no	
Change in appetite	yes	no	specify_____
Change in sleep pattern	yes	no	specify_____
Fever	yes	no	
Changes in pattern of bowel movement or urination	yes	no	

Specify the change _____

Unusual bleeding or discharges	yes	no	specify location_____
Pain resistant to over-the-counter medications	yes	no	
Pain that wakes you at night	yes	no	
Pain that does not change with activity or position	yes	no	

If yes to any of the last three questions above, specify the location of your pain _____

Red streaks	yes	no	specify location_____
Swollen lymph nodes/glands	yes	no	specify location_____
Changes in skin texture	yes	no	specify location_____
Loss of body hair	yes	no	specify location_____
Thickening of nails	yes	no	specify location_____

Figure 21-1. Sample history form. This form is made available to the patient before the first clinical visit to ensure accuracy, especially for list of medications. On clinic visit, review the form with the patient and assess the patient's understanding of the items on the history form.

possible complicating factors that may influence the patient's ability to follow a treatment plan need to be explored. Subsequent visits must have some element of examination, but they are focused more on whether the prognosis developed from the initial visit is still appropriate and gives the clinician the opportunity to explore complications not foreseen during the initial evaluation. General mobility should be evaluated and documented, even if the patient has no mobility. The lack of mobility weighs heavily in the prognosis of certain types of wounds, especially pressure ulcers. The quality of gait is also important, particularly for the person with neuropathic feet. The loss of proprioception leads to unsteady gait, loss of heel-toe progression, and, in extreme cases, a wide-based gait with a slapping of the foot onto the floor. Inability to control the foot and ankle during gait are high-risk factors for the person with neuropathy, as shearing forces on the plantar surface are increased.

Strength, range of motion, sensation, and reflexes need to be addressed. The extent of this aspect of the evaluation needs to be ascertained at the time of the evaluation. Limited range of motion of the foot is also a major prognosticator of neuropathic ulcers. Sensory tests can be done quickly and can distinguish between small and large sensory neuron loss. Reflexes are particularly diagnostic of large neuron deficits in neuropathy but may also be informative for patients with other pathologies. Strength testing of the foot is similarly important, particularly for the individual with peripheral neuropathy. Loss of intrinsic foot muscle strength precedes critical foot deformities.

Ankle-brachial index is considered to be a minimum standard for any patient with lower extremity ulcers. Suspected arterial insufficiency should be quantified this way for referral to a vascular surgeon. A person with diabetes mellitus presenting with neuropathy of the lower extremities is also at risk for arterial insufficiency and should be tested. Moreover, the person with venous insufficiency needs to be tested to rule out arterial insufficiency before initiating compression therapy.

The wound itself and the surrounding skin need to be described thoroughly during the initial evaluation and during each dressing change. For this reason, a section on a hospital chart needs to be devoted to this aspect. Even if the dressing is not changed, the expectation is that at least the dressing be examined during each nursing shift for an inpatient. In settings outside a hospital, documentation of the wound and surrounding skin needs to be done for each visit. If the patient or a caregiver is tending to the wound between visits, the clinician needs to take a report from the patient or caregiver and document the report in the permanent record. The ability of the patient or caregiver to provide necessary care also needs to be documented and the plan of care would then be adjusted as needed.

Information to be documented is discussed thoroughly in Chapters 8 through 11. The type of necessary informa-

tion may vary with the type of wound. The mnemonic CODES was discussed previously. This information is critical for a description with every dressing change. The color of the wound (C) and proportions of the wound consisting of each color must be documented. Odor (O) and drainage (D) can be simply checked or circled on a form. Extent of the wound (E), including length, width, and, if applicable, depth can be documented on a regular basis. In a setting in which the wound is only examined by the clinician periodically, extent should be documented with each visit. In a situation in which the patient is being seen daily, documentation of the extent of the wound may be done less frequently but in compliance with facility policies. Extent also includes any tunneling, undermining, or sinus tracts with documentation of their length and position using clock notation. Surrounding skin condition (S) can usually be documented with a blank or item to check or circle on a form (see examples in Figures 21-2 to 21-6). Any changes in the patient's other abilities from the initial evaluation should be examined on a regular basis by physical examination or interview as set by facility procedures or as deemed necessary by the clinician.

In addition to the physical examination of the wound, the patient should be interviewed, at least briefly, to determine what changes have occurred since the initial evaluation and previous visits in documented information, whether it is physical or related to work, home, recreation, or resources. If the patient or a caregiver is responsible for some aspects of wound management between visits, adherence to the treatment plan should also be documented. The clinician needs to check for signs of nonadherence that might include knowledge of the details of the treatment plan, condition of the wound, condition of dressings, wear on shoes, blood glucose, or other details relevant to the treatment plan.

If the treatment plan outside the clinic is not being followed, modifications are likely to be needed. Nonadherence to the treatment plan that has been documented carefully may be necessary to institute required changes in the treatment plan. If nonadherence is due to physical limitations, the patient may need to be seen more frequently in the outpatient or home health setting. A change from autolytic debridement to sharp debridement may be necessary if the patient is not willing or able to perform the necessary dressing changes or is unable to maintain the integrity of the dressings. The patient may also need to be referred to a social worker to address deficits in social or financial support necessary to follow the treatment plan (Figure 21-7).

PHOTODOCUMENTATION

The phrase, "A picture is worth a thousand words," is frequently used. In the case of open wounds, description of certain wounds and the progression of healing can be inad-

GENERIC INTEGUMENTARY DOCUMENTATION FORM

Patient_____ Age_____ M F   Clinician_____ Date_____

History

Chief complaint_____

Home arrangements_____

Support system_____

Occupation/education/hobbies/home activities_____
_____

Ambulation required for lifestyle_____

Standing required for lifestyle_____

Current lifestyle limitations_____

Medications_____

Past medical history_____

Previous treatment for condition_____

Review of Systems

Neuromuscular_____

Musculoskeletal_____

Cardiopulmonary_____

Integumentary_____

Physical Examination

Wound photo or drawing here:

Color_____ Odor_____ Drainage _____ Extent_____

Shape_____ Tissue in wound   Black_____% Yellow_____%   Red_____%

Surrounding Skin

Texture_____ Temperature_____ Swelling: -   +   ++   +++   ++++

Color_____ Hair/nails_____ Ecchymosis_____ Hemosiderin_____

Demarcation_____ Maceration_____ Epiboly_____

Diagnosis Impaired integumentary integrity with:

_____Risk of injury   _____Superficial injury

_____Partial-thickness injury   _____Full-thickness injury

_____Full-thickness injury and subcutaneous involvement

Prognosis: Within_____days weeks months, and within_____visits, the patient is expected to:

_____

Plan of Care

Patient and family/caregiver education_____

Procedural interventions_____frequency_____ duration_____

_____frequency_____ duration_____

Signature_____ Date_____

Figure 21-2. Generic integumentary documentation form contains a short section for history and physical examination items most directly related to the cause of the wound and several blanks to be filled with words, checks, or "+" signs. The use of this form does not presume any diagnosis or etiology. Instead, the form is a means of keeping the clinician "on track" using the *Guide to Physical Therapist Practice*.[1] The therapist collects data and performs special tests as needed to rule in or rule out the wound's cause. In the diagnosis section, the clinician chooses with a check mark one or more of the five listed diagnoses based on impairments and the guide. The prognosis derives from the diagnosis and the special circumstances of the patient. The plan of care includes patient/family/caregiver education and procedural interventions. To an extent, "goals" are part of the prognosis section; specific documentation requirements may require goals related to functions necessary to the patient (eg, the patient will be able to stand for an 8-hour shift without complaining of pain); the patient will have sufficient range of motion for self-feeding. The final section is only present to allow individuals with a need to know what direct or "procedural" interventions are being performed for the patient, how frequently, and an expected time at which the intervention will no longer be needed. If documentation of functional outcomes is needed, a general initial evaluation form may also need to be used.

SUPPLEMENTAL DATA FOR DIAGNOSIS OF VENOUS ULCERS

Patient_____ Clinician_____ Date_____

Alternatives to standing_____

Location(s)_____

Status of surrounding skin_____

Size of wound(s)	Length_____cm	Width_____cm	Depth	Partial thickness	Full thickness

Ankle brachial index   Right_____   Left_____

Temperature of right foot	normal	increased	decreased
Temperature of left foot	normal	increased	decreased
Capillary refill (right)	normal	sluggish	absent
Capillary refill (left)	normal	sluggish	absent

Foot volume   Right_____   Left_____

Wound bed   % Red_____   % Yellow_____   % Black_____

Color of granulation tissue	red	pink	
Drainage	minimal	moderate	copious

Color of drainage_____

Compression therapy (specify)_____

Signature_____ Date_____

Figure 21-3. Supplemental data for diagnosis of venous ulcers is used for the patient who is determined by the clinician to have venous ulcers. This form is meant to supplement the generic integumentary documentation form. These items are more directly related to venous ulcer risk factors, prevention of recurrence, and appropriate treatment. Note in particular the items to rule out arterial insufficiency. These items include ankle brachial index, foot temperature, capillary refill, and color of granulation tissue. Items used to confirm the suspicion of venous ulcers are also listed and will be illustrated in Figure 21-9.

equate with words. In many cases, a hand-drawn diagram may be adequate; but in others, the quality of the wound needs to be captured more thoroughly. Photography is especially important for the wound containing vast amounts of necrotic tissue. In these cases, wounds frequently become much larger before they can heal. A good photograph can show changes in the quality of the wound and help the clinician explain the need for extended periods of care, increasing wound size, or complications that have led to the need to reevaluate the prognosis or plan of care.

The first question that arises is what type of camera is needed for photodocumentation of wounds. One may choose among digital, 35-mm film, and instant film (Polaroid) cameras. Several advantages exist for each type. Under some circumstances all of them could be useful for a given patient. Polaroids have the distinct advantage of providing an instant permanent record of the wound. Within 1 minute, the clinician knows that the image has been obtained. Polaroids are also simple to operate. All the clinician needs to do is aim and push one button. The cameras focus automatically. However, a standard Polaroid

camera cannot be focused at a suitable distance for most wounds. To allow close-up photography, a special lens system must be attached. Another advantage is special "grid" film available for Polaroid cameras. As the film develops, a grid is formed. In addition, mechanisms for ensuring the same distance from the wound are available. The original adapters for Polaroid cameras only had a retractable line for this purpose. The photographer would hold the camera in one hand and pull the retractable line to the skin's surface to ensure the proper distance and, therefore, standardize the size of the grid. A more recent development is the light-lock system. With this system, nothing touches the patient and the camera can be held with both hands. The light-lock system consists of two beams within the lens adapter that are activated by the press of a button. The camera is then moved to a distance from the subject that causes the two beams to converge. If the camera is held too close or too far from the subject, two separate beams can be seen. On the downside, however, the resolution and color of an instant photograph are usually poor compared with what can be achieved with a 35-mm camera. The cost of an individual photograph is

SUPPLEMENTAL DATA FORM FOR PRESSURE ULCERS

Patient_____   Clinician_____   Date_____

Stage of ulcer (identify location on figure at right with wound number)

Identify location(s) of pressure ulcers

1.	I	II	III	IV	Partially filled	Filled	Covered
2.	I	II	III	IV	Partially filled	Filled	Covered
3.	I	II	III	IV	Partially filled	Filled	Covered
4.	I	II	III	IV	Partially filled	Filled	Covered
5.	I	II	III	IV	Partially filled	Filled	Covered

Size of ulcer (using identification key on right)

1.	Length_____cm	Width_____cm	Depth_____cm
2.	Length_____cm	Width_____cm	Depth_____cm
3.	Length_____cm	Width_____cm	Depth_____cm
4.	Length_____cm	Width_____cm	Depth_____cm
5.	Length_____cm	Width_____cm	Depth_____cm

Tunneling, sinus tracts, undermining

1.	Distance_____cm	Direction_____:00	Drainage_____
2.	Distance_____cm	Direction_____:00	Drainage_____
3.	Distance_____cm	Direction_____:00	Drainage_____
4.	Distance_____cm	Direction_____:00	Drainage_____
5.	Distance_____cm	Direction_____:00	Drainage_____

	1	2	3	4	5
Odor	_____	_____	_____	_____	_____
Drainage	_____	_____	_____	_____	_____
% R, Y, B	_____	_____	_____	_____	_____
Surrounding skin condition	_____	_____	_____	_____	_____

Signature_____   Date_____

Figure 21-4. Supplemental data form for pressure ulcers is used for the patient with pressure ulcers. The first area includes information on the depth and degree of healing of up to five ulcers. Sadly, many patients will have more than five ulcers and a second or third supplemental data form for pressure ulcers may be used. Depth of the ulcer is indicated by using Roman numerals I through IV. As discussed in Chapter 9 and elsewhere in the text, many clinicians have difficulty handling documentation of a healing pressure ulcer. The last three columns of "Stage of ulcer" allow the clinician to document the progress of the wound in addition to the original depth of the injury by which the wound is meant to be staged. To the right, a figure used in Chapter 9 is placed on the form. Note that only a posterior view is used. In this view, wounds on the posterior side of the body and right and left sides can be circled, enumerated, and a line drawn to the circle or ellipse. This view covers a large fraction of pressure ulcers, including the problem areas of the occiput, epicondyles of the elbow, sacrum, ischial tuberosities, and heels. If a wound is located on the anterior surface, a note can be written to indicate that the wound is not on the visible side and give a brief description (eg, chin and a line drawn to the figure to indicate the location on the anterior side). Due to the prevalence of tunneling, sinus tracts, and undermining with pressure ulcers, a section has been devoted to describe them.

expensive (about $1.00 each). Also, no negative is available to make copies or slides, and the film itself is bulky.

The standard for quality photography has been the single lens reflex camera using 35-mm film. The initial costs of quality photographs is rather high and ranges into hundreds of dollars. Lower cost 35-mm cameras are designed for casual consumer use as opposed to medical photography. A single lens reflex camera itself may cost $200 or more and the necessary lenses add to the expense. Ideally, the camera would be equipped with several lenses. For most wounds, a 105-mm lens is appropriate. This size lens allows the photographer to remain at a suitable distance

SUPPLEMENTAL FORM FOR THERMAL INJURY

Anterior
Adult head 4.5%   Child head 8.5%

Adult trunk 18%   Child trunk 18%

Adult upper extremity 4.5%   Child upper extremity 4.5%

Adult and Child 1%

Adult lower extremity 9%   Child lower extremity 6.5%

Posterior
Adult head 4.5%   Child head 8.5%

Adult trunk 18%   Child trunk 18%

Adult upper extremity 4.5%   Child upper extremity 4.5%

Adult lower extremity 9%   Child lower extremity 6.5%

Indicate locations and depths of thermal injuries on the figure to the left.

- - Superficial thickness (1st degree)

//// Superficial partial thickness (2nd degree)

\\\ Deep partial thickness (deep dermal)

xxx Full thickness

	RUE	LUE	RLE	LLE	Anterior trunk	Posterior trunk
Deficits in range of motion	____	____	____	____	_____	_____
Deficits in strength	____	____	____	____	_____	_____
Active exercise	____	____	____	____	_____	_____
Active assisted exercise	____	____	____	____	_____	_____
Passive stretch	____	____	____	____	_____	_____
No movement allowed	____	____	____	____	_____	_____

Deficits in tolerance for bed mobility, bed exercise, position changes, ambulation (specify)_____

_____

Indicate special positioning needs_____

Signature_____   Date_____

Figure 21-5. Supplemental form for thermal injury consists of figures to indicate the extent and depth of thermal injuries, including burns, scalds, and frostbite. This form may also be applicable to chemical and radiation injuries. Different patterns of shading are used to indicate the depth of injury. In some cases, the actual depth may not be certain, especially in the case of distinguishing a deep partial-thickness from a full-thickness wound. A key for the shading is given on the right. The next section is a table with a synopsis of neuromusculoskeletal impairments and appropriate types of movement for the six areas of the body, used as headings for the table. In many cases, thermal injuries are limited to one or two of the segments. For the deficits in range of motion and deficits in strength rows, the clinician may enter a ✓ to indicate a deficit, a Ø to indicate no deficits in that body region, or may explicitly state a movement or muscle group affected. The next four rows of the table use the same six body regions and a ✓ is entered in one of the four rows under each column heading. At a glance, a clinician will know whether active range of motion, active assisted, passive, or no movement is appropriate for the six regions. The clinician may make a note to indicate situations in which different types of movements are appropriate for different areas in one of the six categories given. For example, an injury may create a situation in which active range of motion is required for the hand, passive stretching is appropriate for the elbow, and active range of motion is appropriate for the shoulder. Moreover, certain directions of movement (eg, abduction or flexion) may need to be done in different ways. The next section addresses bed mobility, bed exercise, and ambulation.

SUPPLEMENTAL FORM FOR NEUROPATHIC ULCERS

Patient_____   Clinician_____   Date_____

Location(s): Indicate location of wounds on the diagram below and create a numeric key if there are multiple wounds.

Wound #	1	2	3	4	5
Wagner grade	_____	_____	_____	_____	_____
Size	_____	_____	_____	_____	_____
% red	_____	_____	_____	_____	_____
% yellow	_____	_____	_____	_____	_____
% black	_____	_____	_____	_____	_____

Indicate location of callus on the diagram below with the symbol /////

Reflexes: AJ right   present   diminished   absent   AJ left   present   diminished   absent

Foot deformities (specify)_____

Gait deviations (specify)_____

Pulse (right)   4   3   2   1   0   (specify artery palpated)_____

Pulse (left)   4   3   2   1   0   (specify artery palpated)_____

Capillary refill (right)   normal   sluggish   absent

Capillary refill (left)   normal   sluggish   absent

Ankle brachial index   Right_____   Left_____

Right foot temperature   normal   decreased   increased (specify temperature)

Left foot temperature   normal   decreased   increased (specify temperature)

Sensory testing (indicate on the diagram below + for intact, +/- for diminished, - for absent

Left foot   Right foot

Dorsal   Plantar   Plantar   Dorsal

Signature_____   Date_____

Figure 21-6. Supplemental form for neuropathic ulcers. The term *diabetic foot ulcer* does not recognize that diabetes mellitus can cause both neuropathy and arterial insufficiency. The first item is the Wagner grade, in which 0 is an injury with intact skin; 1 is a shallow ulcer; 2 is a deep ulcer; 3 indicates infection of the wound or surrounding/underlying structures, especially osteomyelitis; 4 pertains to gangrene of the forefoot; and 5 indicates gangrene to most of the foot. The next section is used to document standard tests and measures for neuropathic ulcers and requires the filling of blanks or circling of items. The last item is a map of the feet. Four maps are given. On the left side are views of the plantar and dorsal left foot, and the right foot is on the right. The circles on the foot indicate the standard locations for sensory testing using a monofilament. The plantar foot has nine locations and the dorsal foot only one. In addition to the labels placed on the form, contours on the plantar figure and toenails on the dorsal figure are given to help identify the surface of the foot.

from the subject to avoid distortion of the image and colors that can be produced by photography with smaller lenses. A 35-mm lens allows the entire subject to be photographed, and a 60-mm lens is suitable for large areas of the body. In addition, suitable lights and a light meter are needed. Although the film itself is not expensive, processing can be. One may choose to develop film or send it to a film processor. Processing becomes more expensive per picture if the entire roll of film is not used. A decision to use 35-mm film needs to be based on the volume of photography done. In a clinic where photographic documentation is infrequent, 35-mm photography becomes impractical. The clinic will be faced with the choice of either paying for partial rolls to be processed or a delay in obtaining the photographs. The major risk is the potential loss of information, which increases with the delay between taking the photograph and processing the film. Imagine having 2 weeks of photographs on a roll of film that is taken for processing and none of the photographs develop! Learning to use a single lens reflex camera requires time, patience, and many rolls of film. The novice needs to take practice pictures under a systematic variety of film, lenses, lighting conditions, aperture settings, and film speeds before actual photographs of patients should be taken. Once optimal settings are determined, the photographer can be reasonably sure of good quality photographs in the future.

The newest way of photographing wounds is with the digital camera. Digital cameras combine advantages of instant and 35-mm photographs. The clinician will know immediately if the image is appropriate. A wide range in price and resolution is available. Generally, higher resolution digital cameras are more expensive. A balance needs to be struck between the required resolution and price. A camera with a zoom feature is desirable, especially for smaller wounds. In addition, one must decide on a medium for transferring the picture from the camera. One may choose between cameras with USB connections, floppy disks, or other forms of removable media (memory sticks, etc). Three and one-half-inch floppy disk drives increase the cost of digital cameras, but they are more convenient for transferring images. Floppy disks are limited to 1.44 Mb of files. The number of photographs that fit on a floppy disk is determined by the resolution of the camera. A lower resolution camera may allow as many as 50 photographs on a floppy disk. One must then consider how to store the digital pictures. One may choose to print the picture or upload it to a computerized documentation system. Because the photographs do not require the purchase of film or the cost of film processing, digital photography is the most cost-effective means of photodocumentation. The other major advantage of digital photography is the ability to make as many copies of the picture as needed. In addition, software programs are available to correct color

problems. One may track the progress of a wound by arranging a series of digital photographs in either a video display or hard copy. Lower cost digital cameras will not provide much better quality than a Polaroid, whereas expensive digital cameras can produce pictures that may rival 35-mm film.

General Photography Guidelines

Regardless of the type of camera used, a number of general rules need to be followed to optimize photodocumentation. A photographic release form should always be signed by the patient before photographs are taken. If the patient is a minor, a parent or guardian must sign the photographic release. Identification of the patient, the date, and a scale need to be present on each photograph. The Polaroid grid film provides a standardized grid size provided that the camera is held at the proper distance from the wound. Achieving the proper distance is accomplished easily with either the retractable line or light-lock system. However, this system is inadequate for smaller wounds. For small wounds, the grid may obscure the wound rather than help. A common approach is to use a disposable scale with the patient's initials and the date written on the scale. Even with this approach, the clinician should attempt to keep the camera at the same distance from the subject to better allow an eyeball comparison between photographs of the same wound. The single lens reflex system with interchangeable lenses offers the advantage of sufficient zoom for a range of wound size. For this reason, a digital camera needs to have a sufficient zoom range. For at least the initial evaluation, a photograph needs to be taken that allows the body part to be identified from the wound. The temptation is to fill the entire photograph with the wound. At least one picture should be taken during the initial evaluation to show enough of the patient that the body part can be identified. Generally, the patient's face or anything else that could allow someone else to identify the patient should not be in the photograph unless the wound is on the face. For wounds on the face, zoom only to sufficient detail to identify what part of the face is involved, but minimize the possibility of identifying the subject of the photograph. For subsequent photographs the clinician may choose to zoom in to provide more detail of the wound. In many cases, wounds are slow to heal due to the condition of the surrounding skin; therefore, sufficient surrounding skin needs to be in the photograph.

The background needs to be considered when taking any type of photograph. In many cases, the background will consist only of the patient's intact skin. In cases in which a background other than the patient's surrounding skin exists, avoid white or yellow. These colors reflect too much light and will change the color of the wound. Use blue or green drapes in these cases. Also avoid distracting objects within the photograph. Remove any equipment or

WOUND CARE CHART REVIEW TOOL

Indicators: Clients with wounds will be appropriately cared for as evidenced by the following indicators

Threshold: Goal is 85% on all indicators

Sample size: 100% or 10 charts for clients with a wound per quarter

Year: _____

Quarter: Jan to Mar   Apr to Jun   Jul to Sep   Oct to Dec

	Yes	No	N/A
1. Wound assessment done on admission			
A. Integumentary portion of Outcome and Assessment Information Set (OASIS) filled out	—	—	—
B. Wound assessment sheet initiated	—	—	—
C. Braden scale value computed	—	—	—
D. Integumentary area of point of contact (POC) filled out			
1. If Braden score <12 "Potential for impaired skin integrity demonstrated by" filled out	—	—	—
2. Wounds described in "Problem" section by location, type, stage or partial/full thickness, and size in centimeter	—	—	—
3. Steps of wound care included on "communication with MD" line of OASIS and "perform" section of plan of care. Wound care orders match treatment section of wound assessment sheet, including whether caregiver will be taught	—	—	—
E. Orders for wound care on 485 (plan of care form) includes technique; products, frequency, whether any caregiver will be taught	—	—	—
F. 485 includes "consult to be done by certified wound, ostomy, continence nurse (CWOCN) within 2 weeks"	—	—	—
2. Consistent and accurate wound assessments and wound related teaching documented on skilled nurse visit (SNV) notes			
A. Wound described with each dressing change			
1. Wound bed described	—	—	—
2. Drainage described	—	—	—
3. Surrounding tissue described	—	—	—
4. Signs or infection noted and MD notified or "No s/s infection noted" documented	—	—	—
5. Patient response to wound care noted	—	—	—
6. Wound care steps described	—	—	—
7. Wound location and type described	—	—	—
B. Accurate wound measurements done weekly			
1. L x W x D measured in centimeters to tenths	—	—	—
2. Includes measurement of deepest undermining and where undermining is located	—	—	—
3. Wound described as outlined above in 2A	—	—	—
4. Current wound care described	—	—	—
5. SNV notes evidence of teaching regarding wounds, wound care, products, pressure prevention, and/or skin care as appropriate	—	—	—
3. All changes in wound care and/or frequency done are accompanied by an MD order and Coordination of Care note	—	—	—
4. All MD orders are signed and returned	—	—	—

Figure 21-7. Tool used to ensure complete documentation for home health visits. Developed by Megan Hughes, RN, CWOCN.

personnel that would be in the background. This is more likely to be a problem for the initial photograph showing the body part on which the wound is located. Carefully position the patient to allow the proper amount of light to strike the wound and optimize patient comfort. Insufficient or excessive lighting will obscure the details of the wound and colors will not be true. Also avoid direct flash on the wound or flash too close to the wound. Excessive lighting or flash creates a bright picture with little contrast and will alter the color. Direct flash will be reflected from moist surfaces. If flash is necessary, angle the camera so the flash is not reflected back toward the camera. Insufficient lighting will result in a dark picture with poor contrast and will also change the color of the wound.[2]

DEVELOPING THE DIAGNOSIS

On the initial evaluation and subsequent visits, the type of wound by etiology should be documented. Acute or surgical wounds usually do not present difficulty in diagnosis. Differential diagnosis of lower extremity wounds has been discussed in Chapters 8 to 11. Some facilities use generic forms with either a blank or a series of choices that can be circled to indicate the etiology. Other facilities use forms specific to a given type of wound, especially pressure ulcers, venous insufficiency ulcers, neuropathic ulcers, and burns. The advantage of the etiology-specific forms is the efficiency and readability of forms that contain only information pertinent to the type of wound. For example, a pressure ulcer form may have one of the tools such as the Braden or Norton scale, and a form for neuropathic ulcers would contain the elements of foot screening. Another advantage of an etiology-specific form is that it can usually be printed on a single sheet. A single sheet is more likely to be read by other members of the wound management team and other parties with an interest in the care provided. However, a form should not cram information into a single page and sacrifice the ability of clinicians to find information. As opposed to forms for the initial evaluation, some progress note forms are designed to be used for several days, which also aids in the convenience of communicating the progress in wound healing.

DEVELOPING THE PROGNOSIS

The prognosis part of the documentation should contain an expected outcome and time frame. The time frame may be given in terms of number of visits or unit of times, such as weeks or months. The prognosis needs to be developed based upon patient, family, and caregiver expectations, lifestyle, type of work, and available resources. *The Guide to Physical Therapist Practice*[1] provides a starting

point for prognosis. For each practice pattern in the guide, the prognosis section provides a list of possible outcomes and the time frame expectation for 80% of patients within the practice pattern. A list of potential complications that may hinder attainment of the stated outcomes within the stated time frame is also provided in the prognosis section. Therefore, as discussed above, a good social and work history and physical examination is necessary to develop a meaningful prognosis. A person in overall good health with excellent resources who adheres to the treatment plan and is an active participant in developing the treatment plan is likely to attain a higher level of function and in a shorter time than the individual who has poor health, poor resources, and does not adhere to the treatment plan.

DEVELOPING A LOGICAL PLAN OF CARE

The treatment plan should be a logical extension of the history, physical examination, diagnosis, and prognosis. If these are documented carefully, the details of the treatment plan should be clear to any clinician experienced in wound management who takes over care of the patient, although some details may vary with personal preference of the patient, clinician, or caregiver. The documentation may be in either the well-established SOAP format or some other form, such as a narrative following the language developed in the *Guide to Physical Therapist Practice* (Table 21-1).[1] The subjective portion corresponds roughly with the history taken from the patient. The objective section contains components of the history taken from medical records and the physical examination. The assessment section of a SOAP note will contain elements of diagnosis and sometimes elements of the prognosis. The plan section of a SOAP note contains the treatment plan, although some individuals will place functional objectives and goals with the "P" section.

PROGNOSIS/DEVELOPING AN OUTCOME STATEMENT

Prognosis is done fairly readily based on the *Guide to Physical Therapist Practice*[1] integumentary practice patterns B through E. Practice pattern A is related to prevention of loss of integumentary integrity and some of the pattern's elements may be important for a given patient who already has a wound to prevent either recurrence of the wound or development of a wound in another location. A thorough history and physical examination is necessary to determine if any of the potential complications that may either extend the time frame or lead to a new episode of care are present and how they can be managed.

Table 21-1

COMPARISON OF SOAP NOTE DOCUMENTATION TO *GUIDE TO PHYSICAL THERAPIST PRACTICE* LANGUAGE

SOAP Format	Common Elements	Guide Language
Subjective	Chief complaint; history of complaint; lifestyle, work, school, play	History
Objective	Review of systems; routine screening tests; tests specific to rule in/out suspected diagnosis	Physical examination
Assessment: Diagnosis or a description of the cluster of signs and symptoms; outcomes, functional goals and time frames by some clinicians		Assessment: Mental process, not written, in which information is analyzed critically
		Diagnosis: Identifying a cluster of signs and symptoms, often identified as a practice pattern
		Prognosis: Expected outcomes and time frame for achievement; discussion of complications
Plan: Outcomes, functional goals, and time frames by some clinicians	Specific interventions including patient education, behavior modification, direct interventions (eg, debridement, frequency, and duration)	Plan of care

The clinician needs to assess adherence to the treatment plan constantly and, if necessary, modify it to make adherence achievable. The modifications may either increase or decrease the time frame and may limit some of the outcomes originally expected. An example of a shortened time frame is one in which autolytic debridement was initially proposed; but due to complications, sharp debridement was substituted in the treatment plan.

When developing the prognosis, one must be clear on the clinician's role in the episode of care. In many cases, the clinician in the acute care hospital is not expected to achieve complete healing of a wound but to achieve a clean and stable wound, ready for some type of surgical repair such as grafting or discharge of the patient to the appropriate destination such home with self-care, a caregiver, or to a different type of facility. In other cases, typical of hospital- or resident-based facilities, one type of clinician may work with the patient temporarily and another type of clinician takes over care once characteristics of the wound meet the established criteria. In settings that are not hospital- or resident-based (eg, acute care hospital, rehabilitative facility, skilled nursing facility, nursing home), the clinician will need to vary frequency of visits and discharge the patient from the clinician's care as the characteristics of the wound change. Regardless of the setting, a time frame for complete healing or a prognosis for optimum condition of the wound should be developed. Variance with the final predicted outcome after discharge may be grounds for a new episode of care.

TRANSLATING THE DIAGNOSIS AND HISTORY INTO A PLAN OF CARE

The plan of care needs to flow from the items discussed. Given two patients with identical characteristics, two different plans of care are still likely to be needed. Variances in the plan of care should be viewed as accommodations to the unique combinations of patient characteristics, including physical condition, resources, and lifestyle. The plan of care needs to represent the optimum combination of appropriate wound care and the reality of

Case #1, Generic Integumentary Documentation Form and Supplemental Data Form for Diagnosis of Venous Ulcers (Figures 21-8 and 21-9)

A 42-year-old man (Figure 21-8) was referred with a diagnosis of cellulitis of the distal tibia. Although the true etiology was immediately obvious, the data collection began with a history. During the history, the initial suspicion of venous insufficiency was repeatedly reinforced. The chief complaints of discomfort to mild-moderate pain, the location described by the patient, and discoloration were all consistent with venous ulcers. The six items in Figure 21-8 are designed to help the clinician understand the individual's situation as it may affect prognosis. The patient's domicile and the presence of a small number of steps were not consequential, although numerous combinations of a particular type of domicile and lifestyle could create difficult situations. The patient had several family members at home and all were agreeable to keeping the patient on-track with the treatment plan. Cost issues were not a major concern, which allowed the patient sufficient access to the clinician to ensure that the treatment plan would be carried out to its completion. Although the patient's condition did not prevent the patient from working, he was uncomfortable and sometimes in pain at work, and he rarely engaged in his normal recreational activity. He mostly stayed at home and watched television, which put his cardiopulmonary status at risk. Knowing that the patient was basically on his feet most of the day during his normal routine and how his condition had been limited dictated an aggressive treatment plan and modifications at his place of work.

The review of systems included basic tests as described in the *Guide to Physical Therapist Practice.*[1] This patient was in good health except for the history of hypertension and venous insufficiency. The neuromuscular and musculoskeletal systems were noted to be within normal limits (WNL). Because blood pressure was not completely under control with medications, and venous engorgement was noted in both legs; current BP as well as the venous problem were noted in the cardiopulmonary line. The ulceration and presence of skin changes were noted under integumentary. No integumentary problems were noted elsewhere on the patient.

The observation of the wound was then recorded using the CODES system described earlier in this chapter. This information, in conjunction with the history and condition of the surrounding skin, easily led to the etiology of this ulcer. The impairment-driven diagnoses based on the *Guide to Physical Therapist Practice*[1] could then be chosen. This patient was still at risk of further ulcerations, so this diagnosis was checked in addition to the full-thickness injury. The patient's prognosis was based on his generally good health and apparent willingness to adhere to the treatment plan. This was tempered by the patient's working condition, which is discussed further in the supplemental venous ulcer form. The procedural interventions are listed along with the frequency and duration. The compression bandaging needed to be changed more frequently initially until the venous insufficiency was better controlled and the drainage diminished.

how the plan interacts with the patient. A patient with an acute injury to a toe needs to be treated very differently from a patient with a neuropathic ulcer on the toe with identical characteristics.

To meet the criteria for medical necessity, documentation should support that 1) the treatment is necessary; 2) improvement of the condition is expected; 3) the treatment is being provided by the proper clinician; and 4) the condition will not improve or will become worse if treatment is not provided. Documentation of the treatment plan may be based on the four decision points explored in Chapter 20 with accommodations for circumstances other than characteristics of the wound: 1) presence, suspicion, or reasonable assumption of impending infection; 2) type of debridement needed; 3) subcutaneous tissue loss; and 4) management of drainage and surrounding skin. Although a number of issues were discussed in Chapter 20, a succinct argument framed by the principles of medical necessity should be provided. In many cases, a well-documented initial evaluation that outlines the reasons for the choices made will meet all the goals of documentation, including reimbursement, the ability of other clinicians to understand the treatment plan, and improved clinical decision-making.

SUMMARY

Documentation is important for the obvious reason of maximizing reimbursement, but done well, it provides a road map for the episode of care. Documentation can be done using the old SOAP format or using the language of the *Guide to Physical Therapist Practice.*[1] Certain aspects are common to the two approaches, but a number of items fall into different categories. For example, the information taken from the patient and that taken from medical records go into different parts of the SOAP note, whereas history is a complete section using the guide approach. Information taken from the history section guides the

GENERIC INTEGUMENTARY DOCUMENTATION FORM

Patient__Stan Jones_____ Age_42_ Ⓜ F   Clinician_Linda Smith__ Date _7/4/01__

History

Chief complaint _Discomfort, weeping wound on leg and discoloration around wound_____

Home arrangements_Mobile home, 4 steps with single rail, step mother, 2 teenage brothers, 10-year-old sister live with pt_____

Support system _Relatives living with pt, employer provides health insurance_____

Occupation/education/hobbies/home activities _Cashier in convenience store, hunting, fishing, rebuilding autos_____

Ambulation required for lifestyle _Primarily stands at cash register for 8-hour shift, sometimes with recreational activities___

Standing required for lifestyle _Stands almost entirety of waking hours_____

Current lifestyle limitations _Discomfort to minor pain at work, has curtailed recreational activities_____

Medications _Zoloft, Xanax, Prazosin_____

Past Medical History _Recurrent leg ulcers, anxiety, HTN_____

Previous treatment for condition _W/P, wet-to-dry dressings_____

Review of Systems

Neuromuscular	WNL
Musculoskeletal	WNL
Cardiopulmonary	BP: 130/90, dilated, tortuous superficial leg veins in both legs
Integumentary	Wound on medial, distal right leg, skin changes documented below

Physical Examination

Wound photo or drawing here:

10.2 cm

6.4 cm

Color _red_____ Odor _Ø___ Drainage _copious serous__ Extent _see diagram, full-thickness_____

Shape _irregular___ Tissue in wound: Black _0%_ Yellow _10%_ Red _90%_

Surrounding skin:

Texture _flaky__ Temperature _33.5° C_ Swelling: - + ++ (+++) ++++

Color _brown/yellow_ Hair/nails _WNL_ Ecchymosis _wound edges_ Hemosiderin ✓_

Demarcation _poor_____ Maceration _✓__ Epiboly _Ø_

Diagnosis   Impaired integumentary integrity with:

✓ Risk of injury   __ Superficial injury

__ Partial-thickness injury ✓ Full-thickness injury

__ Full-thickness injury and subcutaneous involvement

Prognosis   Within _3_ days weeks (months) and within _20_ visits, the patient is expected to:

Demonstrate preventive care, have full wound closure

Plan of Care

Patient and family/caregiver education _Causes and care for venous ulcers including self-performance of compression therapy___

Procedural interventions _debridement_____	frequency _3-5 days_	duration _3 weeks_
compression bandaging	frequency _3-5 days_	duration _3 months_
Pt will be fit for custom stockings when leg volume normalizes	frequency _once_____	duration _1 visit___

Signature ___Linda Smith, PT_____   Date_7/4/01_____

Figure 21-8. Example of a generic integumentary documentation form. The forms have been designed to reduce redundancy as much as possible without sacrificing the "at a view" features of the forms.

SUPPLEMENTAL DATA FORM FOR DIAGNOSIS OF VENOUS ULCERS

Patient __Stan Jones_____   Clinician __Linda Smith_____   Date __7/4/01_____

Alternatives to standing __Store manager has agreed to allow pt to rotate between cashier work and stocking__

Location(s) __R medial leg, just proximal to medial malleolus_____

Status of surrounding skin __Hemosiderin staining, flaking, and weeping_____

Size of wound(s):   Length __10.2__ cm Width __6.4__ cm Depth partial-thickness (full-thickness)

Ankle brachial index   Right __1.1__   Left __1.0__

Temperature of right foot   (normal)   increased   decreased

Temperature of left foot   (normal)   increased   decreased

Capillary refill (right)   (normal)   sluggish   absent

Capillary refill (left)   (normal)   sluggish   absent

Foot volume   right __1480__   left __1320__

Wound bed   % red __90__   % yellow __10__   % black __0__

Color of granulation tissue   (red)   pink

Drainage   minimal   moderate   (copious)

Color of drainage   __clear_____

Compression therapy (specify) __4-layer compression bandaging prn, estimate 3 to 5 days between changes ini-__
__tially; fit for custom stocking when volume normalizes_____

Signature_____*Linda Smith, PT*_____   Date ___*7/4/01*_____

Figure 21-9. Example of the venous ulcer form. This form is used if the patient is determined to have venous ulcerations. It is designed to eliminate lengthy descriptions and features components pertinent only to venous ulcers, including preventive measures and treatment specific to venous ulcers. In this example, the location of the wound proximal to the medial malleolus and condition of the surrounding skin are both consistent with venous ulcers. The next items are used to rule out arterial insufficiency. In this patient's case, we can see a normal ankle-brachial index, normal foot temperature, and normal capillary refill so we can assume that compression therapy is appropriate for this patient. Using a foot volumeter to quantify swelling of the lower extremities, clearly the right lower extremity is swollen. As detailed in the generic form, no edema had been observed in the left lower extremity but venous engorgement has. This is a clear sign that the left lower extremity is at risk and the patient should be fitted with a custom stocking if feasible or use one of several alternatives discussed in Chapter 10 to reduce the risk of venous ulcers of the left leg. Note the blank for color of granulation tissue. This is another check for arterial insufficiency. Beefy, red granulation tissue, as in this example, indicates normal arterial inflow to the wound. Pink granulation tissue, on the other hand, is indicative of diminished arterial supply to the wound. Copious drainage is also consistent with uncontrolled venous pressure, although a recent dressing change could deceive the clinician. The clinician must ascertain when the current dressing was applied to estimate the degree of drainage. The last line is complementary to the treatment plan on the generic form. Because of the establishment of venous hypertension as the underlying cause of the wound, the specific form of compression therapy, rather than other forms of intervention described on the generic form, is specified on the supplemental venous ulcer form.

SUPPLEMENTAL DATA FORM FOR PRESSURE ULCERS

Patient __Tom Gray_____ Clinician __Jack Wilson_____ Date __9/30/01____

Stage of ulcer (identify location on figure at right with wound number)

1.	I	II	III	(IV)	partially filled	filled	covered
2.	I	II	III	(IV)	partially filled	filled	covered
3.	I	(II)	III	IV	partially filled	filled	covered
4.	I	II	III	IV	partially filled	filled	covered
5.	I	II	III	IV	partially filled	filled	covered

Size of ulcer (using identification key on right)

1.	Length _5.0_ cm	Width _3.5_ cm	Depth _6.2_ cm
2.	Length _4.6_ cm	Width _3.0_ cm	Depth _1.0_ cm
3.	Length _2.1_ cm	Width _1.7_ cm	Depth _N/A_ cm
4.	Length _____ cm	Width _____ cm	Depth _____ cm
5.	Length _____ cm	Width _____ cm	Depth _____ cm

Tunneling, sinus tracts, undermining

1.	Distance _2.0_ cm	Direction _12_ :00	Drainage _purulent_
2.	Distance _2.8_ cm	Direction _1_ :00	Drainage _gray_
3.	Distance _____ cm	Direction _____ :00	Drainage _____
4.	Distance _____ cm	Direction _____ :00	Drainage _____
5.	Distance _____ cm	Direction _____ :00	Drainage _____

	1	2	3	4	5
Odor	foul	slight	N/A		
Drainage	purulent	min, serosang	N/A		
% R, Y, B	10, 50, 40	10, 80, 10	N/A		
Surrounding skin condition	inflamed	inflamed	WNL		

Signature____Jack Wilson, RN, WOCN_____ Date__9/30/01_____

Figure 21-10. Example of the pressure ulcer form. This is a relatively simple form that takes into account the frequent multiplicity of pressure ulcers. Space for information for five ulcers is available. In the first section, the stage of the ulcer by the National Pressure Ulcer Advisory Panel (NPUAP) (discussed in Chapter 9) and how much healing has occurred are documented.

Case #2, Supplemental Data Form for Pressure Ulcers

The patient described in Figure 21-10 had three ulcers in very common locations and common stages for these locations. The wounds at the left greater trochanter and sacrum had been monitored but not aggressively treated before referral due to the patient's general poor health. Because bone was visible in both, the staging was very straightforward. The epidermis covering the medial epicondyle of the left elbow had been denuded with some injury into the dermis. The elbow ulcer was, therefore, a stage II. This patient was fairly emaciated and fortunate to have only these three ulcerations. This woman had severe contractures of both hips and knees and severely altered mental status. Due to the patient's history and armed with the knowledge of the mechanism of pressure ulcers, the trochanteric and sacral wounds were probed for undermining and tunneling. The undermining would have been drawn on the generic form, and the supplemental form would indicate the size, direction, and drainage with the undermined areas. Both the undermined area and the visible area of the trochanteric ulcer were purulent. Thus, the patient was brought into the hospital for sharp debridement, although the decision had to be made for the patient due to her altered mental status. The sacral wound, on the other hand, was less problematic and the decision was made to treat this wound as well. The sacral wound needed cleaning, as it was filled with old, grayish, necrotic tissue. This residual necrotic tissue was likely the cause of the continued inflammation. The elbow wound was simply cleaned and protected.

SUPPLEMENTAL FORM FOR THERMAL INJURY

Patient __Ray Ator_____   Clinician __Lauren Greene_____   Date __5/5/01_____

Indicate locations and depths of thermal injuries on figure to the left
- - Superficial thickness (1st degree)
//// Superficial partial thickness (2nd degree)
\\\ Deep partial thickness (deep dermal)
XXX Full thickness (3rd degree)

	RUE	LUE	RLE	LLE	Anterior trunk	Posterior trunk
Deficits in range of motion	Ø	✓ all	Ø	Ø	cerv ext	Ø
Deficits in strength	Ø	✓ all	Ø	Ø	Ø	Ø

Appropriate type of exercise

	RUE	LUE	RLE	LLE		
Active exercise	✓	✓	✓	✓	✓	✓
Active assisted exercise						
Passive stretch						
No movement allowed						

Deficits in tolerance for bed mobility, bed exercise, position changes, ambulation (specify) _Guarded, but functional secondary to left upper extremity and neck pain_____

Indicate special positioning needs _Cervical extension, left shoulder abduction and extension_____

Signature_____ _Lauren Greene, OT_____   Date___ _5/5/01_____

Figure 21-11. Example of the thermal injury form.

Case #3, Supplemental Form for Thermal Injury

The patient described in Figure 21-11 received a scald injury from opening the radiator cap after his car overheated. He used a rag to open the radiator cap, thereby avoiding injury to his left hand. The sleeveless undershirt he was wearing protected most of his chest from injury, but exposed his axilla and neck. Although these are critical injuries for functional activity, the depth of injury was superficial and he healed nicely in 2 weeks, regained full function, and returned to work in 3 weeks. Generally speaking, full-thickness injuries are much more likely to result in contractures than partial-thickness injuries. However, superficial partial-thickness injuries are very painful, and the patient could only tolerate small areas of debridement at a time, even with opioid analgesia. The deficits observed in range of motion were due to pain with movement rather than injury to the skin. The patient was encouraged to perform left upper extremity and cervical range of motion exercises. He was only admitted overnight but was seen daily as an outpatient after his discharge. The patient was instructed to maintain his head in extension and alternate between full and 90 degrees of shoulder abduction to prevent taking the neck off stretch.

SUPPLEMENTAL FORM FOR NEUROPATHIC ULCERS

Patient___Brad Smith_____   Clinician___Jim Brown_____   Date__12/7/01__

Location(s): Indicate location of wounds on figure below and create numeric key if multiple wounds

Wound #	1	2	3	4	5
Wagner grade	3				
Size	5.0 cm x 3cm				
% red	90				
% yellow	10				
% black	0				

Indicate location of callus on the diagram below with the symbol /////

Reflexes: AJ right   present   diminished   (absent)   AJ left   present   diminished   (absent)

Foot deformities (specify)___Hammer toes bilaterally_____

Gait deviations (specify)____Nonambulatory_____

Pulse (right)   4   3   2   (1)   0   (specify artery palpated)__DP_____

Pulse (left)   4   3   2   (1)   0   (specify artery palpated)__DP_____

Capillary refill (right)   normal   (sluggish)   absent

Capillary refill (left)   normal   (sluggish)   absent

Ankle brachial index   right__0.5_____   left_0.6_____

Right foot temperature   normal   (decreased)   increased _30.4° C_

Left foot temperature   normal   (decreased)   increased _30.2° C_

Sensory testing (indicate on the diagram below + for intact, +/- for diminished, - for absent

Left foot   Right foot

Dorsal   Plantar   Plantar   Dorsal

Signature__Jim Brown, DPT, CWS_____   Date__12/7/01_____

Figure 21-12. Example of the neuropathic ulcer form.

Case #4, Supplemental Form for Neuropathic Ulcers

The patient described in Figure 21-12 had no sensation on either lower extremity below the knee and eventually required bilateral amputations. The patient had not been ambulatory and was in general poor health, including kidney failure, for which he was receiving hemodialysis. On the generic form, multiple ulcerations including a previous ray amputation on the other foot would have been noted. On this admission, he had osteomyelitis of the second metatarsal, which eventually was amputated. The color of the tissue within the wound was pink instead of red due to his arterial insufficiency, which coexisted with his neuropathy. He had no reflexes, no intrinsic muscle strength (which produced hammer toes), and a weak pulse bilaterally. Moreover, the suspicion of arterial insufficiency was confirmed with the low ankle brachial index, decreased foot temperature, and as would be noted on the generic form, thickened toenails bilaterally. Wound management in this case was limited to preparation of the wound for delayed primary closure following the amputation. This included twice a day W/P and packing with saline-moistened gauze until the surgeon deemed the site ready for closure.

physical examination, and the combined information is assessed by the clinician to develop a diagnosis and prognosis. The diagnosis and prognosis, in turn, guide the plan of care. The plan of care includes patient education and direct interventions. The direct interventions specified in the plan of care follow four hierarchical decision points: infection, debridement, subcutaneous tissue loss, and drainage. The inability of the patient to adhere to the plan of care requires modification of either patient education, direct intervention, or consultation with a social worker to manage resources to allow the patient to adhere to the plan of care. The patient's lifestyle, work, school, and play also need to be accommodated in the plan of care.

STUDY QUESTIONS

1. Why is documentation critical to a good outcome?
2. What is the role of documenting history? How is this important with multiple clinicians working with the same patient?
3. How is physical examination related to history? Explain how the physical examination might differ between a case with an obvious diagnosis and one without a clear diagnosis.
4. Contrast the subjective part of a SOAP note to the history and the objective part to the physical examination.
5. Explain the order of precedence of infection, debridement, subcutaneous tissue loss, and drainage in developing a plan of care.

REFERENCE

1. American Physical Therapy Association. Guide to physical therapist practice. *Physical Therapy.* 1997;77:1177-1619.
2. Classen NS. The basics of medical photography. *Acute Care Perspectives.* 2000;8(2):7-11.

Administrative Concerns

OBJECTIVES

- Discuss Medicare and typical state licensing regulations relevant to wound management.
- Describe how to build a team to optimize wound management.
- Discuss issues related to reimbursement for wound management services.

The issues discussed in this chapter, however contentious and subject to rapid and dramatic change, are important to understand to have a successful practice so that our patients/clients can benefit from the evaluation and direct interventions discussed earlier. Unfortunately, a detailed description of what is optimal or even allowable in terms of reimbursement is likely to be outdated before many readers use this text. Because federal legislation and rules dictated by government agencies such as the Centers for Medicare and Medicaid Services (CMS), prudence dictates that each facility have an individual responsible for analysis of the multitude of health care rules and regulations that may have an impact on reimbursement. Depending on the case mix of individual facilities, these issues may require adjustments of staffing. An attempt will be made to discuss general principles that are unlikely to change in the near future.

REGULATIONS

Appropriately trained and licensed individuals must perform the evaluations and interventions involved in wound management. In some cases, state laws may permit tremendous latitude in assigning personnel to direct patient care. Regardless of the letter of the law, ethical, moral, and risk management issues must be applied to staffing decisions. The potential risk of harm to a patient can never be justified by assigning direct patient care to individuals lacking appropriate training or licensing. Moreover, fee schedules are based on the use of appropriate personnel; therefore, billing for direct patient care provided by an individual lacking the training specified by Medicare requirements could be ruled Medicare fraud with severe consequences.[1]

Medicare regulations, in theory, should apply equally across the United States. The reality of the situation, however, is that the intermediary is often placed in the role of interpreting Medicare regulations. Although only a small number of insurance companies serve the role of Medicare intermediary, staff in different states may have different interpretations of a given Medicare rule, and within a given intermediary different personnel are likely to have different interpretations. This situation is exacerbated by high turnover rates in many states. Individuals working for the intermediary can be educated to understand the role of different interventions for various characteristics of a patient, but the loss of that employee forces the clinician to educate another employee of the intermediary. CMS periodically distributes explicit instructions to intermediaries on certain issues in an attempt to contain costs and improve uniformity.

Medicare payment for sharp debridement is reserved for physical therapists, podiatrists, physicians, and advanced practice nurses with specialized training. Payment under other plans or as part of a diagnosis-related group (DRG) may allow others to perform sharp debridement.

State licensing requirements generally become an issue on two points. First, does the patient have direct access to your services or must the patient be referred, usually through a family practitioner or other medical specialist? The second concern is how the state practice act for the different providers are written in terms of debridement. In Arkansas as of 2000, patients must be referred for wound care and bronchopulmonary hygiene provided by a physical therapist but have direct access to other physical therapy services, and the state practice act for physical therapists makes no direct mention of sharp debridement. Individuals in each state need to determine current regulations for referral and sharp debridement.

REIMBURSEMENT ISSUES

Payments for direct interventions generally include charges for evaluation, debridement, electrical stimulation, and dressing materials but not labor for dressing changes.[2] The American Medical Association (AMA), working with CMS, has developed a coding system for billing for services, termed common procedure terminology (CPT). HCPCS (CMS Common Procedure Coding System) codes for supplies and equipment; temporary or unusual situations are established by CMS itself. Three levels of codes are in existence as of this writing. Level I includes the CPT codes, written by an AMA committee to aid in the administration of Medicare. Level II represents codes developed by CMS itself either on a temporary basis or to handle durable medical equipment (eg, specialty beds or surgical supplies such as wound dressings and compression bandages). Level III is developed to handle unique situations.

The original philosophy for CPT codes was that payment would be based on the service provided, rather than the provider. However, this philosophy has changed first with the codes for evaluation, which are now provider-dependent. Until 2000, debridement codes existed only under the surgical section of the codes. Sharp debridement could be paid under one of the surgical codes 11040-11044 by some intermediaries, but others would not. The major problem with reimbursement under the surgical codes was the cost determined for reimbursing debridement as a surgical procedure and the absence of a code that reflected the lower cost of providing sharp debridement in a nonsurgical environment. In the revisions for 2000, a new HCPCS code, G0169, removal of devitalized tissue without use of anesthesia, was developed to allow appropriate reimbursement for sharp debridement in a setting other than the operating room.

Two new codes were designed for 2001 to replace the temporary code, allowing coding for debridement and related activities in a lower cost environment than surgical debridement by a physician. CPT code 97601 is stated to be for removal of devitalized tissue from wounds by selective debridement without anesthesia. However, specific examples given in the description include pulsatile lavage; selective sharp debridement with scissors, scalpel, and forceps, including topical application(s); wound assessment; and instruction(s) for ongoing care per session. Note that time is immaterial. Moreover, an evaluative component is expected with each session. CPT code 97602 is meant to cover lower cost visits. This code was necessary to allow clinicians other than physicians to re-evaluate wounds on an ongoing basis. Specifically, this code addresses nonselective debridement without anesthesia with specific examples of wet-to-moist dressings, enzymatic debridement, and abrasion and includes application of topical medications, wound assessment, and instructions for ongoing care. Previous to the institution of this code, clinicians such as physical therapists would need to turn care over to another discipline because no reimbursement was available for skilled follow-up care. At the time of this writing, however, no value has been assigned to this code.

Although dressing changes themselves are not billable, dressing materials as well as chemical debriders are billed under the appropriate HCPCS code. Under Medicare Part B, surgical/wound dressings, both primary and secondary are covered under specific criteria: the dressings are medically necessary for the treatment of a wound caused by or treated by a surgical procedure, or when debridement of a wound is medically necessary.[3] Surgical procedures or debridement must be carried out by a licensed health care practitioner under appropriate state law. Surgical dressings can only be ordered by physicians, nurse practitioners, clinical nurse specialists, certified nurse-midwives, or physician's assistants. To be eligible for reimbursement, any type of debridement—sharp, mechanical, chemical, or autolytic—is permissible. No specific time limit is placed on reimbursement. Dressings are not covered for stage I pressure ulcers or first-degree (superficial) burns. No payment is given for skin sealants or barriers, skin cleansers or irrigating solutions, solutions used to moisten gauze, topical antiseptics and topical antibiotics, or enzymatic debriding agents.

Orders must be signed by a health care practitioner with the type of dressing, size, number used each time, frequency of dressing change, and expected duration. New orders are required if a new dressing is added and if the quantity increases. A new order is also required every 3 months for each dressing used. DMERC (durable medical equipment regional carrier) regulations provide for utilization guides; therefore, the frequency of dressing change should match these guidelines when ordered. The guide-

lines are listed in Table 15-4. Consult your DMERC for current guidelines.

MEDICARE DOCUMENTATION REQUIREMENTS

In certain environments, provision of wound care by physical therapists is preferred for economic reasons. Under some guidelines, visits by a nurse are reimbursed at a given rate, regardless of the interventions provided during the visit; whereas under the same conditions, the services provided by a physical therapist are reimbursed. However, interventions must also be chosen prudently. In certain settings, the number of billable units may be limited by classification into categories such as resource utilization groups (RUGs). Time-intensive interventions such as hydrotherapy may not be deemed appropriate. In certain cases, sharp, enzymatic, or autolytic debridement may be necessary because of the classification of a given patient and the number of units of physical therapy allowable for that category.

INDICATIONS AND LIMITATIONS OF COVERAGE AND/OR MEDICAL NECESSITY

According to Medicare standards:[4]

The service of a physical, speech-language pathologist or occupational therapist is a skilled therapy service if the inherent complexity of the service is such that it can be performed safely and/or effectively only by or under the general supervision of a skilled therapist. To be covered, the skilled services must also be reasonable and necessary to the treatment of the patient's illness or injury. It is necessary to determine whether individual therapy services are skilled and whether, in view of the patient's overall condition, skilled management of the services provided is needed although many or all of the specific services needed to treat the illness or injury do not require the skills of a therapist.

The development, implementation management and evaluation of a patient care plan based on the physician's orders constitute skilled therapy services when, because of the patient's condition, those activities require the involvement of a skilled therapist to meet the patient's needs, promote recovery and ensure medical safety. Where the skills of a therapist are needed to manage and periodically reevaluate the appropriateness of a maintenance program because of an identified danger to the patient, such services would be covered even if the skills of a therapist are not needed to carry out the activities performed as part of the maintenance program.

The criteria for reasonable and necessary services are given by Medicare as:[4]

- *The services must be consistent with the nature and severity of the illness or injury, the patient's particular medical needs, including the requirement that the amount, frequency, and duration of the services must be reasonable.*

- *The services must be considered, under accepted standards of medical practice, to be specific, safe, and effective treatment for the patient's condition.*

- *The services must be provided with the expectation, based on the assessment made by the physician of the patient's rehabilitation potential, that:*
  - *The condition of the patient will improve materially in a reasonable and generally predictable period of time; or*
  - *The services are necessary to the establishment of a safe and effective maintenance program.*

Services involving activities for the general welfare of any patient, (eg, general exercises to promote overall fitness or flexibility and activities to provide diversion or general motivation, do not constitute skilled therapy. Those services can be performed by nonskilled individuals without the supervision of a therapist).

- *Services of skilled therapists for the purpose of teaching the patient, family, or caregivers necessary techniques, exercises, or precautions are covered to the extent that they are reasonable and necessary to treat illness or injury. However, visits made by skilled therapists to a patient's home solely to train other HHA staff (eg, home health aides) are not billable as visits since the HHA is responsible for ensuring that its staff is properly trained to perform any service it furnishes. The cost of a skilled therapist's visit for the purpose of training HHA staff is an administrative cost to the agency.*

Based on these guidelines, three key items are needed in Medicare documentation: medical necessity (as this term is applied to physical therapy), progress, and progress relative to the resources used to satisfy Medicare requirements. The first item to document is whether the patient's condition justifies the level of care given. The patient's condition(s), including any complicating factors that weigh in the choice of intervention, should be included. In addition to documenting the need, the documentation should support the intervention(s) based on what is likely to occur if the intervention is not done, that the appropriate person is carrying out the intervention and the likelihood of the intervention being successful. For example, a necrotic wound that is either infected or at risk for infection justifies the intervention of sharp debridement by a physical therapist, advanced practice nurse, podiatrist, or physician. The risks of spreading infection, failure to heal, and possible amputation should also be discussed. Moreover, if more frequent outpatient visits are needed due to limited ability of the patient or patient's caregivers to care for the wound, documentation should be provided to support the great number of visits. Addition of modalities such as ultrasound or electrical stimulation needs to be supported by documented lack of healing despite appropriate wound management.

The second point is how well the patient is responding to the intervention. Patient response to treatment needs to be described in progress reports, as opposed to the initial evaluation. A brief mention that the patient is responding well to treatment is not sufficient. The documented progress should be related directly to the desired outcomes or goals listed on the initial evaluation. The documentation should indicate objective measures of improvement including the removal of necrotic tissue, appearance of the wound bed, drainage, and wound dimensions. Descriptions indicating improved healing or potential for healing such as improvement of the surrounding skin may be necessary. Simple wound measurements may not be sufficient to capture the true improvement in a wound's condition, especially early in the treatment plan, as wounds may actually increase in size with debridement.

The third point is whether the resources used are appropriate for the progress observed. If the treatment plan fails to produce progress, an explanation of why this happened and steps to overcome impediments, including a change in treatment plan need to be documented. For example, if the patient is unable or unwilling to perform required dressing changes or compression therapy, a brief narrative explaining complications and defining a new course needs to be written.

COST-EFFECTIVENESS

This topic is often uncomfortable for clinicians and a seemingly endless battleground between clinicians and administrators. Several studies have indicated, however, that optimal wound care is often more cost-effective than lower cost alternative. For example, Table 4 of the Bolton study[5] shows a range of 53% to 615% greater costs of care to use gauze dressings on various types of ulcers compared to clinically more prudent choices of hydrocolloid dressings. Frequently, the argument for a given type of intervention is based on the cost of materials and not the cost of labor or the likelihood of attaining goals set for the intervention. In particular, the cost of a single application of gauze is much less than a hydrocolloid sheet. The cost of applying gauze to a wound three to four times daily for 5 days is much greater than the single application of a hydrocolloid sheet. Even the cost of the materials can become much greater depending on the number of dressing changes and the quantity of gauze necessary. Several clinical trials are cited by Bolton et al and will not be repeated here.[5]

The larger picture of direct and indirect costs of wound care need to be analyzed for the different possible options. Direct costs include the materials for primary and secondary dressings; materials used for wound cleansing; debridement and dressing change such as bottles of saline; additional gauze, gloves, gowns, masks, shoe covers, tape, and labor involved in these activities including cost of set-up and cleaning, especially when considering whirlpool therapy. Large quantities of water, cost of filling tanks, disinfecting tanks, and quality checks on infection control can become very high relative to other aspects of wound management. Other equipment may include pressure relief/reducing devices, operating room time, surgical procedures, and pharmacy.

Indirect costs need to also be considered. The choice of an alternative with a lower direct cost may drive up indirect costs of a treatment plan to the point that total costs are much greater. These potential indirect costs include prolonged treatment (increased inpatient days, increased home health, or outpatient visits), loss of days of work by the patient, treatment of complications of slower healing, costs of waste disposal driven higher by more frequent dressing changes, and the potential for litigation if a suboptimal plan is followed.

One common example is the comparison of whirlpool therapy to pulsatile lavage with concurrent suction. Although the materials for pulsatile lavage are greater than whirlpool, the much greater cost in clinician's time and possibly slower achievement of the same outcome can make whirlpool therapy much more expensive. Another example is the provision of sharp debridement. One visit for sharp debridement may be more expensive than a single visit for hydrotherapy for debridement, but the faster outcome from sharp debridement can make the cost per outcome achieved much lower for selective sharp debridement compared with serial instrumental debridement using hydrotherapy and either disposable or resterilizable instruments to remove small amounts of necrotic tissue over the course of several days.

Although each clinical unit must make its own decisions regarding cost-effectiveness of treatments, the issues of quality of life must be taken into account along with the more typical issues of decreased wound size, pain relief, debridement, and risk or frequency of infection.

WOUND MANAGEMENT TEAMS

Successful management of patients with wounds, especially those managed by DRGs, require coordination, communication, and cooperation. Teams in an acute care facility typically consist of a physician, physical therapist, clinical dietician, wound ostomy continence nurse (WOCN), and some facilities may also include occupational therapists or other personnel. Each individual on the team plays an important role due to the unique training of the individual within his or her discipline and the individual's experience.[5] The key to success is to determine ahead of time what responsibilities each individual on the team will have. Waiting until the program is underway to assign responsibilities is likely to create hard feelings within the group, perhaps creating a siege mentality and dividing the group. Members need to clearly elaborate what their individual skills are and with what patient populations the individual clinician is familiar. Flow charts designed from this information allow each clinician on the team to determine the next step in the sequence and to refer, when necessary, to a different discipline.

A common pitfall is the assumption of hierarchical knowledge within the team. One individual is unlikely to have all of the knowledge, skills, and abilities (KSA) of the other clinicians. Instead, these could be viewed better as a Venn diagram in which the sum of knowledge about wound management is represented by a circle for each clinician of different disciplines. Certain types of clinicians would display nearly complete overlap of KSA, whereas others might have very little overlap. The hope in developing a team is that each clinician can identify another member of the team with the appropriate KSA for each situation so that any patient would receive all of the necessary evaluations, education, and direct interventions leading to optimal care. KSA can also be viewed as a spectral distribution in which KSA are plotted as graphs. Any given individual clinician on the team would be expected to be high on some KSA and low on others and when the spectral distribution of KSA for the entire team is viewed, a maximum level is reached for all KSA. The planning of the team is then to distribute tasks to the team member with a high level for the KSA of interest.

Every team requires a leader to be functional. Many ways are available to assemble a wound management team. Many automatically assume that the team leader must be a physician. The choice should not be made based on titles alone. In many clinics, the team leader is a physical therapist, nurse, or dietician. The best choice for a team leader is the person who has the desire and skills to lead a team and the respect of the other team members. This person is most likely the person who recognizes how to weed out inefficiency and improve patient satisfaction. A preliminary team representing typical disciplines needs to be assembled, and the perceived roles of members of each discipline need to be shared with the other members. It is often shocking how little members of one discipline understand about the training and experience of other members. "I didn't know you did that!" is a common response to this exercise. Preliminary flow charts identifying what each member will do need to be designed by a small number of members of the team and submitted for approval by the team as a whole. Attempts to design flow charts by the entire team are unlikely to be fruitful. A subgroup of more than four to five individuals is likely to bog down the details, whereas a group smaller than three is likely to miss details. Sharing the work of the subgroup is used to improve the product. Turf battles may still arise; therefore, one of the first agenda items on such committees is a series of team building exercises and establishment of rules of conduct for the meetings. Agreeing to a consensus process as opposed to a majority process may improve the workings of the group as well. In addition, the presence of too many or too few members from a given discipline can create an unhealthy environment. The development of cliques needs to be avoided as well. A perception of "ganging up" will quickly destroy objectivity and undermine any trust built within the group.

Meetings of the committee need to be scheduled regularly with an optimal interval. Often, weekly meetings are used. This time allows individual work to be accomplished between meetings and meaningful reflection to occur. Longer intervals cause members to lose focus and other events to take precedence over the work of the committee.

In any environment, but especially in a DRG environment such as acute care hospitals in which the length of stay may be determined by the effectiveness of the team, cost effectiveness of the team is important. Generally, the DRG environment encourages facilities to discharge patients as rapidly as possible, which may require continued care following discharge. Often, this care takes the form of home health, outpatient physical therapy, or inpatient rehabilitation. Formerly, a patient may have been allowed to stay in an acute care hospital until a wound was completely or nearly completely healed. In many cases this care consisted of BID whirlpool and wet-to-dry dressing changes. More rapid discharge may be accomplished, however, by aggressive sharp debridement or use of pulsatile lavage with concurrent suction to achieve a clean, stable wound that can either be taken over by a surgeon for surgical closure or grafting, or managed with occlusive dressings in a low-cost environment including self-management, home health, outpatient, or inpatient rehabilitation.

Outpatient or home health wound management should be done at regular intervals depending on the risk. The clinician should not rigidly set an interval for follow-up, but should remain flexible. A likely scenario is progressive lengthening as the risk of infection lessens, drainage decreases with diminished wound handling, and the wound begins to heal rapidly. As discussed in Chapter 20, interventions, especially choice of dressing, are selected to allow the appropriate interval of follow-up. Initially, however, the interval may need to be flexible to accommodate variation in the anticipated response to the interventions.

REFERENCES

1. LePostollec M. Making the case for wound care reimbursement. *Advance for Physical Therapists & PT Assistants.* 2000;11(20):8-10

2. Health Care Financing Administration. Your Medicare Handbook 1997: Part A Coverage. Available at: *http://www.hcfa.gov/pubforms/mhbkc02.htm.*

3. Health Care Financing Administration. Your Medicare Handbook 1997: Part B Coverage. Available at: *http://www.hcfa.gov/pubforms/mhbkc03.htm.*

4. Medicare Home Health Agency Manual HCFA Pub. 11 Available at: *http://www.hcfa.gov/pubforms/progman.htm.*

5. Bolton LL, van Rijswijk L, Shaffer FA. Quality wound care equals cost-effective wound care: a clinical model. *Advances in Wound Care.* 1997;10:33-38.

Color Atlas

Selected figures from this text are reproduced in color on the following pages to further benefit our readers' understanding of the material. Please cross-reference these figures with the noted pages for more detail on the content of each image.

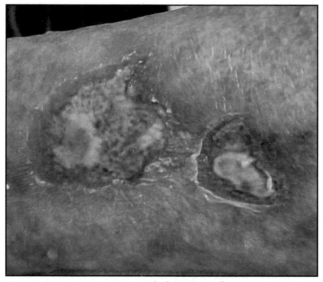

Figure 3-1. Appearance of chronic inflammation. Note the cardinal signs of inflammation in the surrounding skin: redness, swelling, and edema. Also note the presence of necrotic tissue within the wound bed. *(Also shown on page 22.)*

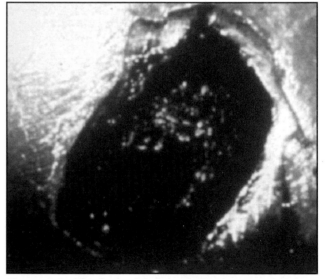

Figure 3-2. The lack of inflammation in a wound covered with black eschar. Also note the desiccation of the surrounding skin. Lack of inflammation prevents the proliferation of epidermal cells and fibroblasts necessary to close this wound. Courtesy of Little Rock Veteran's Administration Hospital. *(Also shown on page 23.)*

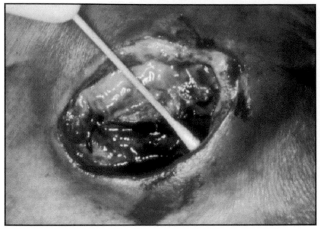

Figure 3-3a. Subcutaneous tissue defects. Undermining is an area of subcutaneous tissue loss beneath the wound edge, as demonstrated by the cotton-tipped applicator, usually in the form of an arc. Also note the presence of rolled edges, known as epiboly. The rolling under the edge prevents closure of the wound. Courtesy of Little Rock Veteran's Administration Hospital. (*Also shown on page 23.*)

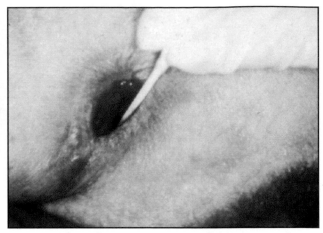

Figure 3-3b. Subcutaneous tissue defects. Tunneling is demonstrated with a cotton-tipped applicator as a linear subcutaneous defect. Courtesy of Little Rock Veteran's Administration Hospital. (*Also shown on page 24.*)

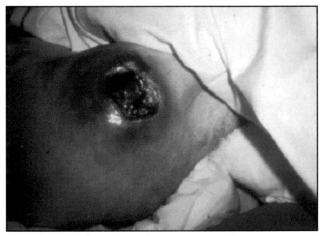

Figure 3-4. Infected trochanteric wound. As compared to the wound in Figure 3-1, inflammation greatly exceeds the edges of the wound and profound edema is present. Also note the presence of necrotic tissue and the emaciated condition of the patient. Courtesy of Little Rock Veteran's Administration Hospital. (*Also shown on page 24.*)

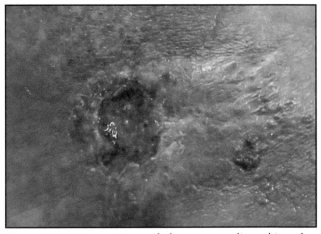

Figure 3-6. Maceration of the surrounding skin of a wound. Note the swollen, bleached out, and very wet appearance of the wound. (*Also shown on page 25.*)

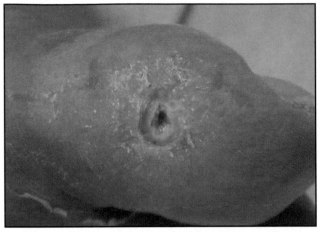

Figure 3-7. Desiccated wound of the great toe of a neuropathic foot. Also note the dryness of the surrounding skin and large margin of callus surrounding the wound, which is characteristic of neuropathic ulcers. (*Also shown on page 25.*)

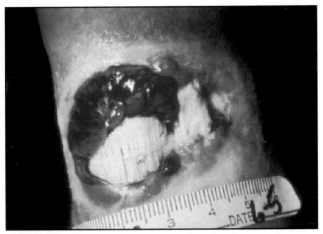

Figure 3-8. Hypergranulation of a tibial wound. Note the maceration of the surrounding skin, the height of the granulation tissue above the surrounding skin, bleeding of the granulation tissue, and the appearance of the tendon in the wound. Courtesy of Little Rock Veteran's Administration Hospital. (*Also shown on page 26.*)

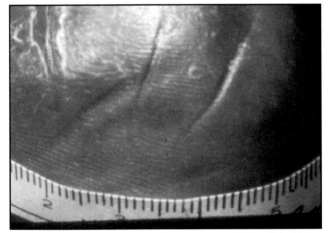

Figure 3-9. Subcutaneous hematoma of the heel. The clinician cannot determine the extent of subcutaneous necrosis in this case. Several authorities have suggested protecting this type of wound as long as it is stable. Courtesy of Little Rock Veteran's Administration Hospital. (*Also shown on page 26.*)

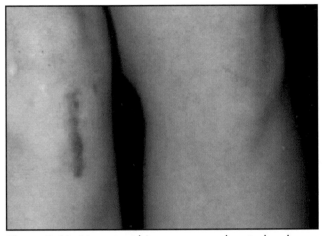

Figure 3-10. Hypertrophic scars secondary to hardware removal several months after arthroscopic surgery for anterior cruciate ligament repair. Note the presence of faint white resolved hypertrophic scars. (*Also shown on page 26.*)

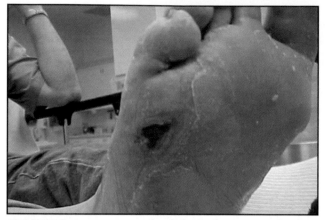

Figure 5-2. Appearance of a diabetic foot. Note the dryness of the skin and thickened nails. (*Also shown on page 41.*)

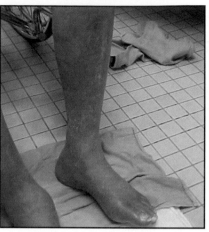

Figure 5-6. Rubor of dependency in an individual with arterial insufficiency. Note the ruddy color of the lower half of both legs; shiny, hairless skin; and the thickened, yellow toenails. (*Also shown on page 45.*)

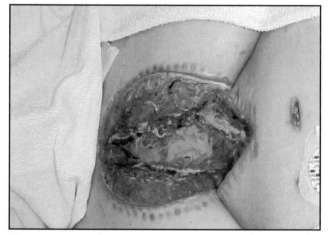

Figure 7-1. Dehiscent sternotomy wound. Note the degree of gapping and inflammation of the suture wounds. (*Also shown on page 62.*)

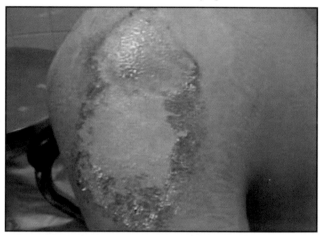

Figure 7-3. Abrasion ("road rash") on the left shoulder. Note the lack of pigmentation of the abraded skin and the darkening of the necrotic epidermis on the edges of the wound. (*Also shown on page 63.*)

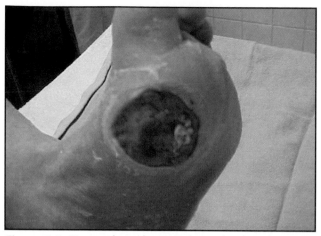

Figure 8-2. Deep ulcer characteristic of a Wagner grade 2 ulcer. Note the thick rim of callus around the wound and the pink, rather than red, color of the granulation tissue caused by concomitant arterial insufficiency. Also note the presence of hammer toes, which increase the shearing forces under the metatarsal heads during gait. (*Also shown on page 74.*)

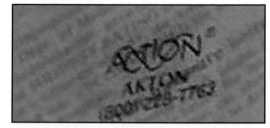

Figure 9-6a. Gel mattress overlay. (*Also shown on page 100.*)

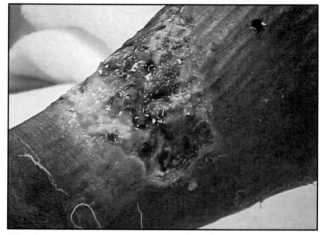

Figure 10-1a. Appearance of venous insufficiency ulcers. Note the irregular borders, location, copious drainage, and red granulation tissue. (*Also shown on page 113.*)

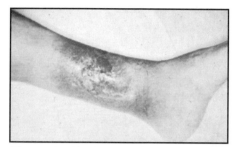

Figure 10-1b. Hemosiderin staining of the lower extremity, characteristic of venous insufficiency. Note, however, that hemosiderin localized to the margins of a wound may occur with wounds caused by mechanical trauma such as pressure ulcers and neuropathic ulcers. Courtesy of Little Rock Veteran's Administration Hospital. (*Also shown on page 113.*)

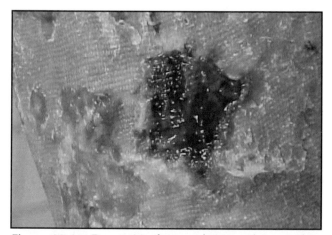

Figure 10-1c. Dermatitis, frequently termed "stasis dermatitis," characteristic of venous insufficiency. Note indentations of skin caused by the weave of the compression bandage. (*Also shown on page 113.*)

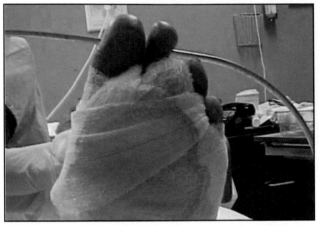

Figure 11-1. Red and green sanguinopurulent drainage of a diabetic foot infected with *Pseudomonas aeruginosa*. (*Also shown on page 127.*)

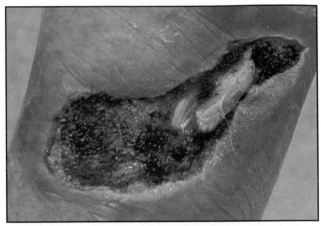

Figure 11-5a. Documenting tissue types. A dorsal foot wound with 100% granulation tissue. Note that much of the granulation tissue has a pink color, indicative of diminished arterial flow. Also note the presence of tendons within the wound bed. Tendons must not be confused with necrotic tissue. (*Also shown on page 129.*)

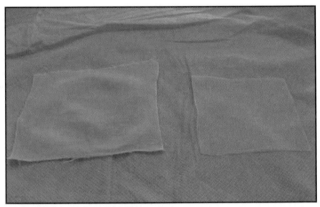

Figure 15-2. Examples of petrolatum gauze. (*Also shown on page 167.*)

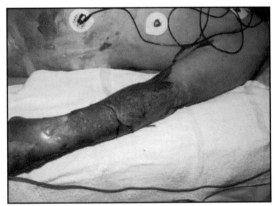

Figure 19-1. Partial-thickness burn caused by flames from an explosion. Courtesy of Arkansas Children's Hospital, Little Rock, Ark. (*Also shown on page 222.*)

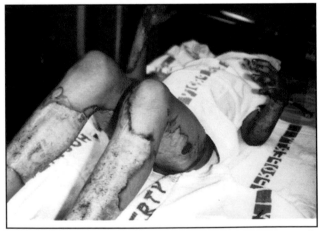

Figure 19-2. Deep partial-thickness burn injury with areas of full-thickness injury. Courtesy of Arkansas Children's Hospital, Little Rock, Ark. (*Also shown on page 222.*)

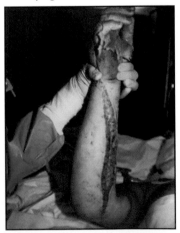

Figure 19-3. Escharotomy to relieve pressure within the forearm and distal arm. Courtesy of Arkansas Children's Hospital, Little Rock, Ark. (*Also shown on page 222.*)

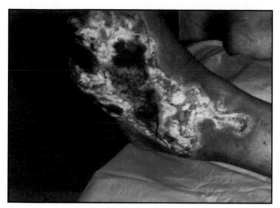

Figure 19-4a. Full-thickness burn caused by contact burn: before debridement. Courtesy of Arkansas Children's Hospital, Little Rock, Ark. (*Also shown on page 223.*)

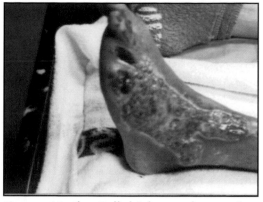

Figure 19-4b. Full-thickness burn after debridement. Note the loss of the fourth and fifth toes to the burn injury. Courtesy of Arkansas Children's Hospital, Little Rock, Ark. (*Also shown on page 223.*)

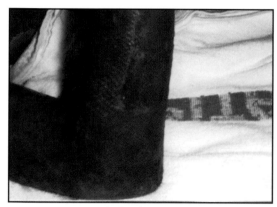

Figure 19-7. Healed split-thickness graft of the forearm and distal arm. (*Also shown on page 226.*)

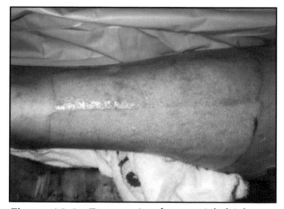

Figure 19-8. Donor site for partial-thickness grafting. Note healing, which will allow this area to be repeatedly harvested for partial-thickness grafting. (*Also shown on page 226.*)

Appendix

AHCPR Guidelines for Intervention

The stated purpose of the AHCPR in developing guidelines is the promotion of effective clinical practice. Although they were developed by a government agency, these guidelines fall short of standards of care. Their legal value lies mainly in any civil action in which a plaintiff may claim that the clinician failed to provide care at a level consistent with other clinicians. Other stated purposes include reducing the costs of care and promoting the scientific basis of clinical care.

An act of congress established AHCPR in 1989 as a part of the Public Health Service. The Office of Forum for Quality and Effectiveness in Health Care was developed to facilitate development and periodic review and updating of clinically-relevant guidelines that may be used by physicians, educators, and health care practitioners to assist in determining how diseases, disorders, and other health care conditions can most effectively and appropriately be prevented, diagnosed, treated, and managed clinically. A number of clinical problems were selected for study. Pressure ulcers were chosen because of their high prevalence and incidence of pressure ulcers in acute and long-term care and among certain populations such as quadriplegia, femoral fractures, and critical care, as well as their high financial cost.

The guidelines were developed by a multidisciplinary, private-sector panel consisting of physicians, nurses, an occupational therapist and a consumer representative. Physical therapists served as consultants, but not as panel members. Evidence was gathered from reviewing the literature, testimony of expert witnesses, and information from consultants. From this evidence, drafts for peer and pilot review were developed. The original intent was to recommend only specific interventions studied with controlled trials. However, some material had not been studied adequately to allow this strategy. Therefore, several recommendations in guidelines exist without trials. These recommendations are based on consultant experience. For each recommendation, a strength of evidence rating is attached.

STRENGTH OF EVIDENCE RATINGS

Each recommendation in the guidelines is given a strength of evidence rating of A, B or C. A rating of A is given if the recommendation is given based on the results of two or more randomized controlled clinical trials on pressure ulcers in humans. Only a few recommendations in the guidelines received this rating. For a recommendation to receive a rating of B, it must be based on the results of two or more controlled clinical trials on pressure ulcers in humans, or two or more controlled trials in an animal model. A rating of C is given based on one of three possibilities: the results of one controlled trial, results of at least two case series/descriptive studies on pressure ulcers in humans or expert opinion.

The target audience for whom the guidelines were developed include clinicians who examine and treat persons who have pressure ulcers, health care administrators, policy analysts and regulatory agencies, third party payers, and patients and families. As conceived, the guidelines were meant to be applicable to palliative as well as restorative care. The prevention guidelines, published in 1992 included recommendations in the following areas: risk assessment tools and risk factors, Skin Care and Early Treatment, Mechanical Loading and Support Surfaces, and Education.

RISK ASSESSMENT TOOLS AND RISK FACTORS

Bed- and chair-bound individuals or those with impaired ability to reposition should be assessed for additional factors that increase risk for developing pressure ulcers. These factors include immobility, incontinence, nutritional factors such as inadequate dietary intake and impaired nutritional status, and altered level of consciousness. Individuals should be assessed on admission to acute care and rehabilitation hospitals, nursing homes, home care programs, and other health care facilities. A systematic risk assessment can be accomplished by using a validated risk assessment tool such as the Braden Scale or Norton Scale. Pressure ulcer risk should be reassessed at periodic intervals. All assessments of risk should be documented.

SKIN CARE AND EARLY TREATMENT

Goal: Maintain and improve tissue tolerance to pressure in order to prevent injury
- All individuals at risk should have a systematic skin inspection at least once a day, paying particular attention to the bony prominences. Results of skin inspection should be documented.
- Skin cleansing should occur at the time of soiling and at routine intervals. The frequency of skin cleansing should be individualized according to need and/or patient preference. Avoid hot water, and use a mild cleansing agent that minimizes irritation and dryness of the skin. During the cleansing process, care should be utilized to minimize the force and friction applied to the skin.
- Minimize environmental factors leading to skin drying such as low humidity (<40%) and exposure to cold. Dry skin should be treated with moisturizers.
- Avoid massage over bony prominences.
- Minimize skin exposure to moisture due to incontinence, perspiration, or wound drainage. When these sources of moisture cannot be controlled, underpads or briefs can be used that are made of materials that absorb moisture and present a quick-drying surface to the skin. Topical agents that act as barriers to moisture can also be used.
- Skin injury due to friction an shear forces should be minimized through proper positioning, transferring, and turning techniques. In addition, friction injuries may be reduced by the use of lubricants (such as corn starch and creams), protective films (such as transparent film dressings and skin sealants), protective dressings (such as hydrocolloids), and protective padding.
- When apparently well-nourished individuals develop an inadequate dietary intake of protein or calories, caregivers should first attempt to discover the factors compromising intake and offer support with eating. Other nutritional supplements or support may be needed. If dietary intake remains inadequate and if consistent with overall goals of therapy, more aggressive nutritional intervention such as enteral or parenteral feedings should be considered. For nutritionally compromised individuals, a plan of nutritional support and/or supplementation should be implemented that meets individual needs and is consistent with the overall goals of therapy.
- If potential for improving mobility and activity status exists, rehabilitation efforts should be instituted if consistent with the overall goals of therapy. Maintaining current activity level, mobility and range of motion is an appropriate goal for most individuals.
- Interventions and outcomes should be monitored and documented.

MECHANICAL LOADING AND SUPPORT SURFACES

Goal: Protect against the adverse effects of external mechanical forces: pressure, friction, and shear.
- Any individual in bed who is assessed to be at risk for developing pressure ulcers should be repositioned at least every 2 hours if consistent with overall patient goals. A written schedule for systematically turning and repositioning the individual should be used.
- For individuals in bed, positioning devices such as pillows or foam wedges should be used to keep bony prominences (for example, knees or ankles) from direct contact with one another, according to a written plan.
- Individuals in bed who are completely immobile should have a care plan that includes the use of devices that totally relieve pressure on the heels, most commonly by raising the heels off the bed. Do not use donut-type devices.
- When the sidelying position is used in bed, avoid positioning directly on the trochanter.
- Maintain the head of the bed at the lowest degree of elevation consistent with medical conditions and other restrictions. Limit the amount of time the head of the bed is elevated.
- Use lifting devices such as a trapeze or bed linen to move (rather than drag) individuals in bed who cannot assist during transfers and position changes.
- Any individual assessed to be at risk for developing pressure ulcers should be placed when lying in bed on

a pressure-reducing device, such as foam, static air, alternating air, gel, or water mattresses.

- Any person at risk for developing a pressure ulcer should avoid uninterrupted sitting in a chair or wheelchair. The individual should be repositioned, shifting the points under pressure at least every hour or be put back to bed if consistent with overall patient management goals. Individuals who are able should be taught to shift weight every 15 minutes.

- For chair-bound individuals, the use of a pressure-reducing device such as those made of foam, gel, air, or a combination is indicated. Do not use donut-type devices.

- Positioning of chair-bound individuals in chairs or wheelchairs should include consideration of postural alignment, distribution of weight, balance and stability, and pressure relief.

- A written plan for the use of positioning devices and schedules may be helpful for chair-bound individuals.

EDUCATION

Goal: Reduce the incidence of pressure ulcers through educational programs

- Educational programs for the prevention of pressure ulcers should be structured, organized, and comprehensive and directed at all levels of health care providers, patients, and family or caregivers.

- The educational program for prevention of pressure ulcers should include information on the following items.
  - Etiology and risk factors for pressure ulcers
  - Risk assessment tools and their application
  - Skin assessment
  - Selection and/or use of support surfaces
  - Development and implementation of an individualized program of skin care
  - Demonstration of positioning to decrease risk of tissue breakdown
  - Instruction on accurate documentation of pertinent data

- The educational program should identify those responsible for pressure ulcer prevention, describe each person's role, and be appropriate to the audience in terms of level of information presented and expected participation. The educational program should be updated on a regular basis to incorporate new and existing techniques or technologies.

- Educational programs should be developed, implemented, and evaluated using principles of adult learning.

A prevention algorithm concludes the prevention guidelines.

The Treatment Guidelines were published in 1994. The categories of recommendation included assessment, managing tissue loads, ulcer care, managing bacterial colonization and infection, operative repair, education and quality improvement. The recommendations are placed in the categories of assessment (16 recommendations), managing tissue loads (17 recommendations), ulcer care (22 recommendations), managing bacterial colonization and infection (11 recommendations), operative repair, and education and quality improvement.

ASSESSING THE PRESSURE ULCER

- Assess the pressure ulcer(s) initially for location, stage, size, sinus tracts, undermining, tunneling, exudate, necrotic tissue, and the presence of absence of granulation tissue and epithelialization.

- Reassess pressure ulcers at least weekly. If the condition of the patient or of the wound deteriorates, reevaluate the treatment plan as soon as any evidence of deterioration is noted.

- A clean pressure ulcer should show evidence of some healing within 2 to 4 weeks. If no progress can be demonstrated, reevaluate the adequacy of the overall treatment plan as well as adherence to this plan, making modifications as necessary.

ASSESSING THE INDIVIDUAL WITH A PRESSURE ULCER

- Perform a complete history and physical examination, because a pressure ulcer should be assessed in the context of the patient's overall physical and psychosocial health.

- Clinicians should be alert to the potential complications associated with pressure ulcers.

- Ensure adequate dietary intake to prevent malnutrition to the extent that this is compatible with the individual's wishes.

- Perform an abbreviated nutritional assessment, as defined by the Nutrition Screening Initiative, at least every 3 months for individuals at risk for malnutrition. These include individuals who are unable to take food by mouth or who experience an involuntary change in weight.

- Encourage dietary intake or supplementation if an individual with a pressure ulcer is malnourished. If dietary intake continues to be inadequate, impractical, or impossible, nutritional support (usually tube feeding) should be used to place the patient into positive nitrogen balance (approximately 30 to 35 calories/kg/day and 1.25 to 1.50 grams of protein/kg/day) according to the goals of care.

- Give vitamin and mineral supplements if deficiencies are confirmed or suspected.

PAIN ASSESSMENT AND MANAGEMENT

- Assess all patients for pain related to the pressure ulcer or its treatment.
- Manage pain by eliminating or controlling the source of pain (eg, covering wounds, adjusting support surfaces, repositioning). Provide analgesia as needed and appropriate.

PSYCHOSOCIAL ASSESSMENT AND MANAGEMENT

- All individuals being treated for pressure ulcers should undergo a psychosocial assessment to determine their ability and motivation to comprehend and adhere to the treatment program. The assessment should include but not be limited to the following:
  - Mental status, learning ability, depression
  - Social support
  - Polypharmacy or overmedication
  - Alcohol and/or drug abuse
  - Goals, values, and lifestyle
  - Sexuality
  - Culture and ethnicity
  - Stressors
- Periodic reassessment is recommended.
- Assess resources (eg, availability and skill of care givers, finances, equipment) of individuals being treated for pressure ulcers in the home.
- Set treatment goals consistent with the values and lifestyle of the individual, family, and care giver.
- Arrange interventions to meet identified psychosocial needs and goals. Follow up should be planned in cooperation with the individual and care giver.

MANAGING TISSUE LOADS

Positioning Techniques While in Bed

- Avoid positioning patients on a pressure ulcer.
- Use positioning devices to raise a pressure ulcer off the support surface. If the patient is no longer at risk for developing pressure ulcers, these devices may reduce the need for pressure-reducing overlays, mattresses and beds. Avoid using donut-type devices.

- Establish a written repositioning schedule.
- Assess all patients with existing pressure ulcers to determine their risk for developing additional pressure ulcers. For those individuals who remain at risk, institute the following measures recommended in Pressure Ulcers in Adults.
- Avoid positioning immobile individuals directly on their trochanters and use devices such as pillows and foam wedges that totally relieve pressure on the heels, most commonly by raising the heels off the bed.
- Use positioning devices such as pillows or foam to prevent direct contact between bony prominences (such as knees or ankles).
- Maintain the head of the bed at the lowest degree of elevation consistent with medical conditions and other restrictions. Limit the amount of time the head of the bed is elevated.

Support Surfaces for Bed

- Assess all patients with existing pressure ulcers to determine their risk for developing additional pressure ulcers. If the patient remains at risk, use a pressure-reducing surface.
- Use a static support surface if a patient can assume a variety of positions without bearing weight on a pressure ulcer and without "bottoming out."
- Use a dynamic support surface if the patient cannot assume a variety of positions without bearing weight on a pressure ulcer, if the patient fully compresses the static support surface, or if the pressure ulcer does not show evidence of healing.
- If the patient has large Stage III or Stage IV pressure ulcers on multiple turning surfaces, a low-air-loss bed or an air-fluidized bed may be indicated.
- When excess moisture on intact skin is a potential source of maceration and skin breakdown, a support surface that provides airflow can be important in drying the skin and preventing additional pressure ulcers.

Positioning Techniques While Sitting

- A patient who has a pressure ulcer on a sitting surface should avoid sitting. If pressure on the ulcer can be relieved, limited sitting may be allowed.
- Consider postural alignment, distribution of weight, balance, stability, and pressure relief when positioning sitting individuals.
- Reposition the sitting individual so the points under pressure are shifted at least every hour. If this schedule cannot be kept or is inconsistent with overall treatment goals, return the patient to bed. Individuals who are able should be taught to shift their weight every 15 minutes.

Support Surfaces for Sitting

- Select a cushion based on the specific needs of the individual who requires pressure reduction in a sitting positions. Avoid donut-type devices.
- Develop a written plan for the use of positioning devices.

ULCER CARE

Debridement

- Remove devitalized tissue in pressure ulcers when appropriate for the patient's condition and consistent with patient goals.
- Select the method of debridement most appropriate to the patient's condition and goals. Sharp, mechanical, enzymatic, and/or autolytic debridement techniques may be used when there is no urgent clinical need for drainage or removal of devitalized tissue. If there is urgent need for debridement, as with advancing cellulitis or sepsis, sharp debridement should be used.
- Use clean, dry dressings for 8 to 24 hours after sharp debridement associated with bleeding; then reinstitute moist dressings. Clean dressings may be used in conjunction with mechanical or enzymatic debridement techniques.
- Heel ulcers with dry eschar need not be debrided if they do not have edema, erythema, fluctuance, drainage.
- Prevent or manage pain associated with debridement as needed.

Wound Cleansing

- Cleanse wounds initially and at each dressing change.
- Use minimal mechanical force when cleansing the ulcer with gauze, cloth, or sponges.
- Do not clean ulcer wounds with skin cleansers or antiseptic agents (eg, povidone iodine, iodophor, sodium hypochlorite solution [Dakin's solution], hydrogen peroxide, acetic acid).
- Use normal saline for cleansing most pressure ulcers.
- Use enough irrigation pressure to enhance wound cleansing without causing trauma to the wound bed. Safe and effective ulcer irrigation pressures range from 4 to 15 psi. Table 3 indicates the irrigation pressure delivered by various clinically available devices.
- Consider whirlpool treatment for cleansing pressure ulcers that contain thick exudate, slough, or necrotic tissue. Discontinue whirlpool when the ulcer is clean.

Dressings

- Use a dressing that will keep the ulcer bed continuously moist. Wet-to-dry dressings should be used only for debridement and are not considered continuously moist saline dressings.
- Use clinical judgment to select a type of moist wound dressing suitable for the ulcer. Studies of different types of moist wound dressings showed no differences in pressure ulcer healing outcomes.
- Choose a dressing that keeps the surrounding intact (periulcer) skin dry while keeping the ulcer bed moist.
- Choose a dressing that controls exudate but does not desiccate the ulcer bed.
- Consider care giver time when selecting a dressing.
- Eliminate wound dead space by loosely filling all cavities with dressing material. Avoid overpacking the wound.
- Monitor dressings applied near the anus, since they are difficult to keep intact.

Adjunctive Therapies

- Consider a course of treatment with electrotherapy for Stage III and IV pressure ulcers that have proved unresponsive to conventional therapy. Electrical stimulation may also be useful for recalcitrant Stage II ulcers.
- The therapeutic efficacy of hyperbaric oxygen, infrared, ultraviolet, and low-energy irradiation, and ultrasound has not been sufficiently established to permit recommendation of these therapies for the treatment of pressure ulcers.
- The therapeutic efficacy of miscellaneous topical agents (eg, sugar, vitamins, elements, hormones, other agents), growth factors, and skin equivalents has not yet been sufficiently established to warrant recommendation of these agents at this time.
- The therapeutic efficacy of systemic agents other than antibiotics has not been sufficiently established to permit their recommendation for the treatment of pressure ulcers.

MANAGING BACTERIAL COLONIZATION AND INFECTION

- Minimize pressure ulcer colonization and enhance wound healing by effective wound cleansing and debridement. If purulence or foul odor is present, more frequent cleansing and possibly debridement are required.
- Do not use swab cultures to diagnose wound infection, because all pressure ulcers are colonized.

- Consider initiating a 2-week trial of topical antibiotics for clean pressure ulcers that are not healing or are continuing to produce exudate after 2 to 4 weeks of optimal patient care (as defined in this guideline). The antibiotic should be effective against gram-negative, gram-positive, and anaerobic organisms (eg, silver sulfadiazine, triple antibiotic).

- Perform quantitative bacterial cultures of the soft tissue and evaluate the patient for osteomyelitis when the ulcer does not respond to topical antibiotic therapy.

- Do not use topical antiseptics (eg, povidone iodine, iodophor, sodium hypochlorite [Dakin's solution], hydrogen peroxide, acetic acid) to reduce bacteria in wound tissue.

- Institute appropriate systemic antibiotic therapy for patients with bacteremia, sepsis, advancing cellulitis, or osteomyelitis. Systemic antibiotics are not required for pressure ulcers with only clinical signs of local infection.

- Protect pressure ulcers from exogenous sources of contamination (eg, feces).

INFECTION CONTROL

- Follow body substance isolation (BSI) precautions or an equivalent system appropriate for the health care setting and the patient's condition when treating pressure ulcers.

- Wear gloves for anticipated contact with blood, secretions, mucous membranes, nonintact skin, and moist body substances for all patients. Change gloves before treating another patient. Handwashing between patients is essential.

- After other types of patient contact, wash the hands for 10 seconds with soap and friction to remove transient microbial flora, and then rinse with running water.

- Wear additional barriers such as gown, plastic aprons, masks, or goggles when moist body substances (secretions, blood, or body fluids) are likely to soil the clothing or the skin or splash in the face. The panel notes that protective eyewear, mask (or a faceshield that covers the eyes and face), gloves, and in some cases protective gowns should be used for pressure ulcer irrigation when there is reasonable expectation that wound secretions might be aerosolized.

- Place soiled reusable articles and linen, as well as trash, in containers that are securely sealed to prevent leaking. Double bagging is not necessary unless the outside of the bag is visibly soiled.

- Place needles (without recapping them) and sharp instruments in puncture-resistant, rigid containers. If such containers are not available, recapping using the one-hand technique is acceptable.

- Assign to private rooms those patients with diseases that could be transmitted by the airborne route (eg, pulmonary tuberculosis) and other diseases listed under precautions for strict isolation in the category-specific isolation. The use of private rooms is also indicated for those patients likely to soil articles in their environment with body substances.

- Use clean gloves for each patient. When treating multiple ulcers on the same patient, attend to the most contaminated ulcer last (eg, in the perianal region). Remove gloves and wash hands between patients.

- Use sterile instruments to debride pressure ulcers.

- Use clean dressings, rather than sterile ones, to treat pressure ulcers, as long as dressing procedures comply with institutional infection-control guidelines.

- Clean dressings may also be used in the home setting. Disposal of contaminated dressings in the home should be done in a manner consistent with local regulations.

When these recommendations are examined, two considerations must be kept in mind. First, these recommendations were made for the prevention and treatment of pressure ulcers, not other types of wounds. Second, these recommendations were written prior to the development of a number of new technologies. Examples include newer kinetic therapy beds, the Isch-dish, platelet-derived growth factor, vacuum-assisted closure, controlled radiant warming to body temperature devices, and ultraviolet C devices. Over time many new devices may become appropriate for treating pressure ulcers and some of the other recommendations may no longer be supported by newer research.

INDEX

Build Your Library

Along with this title, we publish numerous products on a variety of topics. We are sure that you will find the below titles to be an essential addition to your library. Order your copies today or contact us for a copy of our latest catalog for additional product information.

COMPREHENSIVE WOUND MANAGEMENT

Glenn Irion, PhD, PT, CWS

320 pp., Soft Cover, 2002, ISBN 1-55642-477-9, Order #44779, $37.00

Comprehensive Wound Management is written as a multilevel textbook on the management of wounds treated by clinicians. This unique book covers a wide spectrum of both chronic and acute wounds including pressure ulcers, neuropathic ulcers, vascular ulcers, and burn injuries. Full-color photographs of wounds, photographic descriptions of wound management, and line drawings illustrate and reinforce key concepts. These illustrations assist in creating a complete understanding of wound management. The author's seamless flow creates a user-friendly format that is suitable for both students and practicing clinicians of varying wound experience.

PHYSIOLOGY: THE BASIS OF CLINICAL PRACTICE

Glenn Irion, PhD, PT, CWS

432 pp., Hard Cover, 2000, ISBN 1-55642-380-2, Order #43802, $35.00

Physiology: The Basis of Clinical Practice presents an in-depth discussion of clinically related topics in an integrated manner specific to rehabilitation professionals. This book covers important principles of skeletal muscle performance and neurologic control of motor systems. This text presents an in-depth discussion of clinically related topics in an integrated manner specific to rehabilitation professionals. This book covers important principles of skeletal muscle performance and neurologic control of motor systems.

PHYSICAL THERAPY PROFESSIONAL FOUNDATIONS: KEYS TO SUCCESS IN SCHOOL AND CAREER

Kathleen A. Curtis, PhD, PT

304 pp., Soft Cover, 2002, ISBN 1-55642-411-6, Order #44116, $35.00

This user-friendly text begins as the students enter the educational program, offering an introduction to the physical therapy profession and current issues in physical therapy. The author offers practical strategies for students as they progress through professional education including financial considerations, professional behavior, performance expectations, legal and ethical issues, as well as requirements and challenges faced during the transition from school to career. It is also a valuable resource for new graduate physical therapists as they prepare for and begin their careers. Topics that will assist them in this important stage are preparation for the licensure examination, entering the job market, common challenges for new graduate physical therapists, and planning for career development.

Contact us at

SLACK Incorporated, Professional Book Division
6900 Grove Road, Thorofare, NJ 08086
1-800-257-8290/1-856-848-1000, Fax: 1-856-853-5991
E-Mail: orders@slackinc.com or www.slackbooks.com

ORDER FORM

QUANTITY	TITLE	ORDER #	PRICE
	Comprehensive Wound Management	44779	$37.00
	Physiology: The Basis of Clinical Practice	43802	$35.00
	Physical Therapy Professional Foundations	44116	$35.00
	Subtotal		$
	Applicable state and local tax will be added to your purchase		$
	Handling		$4.50
	Total		$

Name _____

Address: _____

City: _____ State:_____ Zip: _____

Phone:_____ Fax_____

Email: _____

- Check enclosed (Payable to SLACK Incorporated)_____

- Charge my: ___ [card] ___ VISA ___ MasterCard

    Account #: _____

    Exp. date: _____ Signature _____

NOTE: Prices are subject to change without notice.
Shipping charges will apply.
Shipping and handling charges are Non-Returnable.

CODE: 328

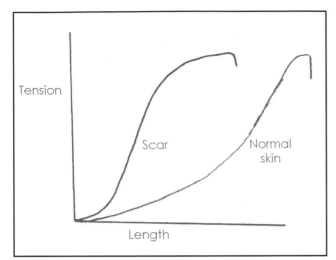

Figure 1-8. Stress-strain relationship of tendon and skin. Note four regions: In the first region, lengthening occurs with little stress. In the second region, a linear relationship between lengthening and stress can be observed. With further stress, fibers are damaged and elasticity is lost. Also note the greater extensibility of skin for a given stress. Scar tissue extensibility is similar to tendon.

characterized by their ability to withstand compression or are more elastic.

Elastic fibers consist of a fibrillar component termed *fibrillin* and an amorphous component named *elastin*. Elastic fibers are characterized by their wavy nature and springlike quality, thereby providing elasticity to skin. In Marfan's syndrome, fibrillin is defective, resulting in the physical characteristics of the disease as well as aortic insufficiency and risk of aortic aneurysm.

Ground Substance

Ground substance refers to the viscoelastic sol-gel of hydrophilic polymers found between cells and fibers of the dermis. The multiple branches of proteins with their charges are able to hold tremendous quantities of interstitial water in place. Overwhelming of the ground substance due to fluid balance derangement (ie, increased capillary pressure due to tissue injury or heart failure) produces free water movement in the interstitial space, manifested as pitting edema. Ground substance both lubricates and separates the fibers of the dermis, allowing them to move freely across each other. The binding of these molecules to collagen fibers also increases the tensile strength of collagen fibers.

Glycosaminoglycans are the primary type of molecule in ground substance. These molecules consist of chains of polysaccharides linked to protein that are metabolized and degraded by fibroblasts. Different proportions of glycosaminoglycans are present in different tissues and contribute to the biomechanical properties of these tissues. The more common glycosaminoglycans are hyaluronic

acid, chondroitin-4 sulfate, dermatan sulfate, and heparan sulfate. Different connective tissues of the body express different proportions of these specific molecules. In normal skin, hyaluronic acid, chondroitin sulfate, and dermatan sulfate represent about 42%, 5%, and 54% of the glycosaminoglycans. In scar tissue, hyaluronic acid decreases dramatically, and chondroitin sulfate increases to proportions similar to those of tendon and bone.

BIOMECHANICS OF SKIN

Skin is much more elastic than the dense connective tissue of bone, ligament, and tendon. Some of the differences are due to the components, and some are due to the arrangements of these components. Tendons are very stiff and elongate very little with applied force. This stiffness is primarily due to the parallel arrangement of very thick bundles of collagen but, as discussed above, tendon has different proportions of glycosaminoglycans than elastic cartilage or skin. In addition to its elastic nature, normal skin has tensile and viscous properties. Much of the elasticity comes from viscous elements; therefore, skin is described as having a viscoelastic property. In a simple model, collagen fibers may be ascribed the role of providing tensile strength (ie, the ability to resist lengthening). However, collagen fibers are both coiled and undulating. As stretch is applied to collagen fibers, they become straightened, and at several points along each bundle of collagen fibers, a number of elastic fibers attach to each other and other collagen bundles. Further stretch straightens the alignment of collagen and elastic fibers. The three-dimensional interaction of collagen fibers and the attachment of elastic fibers made of elastin provide the ability of the skin to recoil when a stretch is applied to it. Ground substance, made of glycosaminoglycans and water, also provides some elasticity to the skin. Dehydration of the skin, as occurs with aging, diminishes skin turgor and allows the fibers of the skin to become lax. This is manifested as tenting, in which a pinch of skin does not recoil when released.

The response of material to an applied force is graphically represented as a stress-strain curve (Figure 1-8). The force applied to the tissue represents the stress (dependent variable on the y axis), and the length of the tissue represents the strain as the independent variable plotted on the x axis. Therefore, these measurements represent a measurement of force across the tissue as its length is changed. Five areas subdivided within two major regions are characteristic of connective tissue. In the elastic region, no permanent change in tissue length occurs with stretch. If force is plotted with both increase and release of the stretch, a somewhat different path is followed. This phenomenon is termed *hysteresis* and is due chiefly to the viscoelastic nature of connective tissue.